Shi

An Introduction to Medical Terminology for Health Care

For Churchill Livingstone:

Senior Commissioning Editor: Sarena Wolfaard
Project Development Manager: Derek Robertson
Project Manager: Andrea Hill
Design Direction: Judith Wright

An Introduction to Medical Terminology for Health Care

A SELF-TEACHING PACKAGE

Andrew R. Hutton

BSc MSc
Lecturer in Life Science
Edinburgh's Telford College, Edinburgh, UK

THIRD EDITION

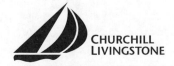

CHURCHILL
LIVINGSTONE

EDINBURGH LONDON NEW YORK OXFORD PHILADELPHIA ST LOUIS SYDNEY TORONTO 2002

CHURCHILL LIVINGSTONE
An imprint of Elsevier Limited

First edition 1993
Second edition 1998
Third edition 2002
  Reprinted 2002 (twice), 2003, 2004, 2005

ISBN 0 443 07079 2

British Library Cataloguing in Publication Data
A catalogue record for this book is available from the British Library

Library of Congress Cataloging in Publication Data
A catalog record for this book is available from the Library of Congress

Note
Medical knowledge is constantly changing. As new information becomes available, changes in treatment, procedures, equipment and the use of drugs become necessary. The author and the publishers have taken care to ensure that the information given in this text is accurate and up to date. However, readers are strongly advised to confirm that the information, especially with regard to drug usage, complies with the latest legislation and standards of practice.

ELSEVIER your source for books,
journals and multimedia
in the health sciences

www.elsevierhealth.com

Working together to grow
libraries in developing countries

www.elsevier.com | www.bookaid.org | www.sabre.org

ELSEVIER   BOOK AID International   Sabre Foundation

The
publisher's
policy is to use
paper manufactured
from sustainable forests

Printed in China
P/06

Contents

About this book

This book is designed to introduce medical terms to students who have little prior knowledge of the language of medicine. Included in the text are simple, nontechnical descriptions of pathological conditions, medical instruments and clinical procedures.

The medical terms are introduced within the context of a body system or medical specialty and each set of exercises provides the student with the opportunity to learn, review and assess new words. Each unit includes a case history exercise that outlines the presentation, diagnosis and treatment of a specific medical condition. Once complete, the exercises will form a valuable reference text.

No previous knowledge of medicine is required to follow the text and, to ensure ease of use, the more complex details of word origins and analysis have been omitted. The book will be of great value to anyone who needs to learn medical terms quickly and efficiently.

Edinburgh 2002   Andrew Hutton

Acknowledgements

We are grateful to Aesculap Ltd incorporating Downs Surgical for permission to reproduce Figures 17, 18, 56 and 57. Figure 23 was redrawn from a catalogue supplied by A.C. Cossor & Son (Surgical) Ltd.

How to use this book

Before you begin working through the units, read through the introduction which explains the basic principles of reading, writing and understanding medical terms.

Once you have understood the elementary rules of medical word building, complete Units 1–21, which are based on different medical topics. The units can be studied in sequence or independently.

For ease of use each unit has the same basic plan and is arranged into:

 WORD EXERCISES

 AN ANATOMY EXERCISE

 A CASE HISTORY

 A WORD CHECK

 A SELF-ASSESSMENT

The different parts of each unit are indicated by icons.

 The word exercise icon indicates a written exercise that can be completed using the Exercise Guide at the beginning of each unit or knowledge acquired during this course of study. The answers to the word exercises are on p. 275.

 The anatomy exercise icon indicates you should complete the anatomy exercise relating to a body system. In this exercise you relate combining forms of medical roots to their position in the body. Check the meanings of the root words using the Quick Reference box.

 The case history icon indicates an account of a medical case history. The purpose of this exercise is to understand the medical terms associated with disease presentation, investigation and treatment. Some of the case histories may seem difficult to follow because of the terminology used when doctors write formal reports. To assist your understanding, a Word Help box is included with each case listing the meanings of difficult or unfamiliar words. In each case history, try to gain an overall picture of the health care required for successful treatment of the patient.

Answers to the exercise that accompanies each case can be found with the answers to the word exercises on p. 275.

The word check icon indicates you should complete the Word Check that lists all prefixes, combining forms and suffixes used in a unit. Try to do this from memory and then correct any errors you have made. Errors can be corrected using the Exercise Guide or the Quick Reference box that follows each Case History. The glossary on p. 319 can also be used.

The self-assessment icon indicates a series of self-assessment tests. Aim to complete the tests using knowledge gained from studying each unit and record your score in the boxes provided with each test. Check your answers on p. 299.

Introduction

Objectives

Once the introduction is complete you should be able to:

- name and identify components of medical words
- split medical words into their components
- build medical words using word components.

Students beginning any kind of medical or paramedical course are faced with a bewildering number of complex medical terms. Surprisingly it is possible to understand many medical terms and build new ones by learning relatively few words that can be combined in a variety of ways. Even the longest medical terms are easy to understand if you know the meaning of each component of the word. For example, you may never have heard of **laryngopharyngitis** but if you learn that **-itis** always means inflammation, **laryng/o** refers to the larynx or voice box and **pharyng/o** refers to the throat or pharynx, its meaning becomes apparent, i.e. inflammation of the pharynx and larynx. Laryngopharyngitis is an inflammation of the upper respiratory tract with symptoms of sore throat and loss of voice.

Most doctors, however, do not use precise medical terminology when conversing with patients. If patients hear a complex medical description of their illness, they may become frightened rather than reassured. Precise medical terms are used when medical records and letters are completed. They are also used when doctors discuss a patient and when medical material is published.

The terms you will use in this book describe common diseases and disorders, instruments, diagnostic techniques and therapies.

The components of medical words

In this introduction you will learn how to split medical terms into their components and deduce their meanings. Skills developed here will enable you to derive the meanings of unfamiliar medical words and improve your ability to understand medical literature.

Let us begin by using a medical word associated with an organ with which you are familiar, the stomach:

Example 1   GASTROTOMY

First we can split the word and examine its individual components:

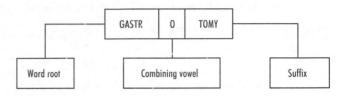

The word root

Roots are the basic medical words. Most are derived from Greek and Roman (Latin) words. Others have their origins in Arabic, Anglo-Saxon and German. Some early Greek words have been retained in their original form whilst others have been latinized. In their migrations throughout Europe and America many words have changed their spelling, meaning and pronunciation.

In our first example we have used the root **gastr** which always means stomach.

The combining vowel

Combining vowels are added to word roots to aid pronunciation and to connect the root to the suffix. In our first example the combining vowel **o** has been added to join the root and suffix. All the combining vowels a, e, i, o and u are used but the most commonly used is o.

In our first example we have added the combining vowel **o** to the root **gastr**.

The suffix

The suffix follows the word root and is found at the end of the word. It also adds to or modifies the meaning of the word root.

In our first example we have used the suffix **-tomy** which always means to form an incision.

We can now fully understand the meaning of our first medical word:

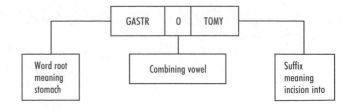

The meaning of gastrotomy is – incision into the stomach. Gastrotomy is a name used by surgeons to describe an operation in which a cut is made into the wall of the stomach.

The combining form

In our first example the root **gastr** can be combined with the vowel **o** to make **gastro**. This word component is called a **combining form** of a word root, i.e.

Word root	+	combining vowel	=	combining form
gastr	+	o	=	gastro

Most combining forms end in o and we will be using many of them in the exercises that follow.

Now we have learnt the meaning of our first root we can use it again with a new word component:

Example 2   EPIGASTRIC

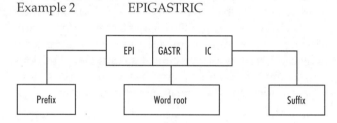

Here we have split the word into its components and we can see it begins with a prefix that appears before the root **gastr**.

The prefix

The prefix precedes the word root and changes its meaning. The prefix **epi-** means upon and so it modifies the word to mean upon or above the stomach. Prefixes, like roots and suffixes, are also derived from Greek and Latin words.

The suffix **-ic** meaning pertaining to was also used in our second example so we can now write the full meaning of epigastric:

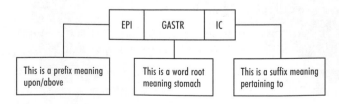

The full meaning of epigastric is – pertaining to above or upon the stomach.

> **Key Point**
> The components of medical words are:
> - prefixes
> - roots
> - suffixes
> - combining vowels
> - combining forms.

The use of prefixes, combining forms and suffixes

There are certain simple 'rules' which need to be applied when building and analysing medical words. To practise using these rules, some new combining forms are introduced. Don't worry about their meanings at the moment, we will study them in a later unit.

Rule 1: Joining a combining form to a suffix

If we add the suffixes **-logy**, meaning study of, and **-algia**, meaning condition of pain, to the combining form gastr/o we can make two new words:

gastr/o	+	-logy	=	gastrology (study of the stomach)
gastr/o	+	-algia	=	gastralgia (condition of pain in the stomach)

Notice that in gastrology the combining vowel o has been left in place whilst in gastralgia it has been dropped. The o has been dropped in gastralgia because -algia begins with a, a vowel. Gastroalgia is not used and it would be more difficult to pronounce.

> **Key Point**
> When a combining form of a root is joined to a suffix, the combining vowel is left in place if the suffix begins with a letter other than a vowel.

Here are some more examples where the vowel is left in place because the suffix begins with a letter other than a vowel:

gastr/o	+	-tomy	=	gastrotomy (incision into the stomach)
gastr/o	+	-scope	=	gastroscope (instrument to view the stomach)

Here are some examples where the vowel is dropped:

gastr/o	+	-itis	=	gastritis (inflammation of the stomach)
gastr/o	+	-ectomy	=	gastrectomy (removal of the stomach)

WORD EXERCISE 1

Use Rule 1 to join the combining forms of word roots and suffixes to make medical words. The meanings of the words will be studied in following units. The first has been completed for you.

Combining form of word root		Suffix		Medical word
(a) gastr/o	+	-pathy	=	gastropathy
(b) gastr/o	+	-scopy	=	gastroscopy
(c) hepat/o	+	-itis	=	hepatitis
(d) hepat/o	+	-megaly	=	hepatomegaly
(e) hepat/o	+	-oma	=	hepatoma.

Rule 2: Joining the combining forms of two word roots

Some medical words contain two or more combining forms of roots, as in Example 3.

Example 3   GASTROENTEROLOGY

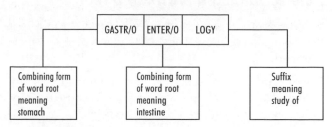

	GASTR/O	ENTER/O	LOGY	
Combining form of word root meaning stomach		Combining form of word root meaning intestine		Suffix meaning study of

The full meaning of gastroenterology is the study of the intestines and stomach. Notice that the vowel between the two roots **gastr** and **enter** is left in place.

> **Key Point**
> When the combining forms of two roots are joined, the combining vowel of the first root is kept in place.

Here are some more examples:

pylor/o + gastr/o + ectomy = pylorogastrec-tomy

duoden/o + enter/o + stomy = duodeno-enterostomy

WORD EXERCISE 2

Use Rules 1 and 2 to join the combining forms of two roots with suffixes to make medical words. The meanings of the words will be studied in following units. The first has been completed for you.

Combining form of word root		Combining form of word root		Suffix		Medical word
(a) duoden/o	+	jejun/o	+	-stomy	=	duodenojejunostomy
(b) trache/o	+	bronch/o	+	-itis	=	tracheobronchitis
(c) gastr/o	+	enter/o	+	-stomy	=	gastroenterostomy
(d) laryng/o	+	pharyng/o	+	-ectomy	=	laryngopharyngectomy
(e) oste/o	+	arthr/o	+	-pathy	=	osteoarthropathy

Note.   There are a few exceptions to this rule which are hyphenated e.g. pharyngo-oral.

Rule 3: Joining a prefix to a root

When a prefix that ends in a vowel is added to a root that begins with a vowel or 'h', the vowel of the prefix is dropped.

If we examine our second example, **epigastric**, again, here the vowel 'i' of **epi-** was retained because the root **gastr** begins with 'g' which is not a vowel.

Consider another example, which may be familiar to you – antacid, a drug used to neutralize stomach acid. This word is made from:

anti   + acid   = antacid
(prefix meaning   (root meaning
against)   acid)

The 'i' is dropped because acid begins with the vowel 'a'.

Here are some more examples, we will learn their meanings later.

Here the vowel of the prefix is retained:

hemi + col/o + ectomy = hemicolectomy

Here the vowel of the prefix is dropped:

endo + arter/i + ectomy = endarterectomy

anti + helminth + ic   = anthelminthic

Note.   This is not a strict rule and there are many exceptions to it, e.g. periosteitis.

> **Key Point**
> When a prefix that ends in a vowel is joined to a root, the vowel of the prefix is dropped if the root begins with a vowel or 'h'.

 WORD EXERCISE 3

Use the rules we have just described to join prefixes, combining forms of roots and suffixes to make medical words. The meanings of the words will be studied in following units. The first has been completed for you.

Prefix	Combining form of word root	Suffix	Medical word
(a) endo-	+ odont/o	+ -ic	= endodontic
(b) prostho-	+ odont/o	+ -ist	= prosthodontist
(c) para-	+ rect/o	+ -al	= pararectal
(d) mono-	+ ocul/o	+ -ar	= monocular
(e) peri-	+ splen/o	+ -itis	= perisplenitis

Reading and understanding medical words

Now you have learnt the basic principle of building medical words, you should be able to deduce the meaning of an unfamiliar word from the meaning of its components. To illustrate this we will use two examples.

Example 1: Gastroenterology

> **First**
>   Split the word into its components gastro/entero/logy.
>
> **Then**
>   Think of or look up the meaning of these components.
>
> **Finally**
>   Read the meaning of the word *beginning with the suffix and reading backwards*:
>   e.g. gastr/o[3], enter/o[2], -logy[1]
>   1 study of
>   2 the intestines and
>   3 the stomach.
>   We read the full meaning of gastroenterology as – the study of the intestines and stomach.

Example 2: Pararectal

Here the prefix *para-* has modified the meaning of the root *rect/* to mean beside the rectum.

> **First**
>   Split the word into its components para/rect/al.
>
> **Then**
>   Think of or look up the meaning of these components.
>
> **Finally**
>   Read the meaning of the word *beginning with the suffix followed by the meaning of the modified root*
>   e.g. pararect[2], al[1]
>   1 pertaining to
>   2 beside the rectum.
>   We read the full meaning of pararectal as pertaining to beside the rectum.

> **Key Point**
> When deducing the meanings of compound medical words, begin with the meaning of the suffix followed by those of the root(s) and prefix (from right to left).

Once you have an understanding of these simple rules you should be able to complete the exercises in Units 1–21. Each unit introduces different medical terms associated with a body system or medical specialty. The units can be completed in an order that complements your studies in anatomy, physiology and health care.

Levels of organization

Objectives

Once you have completed Unit 1 you should be able to:

- understand the meaning of medical words relating to levels of organization

- build medical words relating to levels of organization

- understand medical abbreviations relating to cells and tissues.

Exercise Guide

Use this list of word components and their meanings to complete the word exercises in this unit.

Prefixes

micro-	small

Roots/Combining forms

bi/o	life/living
chem/(istry)	chemicals (study of)
chondr/o	cartilage
erythr/o	red
fibr/o	fibre
granul/o	granule
haem/o	blood
hem/o (Am.)	blood
leuc/o	white
leuk/o (Am.)	white
lymph/o	lymph
melan/o	pigment/melanin
oo	egg/ovum
path/o	disease
spermat/o	sperm
tox/o	poisonous

Suffixes

-blast	immature germ cell/cell that forms ...
-genic	pertaining to formation/genesis
-genesis	formation of
-ic	pertaining to
-ist	specialist
-logist	specialist who studies ...
-logy	study of
-lysis	breakdown/disintegration
-pathy	disease of
-scope	instrument to view/examine
-scopist	specialist who uses viewing instrument
-scopy	technique of viewing/examining
-trophic	pertaining to nourishing

Levels of organization

The human body consists of basic units of life known as **cells**. Groups of cells similar in appearance, function and origin join together to form **tissues**. Different tissues then interact with each other to form **organs**. Finally groups of organs interact to form body **systems**. Thus there are four levels of organization in the human body: cells, tissues, organs and systems. Let us begin by examining the first level of organization.

Cells

The cell is the basic unit of life and the bodies of all plants and animals are built up of cells. Your body consists of millions of very small specialized cells. It is interesting to note that all non-infectious disorders and diseases of the human body are really due to the abnormal behaviour of cells.

Body cells are all built on the same basic plan. Figure 1 represents a model cell.

Cell membrane ————
Cytoplasm ————
Nucleus ————

Figure 1	A cell

Most cells have the same basic components as are shown in the model but they are all specialized to carry out particular functions within the body. In your studies you will come across many terms that relate to different types of cell. Now we will examine our first word root which refers to cells:

Root	Cyt
	*(From a Greek word **kytos**, meaning cell.)*
Combining forms	**Cyt/o,** also used as the suffix **-cyte** *(Remember from our introduction that combining forms are made by adding a combining vowel to the word root.)*

Here we have a word that contains the root cyt:

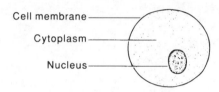

This is a root meaning cell | This is a combining vowel | This is a suffix meaning study of

Reading from the suffix back, cytology means the study of cells.

(Remember when trying to understand medical words, first split the word into its components, then think of the meaning of each component and finally write the meaning beginning with the suffix.)

Cytology is a very important topic in medicine as many diseases and disorders can be diagnosed by studying cells. Cells removed from patients are sent for cytological examination to a hospital cytology laboratory where they are examined with a microscope. (In the word cytological, *-ical* is a compound suffix meaning pertaining to or dealing with.)

The exercises that follow rely on the use of the Exercise Guide which appears at the beginning of this unit; use the guide to look up the meaning of path/o and -pathy and then try Word Exercise 1.

WORD EXERCISE 1

(a) Name the components of the word and give their meanings:

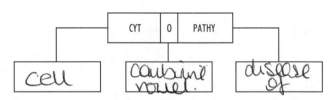

CYT | O | PATHY

cell | combining vowel. | disease of

(b) Reading from the suffix back, the meaning of cytopathy is:

disease of cells.

The root **-path-** can be used at the beginning and in the middle of a compound word as in the next two examples. Write the meaning of these words:

(c) path/o/logy   study of disease

(d) cyt/o/path/o/logy   study of disease of cells

Using the Exercise Guide again find the meaning of -ic, -ist, tox/o, and -lysis and write the meaning of the words below. Remember to read the meaning from the suffix back to the beginning of each word:

(e) cyto/lysis   disintegration of cells.

(f) cyto/tox/ic   pertaining to poisons of cells.

(g) cyto/logist   specialist who studies cells.

In the above examples, **cyt/o** was used at the beginning of words. It can also be used at the end of words in combination with other roots, its meaning remaining the same. Remember, when two roots are joined the combining vowel remains in place.

WORD EXERCISE 2

Here we have an example of two roots joined to make a compound word:

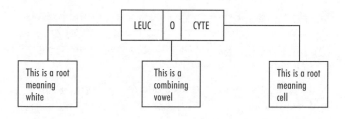

LEUC	O	CYTE
This is a root meaning white	This is a combining vowel	This is a root meaning cell

The meaning of leucocyte is therefore: white cell (actually a type of blood cell) (Am. leukocyte).

(a) Name the components of the following word and use your Exercise Guide to find their meanings.

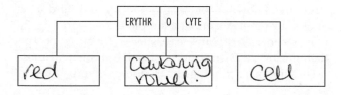

ERYTHR	O	CYTE
red	combining vowel.	cell

(b) The meaning of erythrocyte is: red cell.

WORD EXERCISE 3

Figure 2 and Figure 3 show two specialized cells, each one carrying out a different function.

(i) This cell produces the pigment melanin that gives the dark colour to black or brown skin.

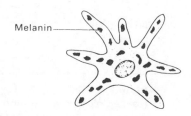

Melanin

Figure 2 A pigment cell

(ii) This cell produces white collagen fibres that give the skin support.

Fibres of collagen

Figure 3 A fibre cell

Use your Exercise Guide to find the combining forms of melanin and fibre to build words that name these cells.

(a) A cell containing melanin   melanocyte

(b) A cell that produces fibres   fibrocyte

(c) Complete the table by looking up the combining forms of the following roots in your Exercise Guide and building words that refer to cell types.

Root	Combining form	Name of cell
oste	osteo	osteocyte (bone cell)
lymph	lympho	lymphocyte lymph cell
spermat	spermato	spermatocyte sperm cell
oo	oo	oocyte - egg cell.
granul	granulo	granulocyte granule cell.
chondr	chondro	chondrocyte cartilage cell.

All of the above examples show how the combining vowel is retained when two roots are joined.

Now we will examine another root that also refers to cells:

Root   **Blast**
(A Greek word meaning bud or germ. It is used to denote an immature stage in cell development or a cell that is forming something.)

Combining forms   **Blast/o**, *also used as the suffix* **-blast**

WORD EXERCISE 4

Without using your Exercise Guide, write the meaning of:

(a) osteo/**blast**   immature bone cell.

(b) fibro/**blast**   immature fibre cell.

Using your Exercise Guide, write the meaning of:

(c) haemo/cyto/**blast** _immature blood cell_.
   (Am. hemo/cyto/blast)

Tissues

As cells become specialized, they form groups of cells known as tissues. A definition of a tissue is a group of cells similar in appearance, function and origin. There are four basic types of tissue: epithelial, muscle, connective and nervous tissue; these form the second level of organization in the body. Figure 4 illustrates how cells form a tissue. Here we can see a cuboidal epithelium from the kidney.

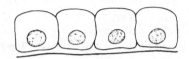

Figure 4	Cuboidal epithelium

The study of tissues is known as histology, the combining form coming from a Greek word *histos* meaning web (web of cells). Histology is an important branch of biology and medicine because it is used to identify diseased tissues. The histology and cytology laboratories are usually sections of the pathology laboratory of a large hospital.

| **Root** | **Hist**
*(From a Greek word **histos**, meaning web. It is used to mean the tissues of the body.)* |
|---|---|
| *Combining forms* | **Hist/i/o** |

 WORD EXERCISE 5

Using your Exercise Guide, find the meaning of:

(a) **histo**/chemistry _____

Without using your Exercise Guide, write the meaning of:

(b) **histo**/patho/logy _____

(c) **histo**/logist _____

(d) **histo**/lysis _____

Cells and tissues are very small and need to be examined using an instrument known as a microscope.

 WORD EXERCISE 6

Using your Exercise Guide, find the meaning of:

(a) **micro**- _____

(b) **micro**/scope _____

(c) **micro**/scopy _____

(d) **micro**/scop/ist _____

Note carefully the differences between **-scope**, **-scopy** and **-scopist**.

(e) **micro**/bio/logy _____

Organs

Groups of different tissues interact to produce larger structures known as organs; these form the third level of organization. A familiar example is the heart (Fig. 5), which consists of muscle tissue, a covering of epithelium, nerve tissue and connective tissue. All these tissues interact so that the heart pumps blood.

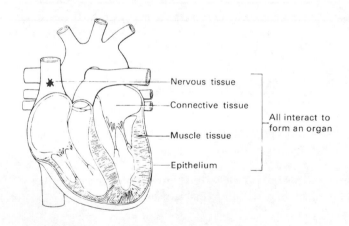

Figure 5	The heart

| **Root** | **Organ**
*(From a Greek word **organon**, meaning tool. Here we are using it to mean body organs).* |
|---|---|
| *Combining forms* | **Organ/o** |

WORD EXERCISE 7

Using your Exercise Guide, find the meaning of:

(a) **organo**/genesis _____
(synonymous with organogeny)

(b) **organo**/genic _____

(c) **organo**/trophic _____

Body systems

Groups of organs interact to form the fourth level of organization, the system, e.g. the stomach, duodenum, colon, etc. interact to form the digestive system that digests and absorbs food. Units 2–17 introduce medical terms associated with the main body systems.

CASE HISTORY 1

The object of this exercise is to understand words associated with a patient's medical history.

To complete the exercise:

• read through the passage on diagnosis of an AIDs related infection; unfamiliar words are underlined and you can find their meaning using the Word Help

• write the meaning of the medical terms shown in bold print.

Diagnosis of an AIDs related infection

Mr A, a 34-year-old <u>HIV positive</u> patient with symptoms of <u>AIDs</u>, was admitted to the unit following a chest X-ray that revealed a left upper lobe <u>mass</u>.

A <u>CT</u> scan confirmed the presence of a mass within the <u>peripheral</u> <u>aspect</u> of the left upper <u>lobe</u>, and a small left <u>pleural</u> <u>effusion</u>. CT guided fine needle <u>aspiration</u> of the left upper lobe mass was performed and the <u>biopsy</u> material sent to the **histology** laboratory for analysis by the duty **pathologist**.

Cytological examination of direct smears using optical **microscopy** revealed a <u>mucoid</u> background, moderate <u>cellularity</u>, <u>polymorphonuclear</u> **leucocytes** (Am. leukocytes), **lymphocytes** and <u>histiocytes</u>. A significant number of oval yeast-like cells were observed which appeared to be <u>budding</u>. No <u>malignant</u> cells were observed.

A sample of the biopsy material was sent for <u>culture and sensitivity</u> testing to the **microbiology** laboratory. The report was positive for <u>encapsulated</u> fungal yeast forms <u>morphologically</u> compatible with **pathogenic** <u>cryptococcus</u> species (*Cryptococcus neoformans*). Mr A's diagnosis was <u>cryptococcosis</u>, a condition seen mainly in AIDs patients and others with <u>compromised</u> immune systems.

WORD HELP

AIDs acquired immune deficiency syndrome

aspect part of a surface facing a designated direction

aspiration withdrawal by suction of a fluid

biopsy removal and examination of living tissue

budding performing asexual reproduction by producing buds that grow into new cells

cellularity state/condition of being made up of cells

compromised lacking the ability to mount an adequate immune response

cryptococcus a yeast-like fungus that causes disease in humans

cryptococcosis abnormal condition of infection with cryptococcus

CT computed tomography, a technique of using X-rays to image a slice or section through the body

culture & sensitivity testing growing microorganisms in the laboratory and testing them for sensitivity to antibiotics

effusion a fluid discharge into a part/escape of fluid into an enclosed space

encapsulated enclosed on a capsule or sheath

histiocytes the word means a tissue cell (actually a large cell found in connective tissue that helps defend against infection)

HIV-positive presence of antibodies to the human immunodeficiency virus in the blood, it indicates the virus has infected the body

lobe a division of an organ into smaller sections, here a lobe of the lung

malignant dangerous, life threatening

mass lump/collection of cohering cells

morphologically referring to the form and structure of an organism

mucoid resembling mucus

peripheral pertaining to the periphery i.e. the surface of an organ

pleural pertaining to the pleura/pleural membranes that surround the lungs

polymorphonuclear pertaining to or having nuclei of many shapes

Now write the meaning of the following words from the case history without using your dictionary lists:

(a) histology _____

(b) pathologist _____

(c) cytological _____

(d) microscopy _____

(e) leucocyte _____
(Am. leukocyte)

(f) lymphocyte _____

(g) microbiology _____

(h) pathogenic _____

(Answers to the case history exercise are given in the Answers to Word Exercises beginning on page 275.)

Quick Reference

Combining forms relating to levels of organization:

Blast/o	immature cell/forming cell
Chondr/o	cartilage
Cyt/o	cell
Granul/o	granule
Hist/i/o	tissue/web
Lymph/o	lymph
Melan/o	pigment/melanin
Oo	egg/ovum
Organ/o	organ
Oste/o	bone
Path/o	disease
Spermat/o	sperm

Abbreviations

Some common abbreviations related to cells and tissues are listed below. Note, some are not standard and their meaning may vary from one health care setting to another. There is a more extensive list for reference on page 307.

Diff	differential blood count (of cell types)
FBC	full blood count (of cells)
GCSF	granulocyte colony stimulating factor
Histo	histology (lab)
HLA	human lymphocyte antigen
Lymphos	lymphocytes
NK	natural killer (cells)
Pap	Papanicolaou smear test (of cervical cells)
PCV	packed cell volume
RBC	red blood count/red blood cell
RCC	red cell count
WBC	white blood cell/white blood count

 NOW TRY THE WORD CHECK ◁

 WORD CHECK

This self-check exercise lists all the word components used in this unit. First write down the meaning of as many word components as you can. Then check your answers using the Exercise Guide and Quick Reference box or the Glossary of Word Components (pp. 319–341).

Prefixes

micro- _____

Combining forms of word roots

bi/o _____

blast/o _____

chem/o _____

chondr/o _____

cyt/o _____

erythr/o _____

fibr/o _____

granul/o _____

hist/i/o _____

leuc/o _____

lymph/o _____

melan/o _____

oo- _____

organ/o _____

oste/o _____

path/o _____

spermat/o _____

tox/o _____

Suffixes

-blast _____

-genic _____

-genesis _____

-ic _____

-ical _____

-ist _____

-log(ist) _____

-logy _____

-lysis _____

-pathy _____

-scope _____

-scop(ist) _____

-scopy _____

-tox(ic) _____

-trophic _____

> **NOW TRY THE SELF-ASSESSMENT** <

SELF-ASSESSMENT

Test 1A

Prefixes, suffixes and combining forms of word roots

Match each word component in Column A with a meaning in Column C by inserting the appropriate number in Column B.

Column A	Column B	Column C
(a) chem/o	_____	1. egg
(b) cyt/o	_____	2. bone
(c) erythr/o	_____	3. white
(d) granul/o	_____	4. study of
(e) hist/i/o	_____	5. pigment (black)
(f) leuc/o	_____	6. sperm cells
(g) -log(ist)	_____	7. chemical
(h) -logy	_____	8. tissue
(i) lymph/o	_____	9. person who studies (specialist)
(j) -lysis	_____	10. small
(k) melan/o	_____	11. specialist who views/examines
(l) micro-	_____	12. breakdown/ disintegration
(m) oo-	_____	13. poisonous/ pertaining to poison
(n) oste/o	_____	14. cell
(o) -pathy	_____	15. visual examination
(p) -scope	_____	16. disease
(q) -scop(ist)	_____	17. lymph
(r) -scopy	_____	18. red
(s) spermat/o	_____	19. granule
(t) -tox(ic)	_____	20. viewing instrument

Score

20
20

Test 1B

Write the meaning of:

(a) chondrolysis _____

(b) leucocytolysis _____

(c) histotoxic _____

(d) osteopathy _____

(e) lymphoblast _____

Score

5
5

Test 1C

This type of test may seem difficult at first but as the terms become familiar you will improve.

Build words that mean:

(a) small cell _____

(b) person who specializes in the study of disease _____

(c) person who specializes in the study of disease of cells _____

(d) scientific study of cartilage _____

(e) pertaining to disease of cells _____

Score

5
5

Check answers to Self-Assessment Tests on page 299.

The digestive system

Objectives

Once you have completed Unit 2 you should be able to:

- understand the meaning of medical words relating to the digestive system

- build medical words relating to the digestive system

- associate medical terms with their anatomical position

- understand medical abbreviations relating to the digestive system.

Exercise Guide

Use this list of word components and their meanings to complete the word exercises in this unit.

Prefixes

a-	without
endo-	inside/within
epi-	upon/above
mega-	large
para-	beside
peri-	around

Suffixes

-aemia	condition of blood
-al	pertaining to
-algia	condition of pain
-clysis	infusion/injection into
-ectomy	removal of
-emia (Am.)	condition of blood
-gram	X-ray/tracing/recording
-graphy	technique of recording/making X-ray
-ia	condition of
-iasis	abnormal condition
-ic	pertaining to
-ist	specialist
-itis	inflammation of
-lith	stone
-lithiasis	abnormal condition of stones
-logist	specialist who studies …
-logy	study of
-lysis	breakdown/disintegration
-megaly	enlargement
-oma	tumour/swelling
-pathy	disease of
-scope	instrument to view/examine
-scopy	technique of viewing/examining
-stomy	formation of an opening into …
-tomy	incision into
-toxic	pertaining to poisoning
-uria	condition of the urine

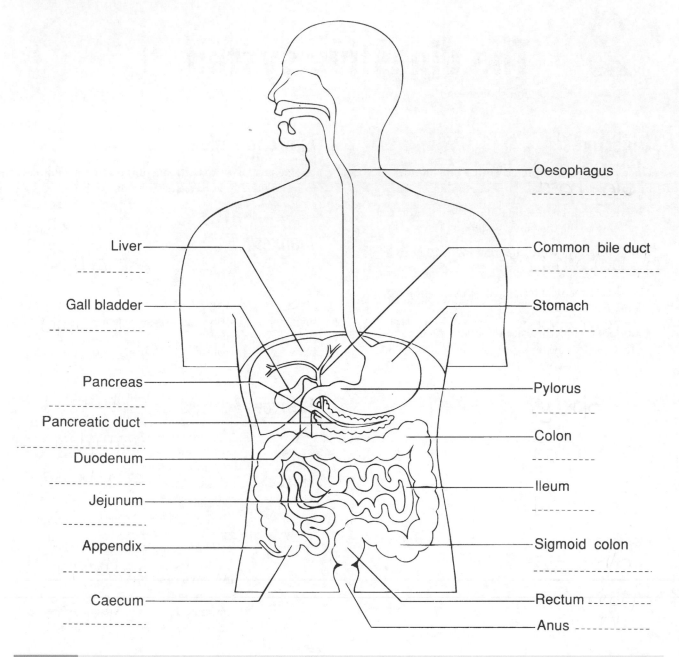

Oesophagus

Liver

Common bile duct

Gall bladder

Stomach

Pancreas

Pylorus

Pancreatic duct

Colon

Duodenum

Ileum

Jejunum

Appendix

Sigmoid colon

Caecum

Rectum

Anus

Figure 6 The digestive system

ANATOMY EXERCISE

When you have finished Word Exercises 1–12, look at the word components listed below. Complete Figure 6 by writing the appropriate combining form on each dotted line. (You can check their meanings in the Quick Reference box on page 23.)

Appendic/o	Gastr/o	Pancreatic/o
Caec/o, Cec/o (Am.)	Hepat/o	Proct/o
Cholecyst/o	Ile/o	Pylor/o
Choledoch/o	Jejun/o	Rect/o
Col/o	Oesophag/o, Esophag/o (Am.)	Sigmoid/o
Duoden/o	Pancreat/o	

The digestive system

The organs that compose the digestive system digest, absorb and process nutrients taken in as food. Materials not absorbed into the lining of the intestine form the faeces and leave the body through the anus.

Our study of the digestive system begins at the point where food leaves the mouth and enters the gullet or oesophagus.

Use the Exercise Guide at the beginning of this unit to complete Word Exercises 1–12 unless you are asked to work without it.

Root	Oesophag
	*(From a Greek word **oisophagos**, meaning oesophagus or gullet.)*
Combining forms	**Oesophag/o**
	Esophag/o *(Am.)*

WORD EXERCISE 1

Using your Exercise Guide, find the meaning of:

(a) **oesophago**/scope _____
     (Am. esophago/scope)

Remember that, to understand the meaning of these medical terms, we read the components from the suffix towards the beginning of the word.

(b) **oesophag**/ectomy _____
     (Am. esophag/ectomy)

(c) **oesophago**/tomy _____
     (Am. esophago/tomy)

(d) **oesophag**/itis _____
     (Am. esophag/itis)

Once you have learnt the suffixes in Word Exercise 1, it is easy to work out the meaning of other words with similar endings. Now we will use the same suffixes again with a different word root.

Root	Gastr
	*(From a Greek word **gaster**, meaning belly or stomach.)*
Combining forms	**Gastr/o**

WORD EXERCISE 2

Without using your Exercise Guide, write the meaning of:

(a) **gastro**/scope _____

(b) **gastr**/ectomy _____

(c) **gastro**/tomy _____

(d) **gastr**/itis _____

Using your Exercise Guide, build words that mean:

(e) disease of the stomach _____

(f) study of the stomach _____

(g) pertaining to upon/above
     the stomach _____

Remember, when building words the combining vowel is usually dropped if the suffix begins with a vowel.

Note.   A naso **gastr**ic tube (nas/o meaning nose) that passes through the nose to the stomach can be used for suction, irrigation or feeding.

Root	Enter
	*(From a Greek word **enteron**, meaning intestine or gut.)*
Combining forms	**Enter/o**

WORD EXERCISE 3

Without using your Exercise Guide, write the meaning of:

(a) **enter**/itis _____

(b) **entero**/pathy _____

(c) **entero**/tomy _____

Using your Exercise Guide, find the meaning of:

(d) **entero**/stomy _____

Here you need to note the difference between:

> **-stomy**
> This means a mouth or opening. Usually a stoma is formed by surgery, e.g. a colostomy is an opening or the formation of an opening into the colon. This word component is also used in anastomosis, an operation to form an opening/communication between two parts (Fig. 7). A stoma can be temporary or permanent.
>
> **-tomy**
> Means an incision as at the beginning of an operation.

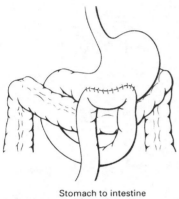

Stomach to intestine
(side to side)

Intestine to intestine
(side to end)

Figure 7   Surgical anastomoses

(e) **entero**/lith _____

Without using your Exercise Guide, build words that mean:

(f) study of the intestine _____

(g) a person who studies the intestines _____

Now we can put two roots together to make a larger word. Although these words look complicated it is now quite easy to understand their meaning.

Without using your Exercise Guide, write the meaning of:

(h) gastro/**entero**/logy _____

(i) gastro/**entero**/pathy _____

(j) gastro/**enter**/itis _____

(k) gastro/**entero**/scopy _____

Note.   When the two roots **gastr/o** and **enter/o** are joined the combining vowel of the first root is retained.

Between the stomach and the small intestine there is a sphincter muscle known as the **pylorus**. This acts as a valve which opens periodically to allow digested food to leave the stomach.

 Root   **Pylor**
(From a Greek word **pylouros**, *meaning gate-keeper. It is used to mean the pylorus.)*

Combining forms   **Pylor/o**

WORD EXERCISE 4

Without using your Exercise Guide, write the meaning of:

(a) **pyloro**/gastr/ectomy _____

(b) **pyloro**/scopy _____

The small intestine

Now let us examine the small intestine which consists of three parts, the **duodenum**, **jejunum** and **ileum**. The duodenum is concerned mainly with digestion of food while the jejunum and ileum are specially adapted for the absorption of nutrients.

Note.   Although the root **enter** refers generally to intestines, it is often used to mean the small intestine. However, there are special roots that describe the different regions of the intestine. We shall use these in the next three exercises.

Root   **Duoden**
(From a Latin word **duodeni**, *meaning twelve. It refers to the duodenum, which is the first 12 inches of the small intestine.)*

Combining forms   **Duoden/o**

Root   **Jejun**
(From a Latin word **jejunus**, *meaning empty. It refers to the jejunum, part of the intestine between the duodenum and ileum approx 2.4 m in length.)*

Combining forms   **Jejun/o**

Ile
*(From a Latin word **ilia**, meaning flanks. We use it here to mean the lower three-fifths of the small intestine.)*

Combining forms   **Ile/o**

WORD EXERCISE 5

Without using your Exercise Guide, write the meaning of:

(a) **duodeno**/entero/stomy _____

(b) **jejuno**/jejuno/stomy _____

Using your Exercise Guide, find the meaning of:

(c) **duodeno**/jejun/al _____

Without using your Exercise Guide, build words that mean:

(d) formation of an opening into the ileum _____

(e) inflammation of the ileum _____

(Exception – two vowels together.)

A permanent opening or **ileostomy** is made when the whole of the large intestine has been removed. This acts as an artificial anus. The ileum opens directly on to the abdominal wall and the liquid discharge from it is collected in a plastic **ileostomy bag** (Fig. 8).

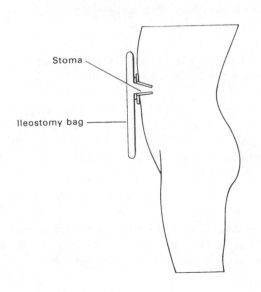

Stoma

Ileostomy bag

| Figure 8 | Ileostomy |

After passing through the small intestine, any remaining material passes into the large intestine or large bowel.

The large intestine

The large intestine has a wider diameter than the small intestine and it is shorter. Its main function is to absorb water from the materials that remain after digestion and eject them from the body as faeces (Am. feces) during defaecation. The large intestine is made up of the **caecum** (Am. cecum), **appendix**, **colon**, **rectum** and **anus** (Fig. 9).

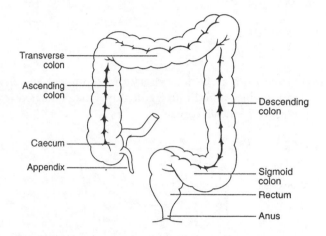

Transverse colon
Ascending colon
Descending colon
Caecum
Appendix
Sigmoid colon
Rectum
Anus

| Figure 9 | The large intestine |

The next six roots refer to the large intestine:

Caec
*(From a Latin word **caecus** meaning blind. It refers to a blindly ending pouch, the caecum attached to the vermiform appendix and separated from the ileum by a valve, the ileocaecal valve.)*

Combining forms   **Caec/o**
                   Cec/o (Am.)

Append
*(From a Latin word **appendix**, meaning appendage, the root refers to the appendix, a blindly ending sac attached to the caecum.)*

Combining forms   **Appendic/o**
                   Append/o (Am.)

Col
*(From a Greek word **kolon**, meaning colon, the large bowel extending from caecum to rectum.)*

Combining forms   **Col/o, colon/o**

WORD EXERCISE 6

Using your Exercise Guide, find the meaning of:

(a) mega/**colon** _____

Without using your Exercise Guide, write the meaning of:

(b) **appendic**/itis _____

(c) **col**/ectomy _____

(d) **colo**/stomy _____
     (see Fig. 10)

A colostomy may be temporary or permanent and its effluent is discharged into a **colostomy bag** attached to the surface of the abdomen.

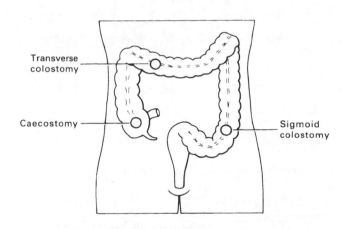

Transverse colostomy

Caecostomy

Sigmoid colostomy

Figure 10	Common sites of stomas of large bowel

Without using your Exercise Guide, build words that mean:

(e) formation of an opening into _____
     the caecum (Am. cecum)

(f) removal of the appendix _____

(g) formation of an opening _____
     (anastomosis) between the colon
     and stomach

Root	**Sigm** *(From a Greek word* **sigma**, *meaning the letter S. It refers to the last part of the descending colon that resembles an S-shape and is called the sigmoid colon.)*

Combining forms   **Sigmoid/o**

Root	**Rect** *(From a Latin word* **rectus**, *meaning straight. Here it refers to the last part of the large intestine, the rectum, which is straight.)*

Combining forms   **Rect/o**

Root	**Proct** *(From a Greek word* **proktos**, *meaning anus. It is used to mean the anus or rectum.)*

Combining forms   **Proct/o**

WORD EXERCISE 7

Using your Exercise Guide, find the meaning of:

(a) **sigmoido**/scopy _____

(b) para/**rect**/al _____

(c) peri/**proct**/itis _____

(d) **procto**/clysis _____

(e) **proct**/algia _____

Without using your Exercise Guide, build words that mean:

(f) instrument to view anus/rectum _____

(g) formation of an opening between _____
     the caecum and anus

(h) formation of an opening between _____
     the sigmoid colon and caecum

Sometimes the lining of the intestine develops enlarged pouches or sacs. Each is known as a **diverticulum** (pl. **diverticulae**). These can become inflamed as in **diverticul**itis and may have to be removed by **diverticul**ectomy.

The outer layer of the intestines and the lining of the cavity in which they lie consist of serous membrane. This secretes a serum-like fluid, serous fluid, that acts as a lubricant. A film of serous fluid allows organs to slide over each other as they move by peristalsis.

Peritone
*(From Greek words **peri**, meaning around, and **teinein**, meaning to stretch. It refers to the peritoneum, the serous membrane lining the abdominal and pelvic cavities and covering all abdominal organs.)*

Combining forms   **Periton/e/o**

WORD EXERCISE 8

Without using your Exercise Guide, write the meaning of:

(a) **periton**/itis _____

(b) **peritoneo**/clysis _____

Accessory organs of the digestive system

The pancreas

This gland is found beneath the stomach (see Fig. 6). Its function is to produce **pancreatic juice** that is passed to the duodenum where it neutralizes acid and digests food. It can also produce the hormones **insulin** and **glucagon** which are secreted directly into the blood.

Pancreat
*(From a Greek word **pankreas**, meaning the pancreas.)*

Combining forms   **Pancreat/o**
*A combining form **pancreatic/o** is also derived from this root. It is used to mean pancreatic duct. This duct transfers pancreatic juice containing digestive enzymes from the pancreas to the duodenum.*

The liver

The liver is the largest abdominal organ (Fig. 11). It is located just beneath the diaphragm. It processes nutrients which it receives from the intestine, stores materials and excretes wastes in the form of **bile** back into the intestine.

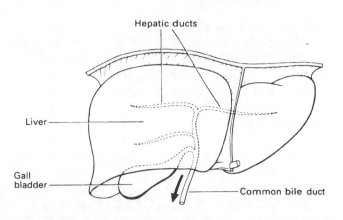

Hepatic ducts

Liver

Gall bladder

Common bile duct

The liver and bile ducts

Hepat
*(From a Greek word **hepatos**, meaning the liver.)*

Combining forms   **Hepat/o**
*A combining form **hepatic/o** is also derived from this root and is used to mean the hepatic duct.*

WORD EXERCISE 9

Using your Exercise Guide, find the meaning of:

(a) **pancreato**/lysis _____

(b) **hepato**/megaly _____

(c) **hepat**/oma _____

(d) **hepato**/toxic _____

Without using your Exercise Guide, write the meaning of:

(e) **hepatico**/gastro/stomy _____

(f) **pancreatico**/duoden/al _____

Chol
*(From a Greek word **chole**, meaning bile.)*

Combining forms   **Chol/e**

Liver cells produce a yellowish-brown waste known as bile. This drains through small canals and hepatic ducts into a sac known as the gall bladder. Bile leaves the gall bladder through the common bile duct and enters the intestine. Although bile is a waste product, the bile salts it contains help to emulsify lipids (fats) in the intestine. The structures in which bile is transported are referred to as the **biliary** system (*bili-* meaning bile, *-ary* meaning pertaining to).

WORD EXERCISE 10

Using your Exercise Guide, find the meaning of:

(a) a/**chol**/ia   _____

(b) **chole**/lith   _____

(c) **chole**/lith/iasis   _____

(d) **chol**/aemia (Am. chol/emia)   _____

(e) **chol**/uria   _____

A word root commonly combined with **chol/e** is **cyst/o**, meaning bladder. **Cholecyst/o** refers specifically to the bile bladder, commonly called the gall bladder.

Without using your Exercise Guide, write the meaning of:

(f) **cholecysto**/tomy   _____

(g) **cholecyst**/ectomy   _____

(h) **cholecysto**/lithiasis   _____

A second word root often combined with **chol/e** is **angi/o** meaning vessel. **Cholangi/o** therefore refers to the bile vessels/ducts.

Using your Exercise Guide, find the meaning of:

(i) **cholangio**/gram   _____

(j) **cholangio**/graphy   _____

A third word root often combined with **chol/e** is **doch/o**, meaning to receive. **Choledoch/o** refers to the common bile duct, i.e. that which receives the bile.

Without using your Exercise Guide, write the meaning of:

(k) **choledocho**/lithiasis   _____

(l) **choledocho**/litho/tomy   _____

Here we need to distinguish between three suffixes that often cause some confusion:

> **-gram**
> This refers to a tracing. In practice in medicine it usually refers to an X-ray picture, paper recording or to a trace on a screen.
>
> **-graphy**
> This refers to the technique or process of making a recording, e.g. an X-ray or tracing. It can also refer to a written description.
>
> **-graph**
> This means a description or writing but more often it is used in medicine for the name of an instrument that carries out a recording. Occasionally it is used to mean the recording itself.

Root   **Lapar**
*(From a Greek word **lapara**, meaning soft part between the ribs and hips, i.e. the flank/abdomen.)*

Combining forms   **Lapar/o**

WORD EXERCISE 11

Without using your Exercise Guide, write the meaning of:

(a) **laparo**/scopy   _____

(b) **laparo**/tomy   _____

Laparotomy is an exploratory operation performed when the diagnosis of an abdominal problem is uncertain. With advances in diagnostic procedures such as CT scanning, ultrasonography and laparoscopy, it has become less common.

Laparoscopy is performed using a laparoscope, a device consisting of a thin tube containing a lens system that can be passed through a small hole into the abdominal cavity. The laparoscope allows the internal organs (viscera) to be viewed and manipulated by a surgeon.

Medical equipment and clinical procedures

In this unit we have named several instruments. Let us review their names:

gastroscope
gastroenteroscope
sigmoidoscope

colonoscope
proctoscope
laparoscope

All of these instruments are used to view various parts of the digestive system. Now fibreoptic endoscopes have replaced some of the original viewing instruments. Endoscope means an instrument to view inside (**endo-** within/inside).

Endoscopes utilize flexible/fibreoptic tubes (Fig. 12) that can be inserted into body cavities or into small incisions made in the body wall. Each is provided with illumination and a system of lenses which enables the operator to view the inside of the body. The inclusion of electronic chips at the end of the fibreoptic tube allows the view to be transmitted to a video screen. Sometimes the endoscope is used for photography and it is then known as a photoendoscope.

The endoscope can be adapted to view particular areas of the body. In the case of the digestive system, the fibreoptic tube can be passed into the mouth to examine the oesophagus, stomach and intestine. Alternatively it can be passed into the anus to view the rectum and colon. Note that when an endoscope is adapted to examine the stomach it may be referred to as a gastroscope.

Often endoscopes are used to examine the oesophagus, stomach and duodenum at the same examination. This procedure is **pan**endoscopy (**pan-** means all, i.e. all the upper digestive system). Similarly, panendoscopy could be performed on all of the large intestine via the anus.

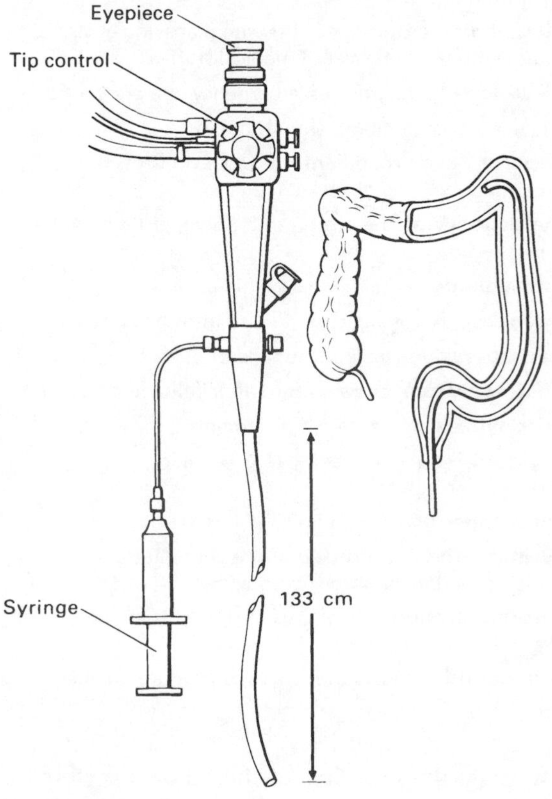

In addition to viewing cavities, endoscopes can be fitted with a variety of attachments, such as forceps and catheters, and they can then be used for special applications. One such procedure is:

ERCP or **endoscopic, retrograde, cholangiopancreatography**

Let us examine the words separately:

endoscopic	referring to an endoscope
retrograde	going backwards
chol	bile
angio	vessel
pancreato	pancreas
graphy	technique of making a tracing/X-ray recording

Although we cannot deduce the exact meaning from the words we can see why they have been used. Here is the meaning of ERCP:

A technique of making an X-ray (graphy) of the pancreatic vessels and bile duct (pancreat/chol/angio), by passing a catheter (tube) backwards (retrograde) into them using an endoscope. Dye is injected through the catheter to outline the vessels and ducts on the X-ray.

WORD EXERCISE 12

Match each term in Column A with a description from Column C by placing an appropriate number in Column B.

Column A	Column B	Column C
(a) enteroscope	_____	1. instrument to view rectum
(b) endoscope	_____	2. technique of taking photographs using an endoscope
(c) enteroscopy	_____	3. visual examination of the colon
(d) endoscopy	_____	4. instrument to view the intestine
(e) endoscopist	_____	5. visual examination of all cavities, e.g. oesophagus, stomach and duodenum
(f) colonoscopy	_____	6. instrument to view body cavities
(g) proctoscope	_____	7. visual examination of the intestine
(h) sigmoidoscopy	_____	8. person who operates an endoscope

Eyepiece

Tip control

Syringe

133 cm

Figure 12 Fibreoptic endoscope used to view the colon

Column A	Column B	Column C
(i) panendoscopy	_____	9. visual examination of body cavities
(j) photoendoscopy	_____	10. visual examination of S-colon

ANATOMY EXERCISE

Now complete the Anatomy Exercise on page 14.

CASE HISTORY 2

The object of this exercise is to understand words associated with a patient's medical history. To complete the exercise:

- read through the passage on gallstones; unfamiliar words are underlined and you can find their meaning using the Word Help

- write the meaning of the medical terms shown in bold print.

Gallstones (Cholelithiasis)

Miss B, a 35-year-old, presented to her general practitioner complaining of pain emanating from the **epigastric** and right hypochondrial regions radiating to the back. The pain lasted for about 3 hours following each meal and was accompanied by nausea and occasional vomiting. Her GP's initial diagnosis was **biliary** colic, and he prescribed the analgesic pethidine. The pain did not resolve and she was admitted to the **gastroenterology** unit.

Initial ultrasound investigations revealed multiple stones in the gall bladder and a dilated common bile duct. A date was set for early elective **laparoscopic cholecystectomy.** Miss B was counselled on her perioperative drug regimen and was introduced to the concept of patient controlled analgesia (PCA) using a syringe driver. Unfortunately, her elective procedure was delayed by an episode of acute **cholecystitis**.

Once recovered Miss B was admitted again but, due to her excessive weight, laparoscopy was deemed inappropriate by the surgeon and she was advised of the associative risks of an alternative procedure.

Vital signs on admission

Pulse 90/minute	Oral temp 37°C	BP 140/70
Height 1.52 m	Weight 85 kg	Smoker 25/day
Moderate drinker	Medication None	

An open cholecystectomy was performed and the inflamed gall bladder found to contain three gallstones each approximately 1.5 cm in diameter. A bile sample was sent for culture and sensitivity testing and a **nasogastric** tube passed. Antibiotic prophylaxis (cefuroxime) was administered prior to her operation and continued for 48 hours. Miss B also received low dose subcutaneous heparin injections as part of her thromboembolic prophylaxis.

The patient tolerated surgery well, PCA controlled her pain and she was apyrexial. In the immediate postoperative period she received an intravenous (i.v.) infusion of dextrose 4%, NaCl 0.18%, KCl 0.05% at a rate of 125 ml/hour.

On day four following her operation, the nasogastric tube and wound drains were removed and i.v. fluid replacement ceased. Miss B left the unit on day six and was provided with diclofenac 50 mg analgesic tablets to be taken up to 3 times daily when required. She agreed to an appointment with the dietician to discuss the desirability of reducing her weight.

WORD HELP

analgesic pain relieving drug

apyrexial absence of fever

culture and sensitivity testing growing microorganisms in the laboratory and testing them for sensitivity to antibiotics

dietician/dietitian specialist who plans and advises on diet with the approval of medical staff

elective voluntary/not an emergency/at a planned date

GP general practitioner (family doctor)

heparin an anticoagulant drug that prevents blood clotting

hypochondrial the region to the side, just below the ribs

intravenous pertaining to within a vein

open surgery via an incision (here into the abdomen)

peri-operative around the time of operation

post-operative pertaining to after/following operation

prophylaxis preventative treatment

regimen regulated scheme (e.g. of taking drugs/medication)

subcutaneous pertaining to under the skin

syringe driver motorized device that injects medication/drugs into the body

thromboembolic thrombus or clot moving and blocking another blood vessel

ultrasound using sound waves to produce an image

Now write the meaning of the following words from the case history without using your dictionary lists:

(a) cholelithiasis _____

(b) epigastric _____

(c) biliary _____

(d) gastroenterology _____

(e) laparoscopic _____

(f) cholecystectomy _____

(g) cholecystitis _____

(h) nasogastric _____

(Answers to the case history exercise are given in the Answers to Word Exercises beginning on page 275).

Quick Reference

Combining forms relating to the digestive system:

Appendic/o	appendix
Bil/i	bile
Caec/o	caecum
Cec/o (Am.)	cecum
Chol/e	bile
Cholangi/o	bile vessel/duct
Cholecyst/o	gall bladder
Choledoch/o	common bile duct
Col/o	colon
Colon/o	colon
Diverticul/o	diverticulum
Duoden/o	duodenum
Enter/o	intestine
Esophag/o (Am.)	esophagus
Gastr/o	stomach
Hepat/o	liver
Hepatic/o	hepatic duct
Ile/o	ileum
Jejun/o	jejunum
Lapar/o	flank/abdominal wall
Oesophag/o	oesophagus
Pancreat/o	pancreas
Pancreatic/o	pancreatic duct
Peritone/o	peritoneum
Proct/o	anus/rectum
Pylor/o	pyloric sphincter
Rect/o	rectum
Ser/o	serous/serum
Sigmoid/o	sigmoid colon

Abbreviations

Some common abbreviations related to the digestive system are listed below. Note, some are not standard and their meaning may vary from one health care setting to another. There is a more extensive list for reference on page 307.

Abdo	abdomen
CD	Crohn's disease
DU	duodenal ulcer
GI	gastrointestinal
GU	gastric ulcer
IUC	idiopathic ulcerative colitis
LLQ	left lower quadrant
pr/PR	per rectum
PU	peptic ulcer
RE	rectal examination
UC	ulcerative colitis
UGI	upper gastrointestinal

> ## NOW TRY THE WORD CHECK <

WORD CHECK

This self-check exercise lists all the word components used in this unit. First write down the meaning of as many word components as you can. Then check your answers using the Exercise Guide and Quick Reference box or the Glossary of Word Components (pp. 319–341).

Prefixes

a- _____

endo- _____

epi- _____

mega- _____

pan- _____

para- _____

peri- _____

retro- _____

Combining forms of word roots

angi/o

appendic/o

bil/i

caec/o
(Am. cec/o)

chol/e

choledoch/o

col/o

colon/o

cyst/o

diverticul/o

duoden/o

enter/o

gastr/o

hepat/o

hepatic/o

ile/o

jejun/o

lapar/o

nas/o

oesophag/o
(Am. esophag/o)

pancreat/o

pancreatic/o

peritone/o

proct/o

pylor/o

rect/o

ser/o

sigmoid/o

tox/o

Suffixes

-aemia
(Am. -emia)

-al

-algia

-ary

-clysis

-ectomy

-grade

-gram

-graph

-graphy

-ia

-iasis

-ic

-ist

-itis

-lith

-lithiasis

-logist

-logy

-lysis

-megaly

-oma

-pathy

-scope

-scopy

-stomy

-tomy

-toxic

-uria

 NOW TRY THE SELF-ASSESSMENT

SELF-ASSESSMENT

Test 2A

Below are some combining forms that refer to the anatomy of the digestive system. Indicate which part of the system they refer to by putting a number from the diagram (Fig. 13) next to each word. You can use a number more than once.

(a) pylor/o _____

(b) gastr/o _____

(c) proct/o _____

(d) hepat/o _____

(e) appendic/o _____

(f) choledoch/o _____

(g) col/o _____

(h) pancreat/o _____

(i) sigmoid/o _____

(j) oesophag/o
    (Am. esophag/o) _____

(k) cholecyst/o _____

(l) ile/o _____

(m) caec/o
    (Am. cec/o) _____

(n) duoden/o _____

(o) rect/o _____

Score

15 / 15

Test 2B

Prefixes and suffixes

Match each prefix or suffix in Column A with a meaning in Column C by inserting the appropriate number in Column B.

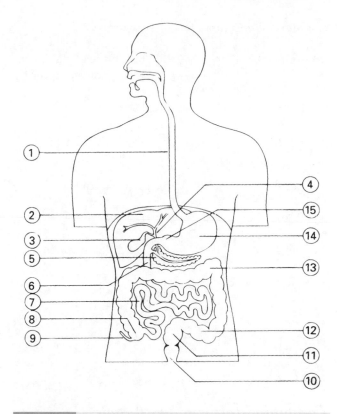

Figure 13 The digestive system

Column A	Column B	Column C
(a) a-	_____	1. enlargement
(b) -aemia (Am. -emia)	_____	2. condition of pain
(c) -algia	_____	3. study of
(d) -clysis	_____	4. around
(e) -ectomy	_____	5. injection/infusion
(f) endo-	_____	6. X-ray/tracing
(g) -gram	_____	7. inflammation
(h) -graph	_____	8. condition of urine
(i) -graphy	_____	9. within/inside
(j) -itis	_____	10. beside/near
(k) -lithiasis	_____	11. tumour
(l) -logy	_____	12. abnormal condition of stones
(m) mega-	_____	13. all
(n) -megaly	_____	14. without

Column A	Column B	Column C
(o) -oma	_____	15. technique of making an X-ray/tracing/record
(p) pan-	_____	16. large
(q) para-	_____	17. instrument which records
(r) peri-	_____	18. incision into
(s) -tomy	_____	19. removal of
(t) -uria	_____	20. condition of blood

Score

20
20

Test 2C

Combining forms of word roots

Match each combining form of a word root from Column A with a meaning from Column C by inserting the appropriate number in Column B.

Column A	Column B	Column C
(a) angi/o	_____	1. pylorus
(b) appendic/o	_____	2. sigmoid colon
(c) caec/o (Am. cec/o)	_____	3. peritoneum
(d) chol/e	_____	4. jejunum
(e) choledoch/o	_____	5. intestine
(f) colon/o	_____	6. vessel
(g) cyst/o	_____	7. duodenum
(h) duoden/o	_____	8. colon
(i) enter/o	_____	9. rectum
(j) gastr/o	_____	10. rectum/anus
(k) hepat/o	_____	11. bladder
(l) jejun/o	_____	12. stomach
(m) lapar/o	_____	13. oesophagus
(n) oesophag/o (Am. esophag/o)	_____	14. bile

Column A	Column B	Column C
(o) pancreat/o	_____	15. abdomen/flank
(p) peritone/o	_____	16. common bile duct
(q) proct/o	_____	17. caecum
(r) pylor/o	_____	18. pancreas
(s) rect/o	_____	19. liver
(t) sigmoid/o	_____	20. appendix

Score

20
20

Test 2D

Write the meaning of:

(a) gastroenterocolitis _____

(b) hepatography _____

(c) ileorectal _____

(d) proctosigmoidoscope _____

(e) pancreatomegaly _____

Score

5

Test 2E

Build words that mean:

(a) inflammation of the duodenum _____

(b) condition of pain in the stomach _____

(c) incision into the liver _____

(d) study of the anus/rectum _____

(e) formation of an opening/ anastomosis between the anus and the ileum _____

Score

5

Check answers to Self-Assessment Tests on page 299.

3 The breathing system

Objectives

Once you have completed Unit 3 you should be able to:

- understand the meaning of medical words relating to the breathing system

- build medical words relating to the breathing system

- associate medical terms with their anatomical position

- understand medical abbreviations relating to the breathing system.

Exercise Guide

Use this list of word components and their meanings to complete the word exercises in this unit.

Prefixes

a-	without
dys-	difficult/painful
hyper-	above/excessive
hypo-	below/low
inter-	between
tachy-	fast

Roots/Combining forms

chondr/o	cartilage
esophag/o (Am.)	esophagus
gastr/o	stomach
haem/o	blood
hem/o (Am.)	blood
hepat/o	liver
myc/o	fungus
oesophag/o	oesophagus
radi/o	radiation/X-ray

Suffixes

-al	pertaining to
-algia	condition of pain
-ary	pertaining to
-centesis	surgical puncture to remove fluid
-desis	fixation/bind together by surgery/sticking together
-dynia	condition of pain
-eal	pertaining to
-ectasis	dilatation/stretching
-ectomy	removal of
-genic	pertaining to formation/originating in
-gram	X-ray/tracing/recording
-graphy	technique of recording/making X-ray
-ia	condition of
-ic	pertaining to
-itis	inflammation of
-logy	study of
-meter	measuring instrument
-metry	process of measuring
-osis	abnormal condition/disease of
-pathy	disease of
-plasty	surgical repair/reconstruction
-pexy	surgical fixation/fix in place
-plegia	condition of paralysis
-rrhaphy	suture/stitch/suturing
-rrhea (Am.)	excessive discharge/flow
-rrhoea	excessive discharge/flow
-scope	an instrument to view/examine
-scopy	technique of viewing/examining
-spasm	involuntary contraction
-stenosis	abnormal condition of narrowing
-stomy	formation of an opening into …
-tomy	incision into
-us	thing/a structure (indicates an anatomical part)

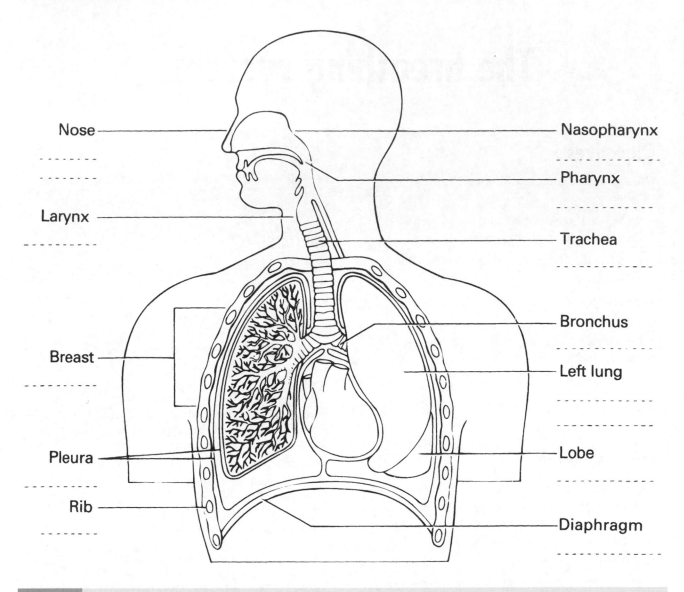

Nose ——————————

- - - - - - -

- - - - - - - -

Larynx ——————————

- - - - - - - -

Breast ——————————

- - - - - - - -

Pleura ——————————

- - - - - - - -

Rib ——————————

- - - - - - - -

Nasopharynx ——————————

- - - - - - - - - - -

Pharynx ——————————

- - - - - - - - - -

Trachea ——————————

- - - - - - - - - - -

Bronchus ——————————

- - - - - - - -

Left lung ——————————

- - - - - - - -

- - - - - - - - -

Lobe ——————————

- - - - - - - - - -

Diaphragm ——————————

- - - - - - - - - - -

Figure 14 The breathing system

ANATOMY EXERCISE

When you have finished Word Exercises 1–16, look at the word components listed below. Complete Figure 14 by writing the appropriate combining form on each dotted line – more than one component may relate to the same position. (You can check their meanings in the Quick Reference box on p. 35.

Bronch/o	Nasopharyng/o	Pulmon/o
Cost/o	Pharyng/o	Rhin/o
Laryng/o	Phren/o	Steth/o
Lob/o	Pleur/o	Trache/o
Nas/o	Pneumon/o	

The breathing system

Humans breathe air into paired lungs through the nose and mouth during inspiration. Whilst air is in the lungs gaseous exchange takes place; in this process oxygen enters the blood in exchange for carbon dioxide. During expiration, air containing less oxygen and more carbon dioxide leaves the body. The oxygen obtained through gaseous exchange is required by body cells for cellular respiration, a process that releases energy from food.

Our study of the breathing system begins at the point where air enters the body, the nose.

Use the Exercise Guide at the beginning of this unit to complete Word Exercises 1–16 unless you are asked to work without it.

Root	**Rhin** *(From a Greek word* **rhinos**, *meaning nose.)*
Combining forms	**Rhin/o**

WORD EXERCISE 1

Using your Exercise Guide, find the meaning of:

(a) **rhino**/scopy _____

(b) **rhino**/pathy _____

(c) **rhin**/algia _____

(d) **rhin**/itis _____

(e) **rhino**/rrhoea
(Am. rhino/rrhea) _____

(f) **rhino**/plasty _____

Root	**Nas** *(From a Latin word* **nasus**, *meaning nose.)*
Combining forms	**Nas/o**

WORD EXERCISE 2

Using your Exercise Guide, find the meaning of:

(a) **naso**/gastr/ic tube _____

(b) **naso**-oesophag/eal tube
(Am. naso-esophag/eal) _____

Root	**Pharyng** *(From a Greek word* **pharynx**, *meaning throat, here it is used to mean the pharynx.)*
Combining forms	**Pharyng/o**

WORD EXERCISE 3

Without using your Exercise Guide, write the meaning of:

(a) **pharyng**/algia _____

(b) **pharyngo**/rrhoea
(Am. pharyngo/rrhea) _____

Without using your Exercise Guide, build words that mean:

(c) surgical repair of the pharynx _____

(d) inflammation of the nose and pharynx (use rhin/o) _____

Root	**Laryng** *(From a Greek word* **larynx** *that refers to the voice box, here it is used to mean the larynx.)*
Combining forms	**Laryng/o**

WORD EXERCISE 4

Using your Exercise Guide, find the meaning of:

(a) **laryngo**/logy _____

(b) **laryngo**/pharyng/ectomy _____

Without using your Exercise Guide, build words that mean:

(c) technique of viewing the larynx _____

(d) the study of the nose and larynx (use rhin/o). _____

When swallowing, food is prevented from falling into the larynx by the **epiglottis**, a thin flap of cartilage lying above the glottis and behind the tongue. When the epiglottis moves, it covers the opening into the larynx and sound-producing glottis. **Epiglott/o** is the combining form derived from epiglottis; inflammation of the epiglottis may produce **epiglott**itis and tumours may be removed by **epiglott**ectomy.

Root

Trache
*(From Greek **tracheia**, meaning rough. Note that it refers to the rough appearance of the rings of cartilage in the windpipe. It is used to mean trachea or windpipe.)*

Combining forms **Trache/o**

WORD EXERCISE 5

Using your Exercise Guide, find the meaning of:

(a) **tracheo**/tomy _____

(b) **tracheo**/stomy (operation _____
used to maintain the airway; see Fig. 15)

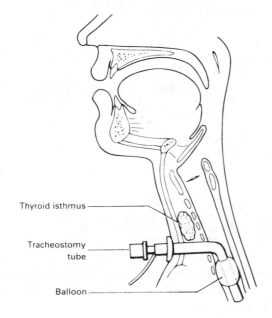

Thyroid isthmus

Tracheostomy
tube

Balloon

Figure 15 Tracheostomy

 Root

Bronch
*(From a Greek word **bronchos**, meaning bronchus or windpipe.)*

Combining forms **Bronch/i/o**

WORD EXERCISE 6

Using your Exercise Guide, build words that mean:

(a) discharge/excessive flow of mucus _____
from bronchi

(b) an X-ray of the bronchus _____

(c) technique of making an X-ray of _____
the bronchi

(d) an instrument for the visual _____
examination of the bronchi

Using your Exercise Guide, find the meaning of:

(e) **bronch**/us _____

(f) **broncho**/plegia _____

(g) **broncho**/rrhaphy _____

(h) **bronchi**/ectasis _____

(i) **broncho**/myc/osis _____

(j) **broncho**/genic _____

(k) **broncho**/spasm _____

(l) tracheo/**bronchi**/al _____

Without using your Exercise Guide, write the meaning of:

(m) laryngo/tracheo/**bronch**/itis _____

(n) **bronch**/oesophago/stomy _____
(Am. bronch/esophago/stomy)

Note. The combining form **bronchiol/o** is used when referring to the very small subdivisions of the bronchi known as **bronchioles**, e.g. **bronchiol**itis for inflammation of the bronchioles.

The smallest bronchioles end in microscopic air sacs known as **alveoli** (from Latin *alveus*, meaning hollow cavity). Alveoli form a large surface area of the lungs across which the gases oxygen and carbon dioxide are exchanged and therefore play an essential role in maintaining life. The combining form is **alveol/o**, but few terms are in use, e.g. **alveol**itis.

At the alveolar surface oxygen diffuses into the blood from the cavities of the alveoli, carbon dioxide diffuses in the opposite direction and is lost from the body in expired air. Disorders of the breathing and cardiovascular systems can affect gaseous exchange and therefore the concentration of these gases in the blood. **Hypoxia** is a condition of deficiency of oxygen in the tissues (*hypo-* meaning below/low, *-oxia* meaning condition of oxygen). **Hypercapnia** is a condition of too much carbon dioxide in the blood (*hyper-* meaning above/excessive, *-capnia* meaning a condition of carbon dioxide).

Poor oxygenation also results in the presence of large amounts of unoxygenated haemoglobin

(Am. hemoglobin) in the blood. This produces **cyanosis**, an abnormal condition in which unoxygenated haemoglobin gives a blue tinge to the skin, lips and nail beds (*cyan/o* meaning blue, *-osis* meaning abnormal condition).

Root	Pneumon
	(A Greek word, meaning lung.)

Combining forms   **Pneumon/o**

WORD EXERCISE 7

Without using your Exercise Guide, write the meaning of:

(a) **pneumono**/tomy   _____

(b) **pneumono**/rrhaphy   _____

(c) **pneumon**/osis   _____

Note. Pneumonia means a condition of the lungs. It refers to an inflammation of the lungs with exudation caused by infection. (The exudate is a fluid that has escaped from capillaries lining the lungs).

Without using your Exercise Guide, build words that mean:

(d) removal of a lung   _____

(e) disease of a lung   _____

Using your Exercise Guide, find the meaning of:

(f) **pneumono**/centesis   _____

(g) **pneumono**/pexy   _____

Root	Pneum
	*(From a Greek word **pneumatos**, meaning breath, air, gas and lung. Here we are using it to mean gas/air.)*

Combining forms   **Pneum/a/o, Pneumat/o**

At this point we need to introduce the word **pneumothorax**. The components of this word refer to air and thorax (chest) but the meaning of the word is not obvious. It means air or gas in the pleural cavity, i.e. the space between the wall of the thorax and the lungs.

A pneumothorax is formed by puncture of the chest wall; this can be caused by a stab wound or made as part of a surgical procedure.

WORD EXERCISE 8

Using your Exercise Guide, find the meaning of:

(a) **pneumo**/haemo/thorax   _____
    (Am. pneumo/hcmo/thorax; see Fig. 16)

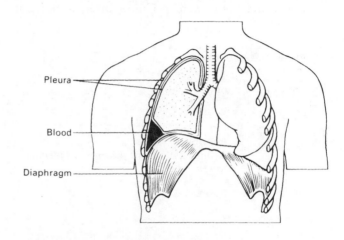

| Figure 16 | Haemothorax (Am. hemothorax) |

(b) **pneumo**/radio/graphy   _____
    (This term does not refer specifically to the breathing system. It is a technique used to enhance the contrast of X-rays of body cavities by injecting air into them.)

A combining form **-pnoea**, meaning breathing, is also derived from this root (Am. -pnea).

Using your Exercise Guide, find the meaning of:

(c) a/**pnoea**   _____
    (Am. a/pnea)

(d) dys/**pnoea**   _____
    (Am. dys/pnea)

(e) hyper/**pnoea**   _____
    (Am. hyper/pnea)

(f) hypo/**pnoea**   _____
    (Am. hypo/pnea)

(g) tachy/**pnoea**   _____
    (Am. tachy/pnea)

Root   **Lob**
*(From a Greek word **lobos**, meaning a rounded section of an organ. In the lungs, lobes are formed by fissures or septa that divide the right lung into three lobes and the left lung into two. Note that other organs in the body are lobar.)*

Combining forms   **Lob/o**

 WORD EXERCISE 9

Without using your Exercise Guide, build words that mean:

(a) incision into a lobe _____

(b) removal of a lobe _____

Root   **Pulmon**
*(From a Latin word **pulmonis**, meaning lung.)*

Combining forms   **Pulmon/o**

 WORD EXERCISE 10

Using your Exercise Guide, find the meaning of:

(a) **pulmon**/ic _____

(b) **pulmon**/ary _____

Root   **Pleur**
*(From a Greek word **pleura**, meaning rib or side. It is used to mean pleura, the shiny membranes covering the lungs and internal surfaces of the thorax. The space in between the membranes is the pleural cavity.)*

Combining forms   **Pleur/o**

 WORD EXERCISE 11

Without using your Exercise Guide, write the meaning of:

(a) **pleur**/itis (also called pleurisy) _____

(b) **pleuro**/centesis _____

Without using your Exercise Guide, build a word that means:

(c) technique of making an X-ray _____
     of pleural cavity

Using your Exercise Guide, find the meaning of:

(d) **pleuro**/dynia _____

(e) **pleuro**/desis _____

Root   **Phren**
(A Greek word, meaning midriff or diaphragm.)

Combining forms   **Phren/o**

 WORD EXERCISE 12

Using your Exercise Guide, find the meaning of:

(a) **phreno**/gastr/ic _____

(b) **phreno**/hepat/ic _____

(c) **phreno**/pleg/ia _____

Root   **Thorac**
*(From a Greek word **thorax**, meaning chest.)*

Combining forms   **Thorac/o**, also **-thorax** used as a suffix

 WORD EXERCISE 13

Without using your Exercise Guide, build words that mean:

(a) any disease of thorax _____

(b) incision into chest _____

Without using your Exercise Guide, write the meaning of:

(c) **thoraco**/centesis _____

(d) **thoraco**/scope _____

Using your Exercise Guide, find the meaning of:

(e) **thoraco**/stenosis _____

Root   Cost
          *(From a Latin word **costa**, meaning rib.)*

Combining forms   **Cost/o**

WORD EXERCISE 14

Using your Exercise Guide, find the meaning of:

(a) inter/**cost**/al   _____

(b) **costo**/genic   _____

(c) **costo**/chondr/itis _____

Medical equipment and clinical procedures

In this unit we have named several instruments used to examine the breathing system. Some of those mentioned may be modified fibreoptic endoscopes. Let us review their names:

  rhinoscope
  pharyngoscope
  laryngoscope
  bronchoscope
  thoracoscope

The nose and pharynx can be superficially examined using a source of illumination with a tongue depressor and a nasal speculum (Figs 17 and 18).

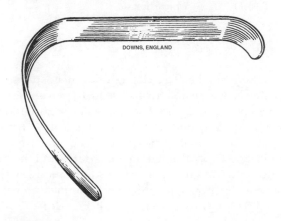

Figure 17   Tongue depressor

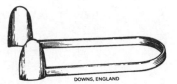

Figure 18   Nasal speculum

Note.   The word **speculum** refers to an instrument used to hold the walls of a cavity apart so that the interior can be examined visually.

Other instruments used to investigate the breathing system include:

Stethoscope
  (From a Greek word **stethos**, meaning breast, and **skopein**, meaning to examine.) Although this word ends in scope, which usually refers to an instrument for visual examination, it is used to listen to the sounds from the chest.

Spirograph
  (From a Latin word **spirare**, meaning to breathe.) An instrument that records breathing movements of lungs.

Spirometer
  An instrument that measures the capacity of the lung. The technique for using this instrument is spirometry (synonymous with pneumatometry).

We also need to distinguish between the suffixes:

-meter
  an instrument that measures.

-metry
  the technique of measuring, i.e. using a measuring instrument.

Now revise the names and uses of all instruments and examinations mentioned in this unit and then try Exercises 15 and 16.

WORD EXERCISE 15

Match each term in Column A with a description from Column C by placing an appropriate number in Column B.

Column A	Column B	Column C
(a) bronchoscope	_____	1. person who may use a nasal speculum

Column A	Column B	Column C
(b) laryngoscopy	_____	2. instrument to examine the vocal cords
(c) rhinoscope	_____	3. instrument to examine the bronchi
(d) pharyngoscope	_____	4. visual examination of the vocal cords
(e) bronchoscopy	_____	5. device used to allow air through the tracheal wall
(f) rhinologist	_____	6. instrument to view the back of the mouth
(g) tracheostomy tube	_____	7. visual examination of the bronchi
(h) laryngoscope	_____	8. instrument to view nasal cavities

WORD EXERCISE 16

Match each term in Column A with a description from Column C by placing an appropriate number in Column B.

Column A	Column B	Column C
(a) thoracoscope	_____	1. instrument to open the nostrils
(b) stethoscope	_____	2. technique of making an X-ray of pleura
(c) spirometer	_____	3. technique of recording breathing movements
(d) spirography	_____	4. technique of measuring lung capacity
(e) nasal speculum	_____	5. instrument to view the thorax
(f) nasogastric tube	_____	6. instrument that measures lung capacity
(g) pleurography	_____	7. instrument to examine/listen to the breast
(h) spirometry	_____	8. tube inserted into the stomach via nose

ANATOMY EXERCISE

Now complete the Anatomy Exercise on page 28.

CASE HISTORY 3

The object of this exercise is to understand words associated with a patient's medical history.

To complete the exercise:

- read through the passage on chronic obstructive pulmonary disease; unfamiliar words are underlined and you can find their meaning using the Word Help

- write the meaning of the medical terms shown in bold print.

Chronic obstructive pulmonary disease

Mr C is 56 years of age and has a long history of chronic obstructive **pulmonary** disease (COPD). He began smoking at the age of 14 and until 6 years ago smoked approximately 25–30 cigarettes per day but now only smokes 2 or 3 per week. Five years ago he developed a squamous cell carcinoma and had a right upper **lobectomy.**

Mr C has had two acute exacerbations of bronchitis in the past year. His wife says that over the last few days he has become increasingly out of breath and has difficulty in walking, speaking and eating. He was seen in casualty with increasing **dyspnoea**, **cyanosis** and a productive, purulent sputum.

Vital signs on admission

Pulse 100/min	Oral temp 38 °C	BP 150/95
Medication	Home oxygen therapy	salbutamol 5 mg nebulized q.i.d prednisolone 30 mg/day

Blood Gas Analysis

paCO₂ 8.90 kPa (4.5–6.1)	Standard bicarbonate 29.2 (22–28)	PEFR 180 L/min
paO₂ 4.5 kPa (12–15)	Blood pH 7.05 (7.32–7.42)	

On examination he had a degree of **bronchospasm** and was showing signs of **hypoxia** and **hypercapnia**. His serious condition required his immediate transfer to the intensive therapy unit (ITU) for mechanical ventilatory support. An arterial catheter for blood gas sampling was inserted via the left radial artery, and he was sedated. He was given a muscle relaxant intravenously to enable tracheal intubation and commencement of intermittent positive pressure ventilation (IPPV).

Mr C was initially diagnosed as having basal **pneumonia** in the right lung complicating his COPD.

He was administered one <u>intravenous</u> dose of 500 mg of ampicillin followed by 500 mg amoxicillin 8-hourly.

WORD HELP

acute symptoms/signs of short duration

carcinoma malignant growth from epidermal cells/a cancer

catheter a tube inserted into the body

chronic lasting/lingering for a long time

exacerbations acute increased severity of symptoms

intravenous pertaining to within a vein

intubation insertion of a tube into a hollow organ in this case the trachea

productive producing e.g. producing mucus/sputum

purulent resembling pus/infected

sedated state of reduced activity usually as a result of medication

sputum material expelled from the respiratory passages by coughing or clearing the throat

squamous pertaining to scale-like/from squamous epithelium

Now write the meaning of the following words from the case history without using your dictionary lists:

(a) pulmonary   _____

(b) lobectomy   _____

(c) dyspnoea   _____

(d) cyanosis   _____

(e) bronchospasm   _____

(f) hypoxia   _____

(g) hypercapnia   _____

(h) pneumonia   _____

(Answers to the case history exercise are given in the Answers to Word Exercises beginning on page 275.)

Quick Reference

Combining forms relating to the breathing system:

Alveol/o	alveolus
Bronch/o	bronchus
Bronchiol/o	bronchiole
Chondr/o	cartilage

Quick Reference (contd.)

Combining forms relating to the breathing system:

Cost/o	rib
Epiglott/o	epiglottis
Laryng/o	larynx
Lob/o	lobe
Nas/o	nose
Nasopharyng/o	nasopharynx
Pharyng/o	pharynx
Phren/o	diaphragm
Pleur/o	pleura
Pneum/o	gas/air/lung
Pneumon/o	lung/air
-pnoea	breathing
-pnea (Am.)	breathing
Pulmon/o	lung
Rhin/o	nose
Spir/o	to breathe
Steth/o	breast
Thorac/o	thorax
Trache/o	trachea

Abbreviations

Some common abbreviations related to the breathing system are listed below. Note, some are not standard and their meaning may vary from one health care setting to another. There is a more extensive list for reference on page 307.

BRO	bronchoscopy
COPD	chronic obstructive pulmonary disease
CXR	chest X-ray
ET	endotracheal
FVC	forced vital capacity
LLL	left lower lobe
PE	pulmonary embolism
PEFR	peak expiratory flow rate
PFts	pulmonary function tests
RSV	respiratory syncytial virus
SOBE	shortage of breath on exertion
URTI	upper respiratory tract infection

 NOW TRY THE WORD CHECK

WORD CHECK

This self-check lists all the word components used in this unit. First write down the meaning of as many word components as you can. Then check your answers using the Exercise Guide and Quick Reference box or the Glossary of Word Components (pp. 319–341).

Prefixes

a- _____

dys- _____

hyper- _____

hypo- _____

inter- _____

tachy- _____

Combining forms of word roots

alveol/o _____

bronch/o _____

bronchiol/o _____

chondr/o _____

cost/o _____

cyan/o _____

epiglott/o _____

gastr/o _____

haem/o
(Am. hem/o) _____

hepat/o _____

laryng/o _____

lob/o _____

myc/o _____

nas/o _____

oesophag/o
(Am. esophag/o) _____

pharyng/o _____

phren/o _____

pleur/o _____

pneum/o _____

pneumon/o _____

pnoea
(Am. pnea) _____

pulmon/o _____

radi/o _____

rhin/o _____

spir/o _____

sten/o _____

thorac/o _____

trache/o _____

Suffixes

-al _____

-algia _____

-ary _____

-capnia _____

-centesis _____

-desis _____

-dynia _____

-ectasis _____

-ectomy _____

-genic _____

-gram _____

-graphy _____

-ia _____

-ic _____

-itis _____

-logy   _____

-meter   _____

-metry   _____

-osis   _____

-oxia   _____

-pathy   _____

-pexy   _____

-plasty   _____

-plegia   _____

-rrhaphy   _____

-rrhoea
(Am. rrhea)   _____

-scope   _____

-scopy   _____

-spasm   _____

-stomy   _____

-tomy   _____

-us   _____

(e) pleur/o   _____

(f) pneum/o   _____

(g) trache/o   _____

(h) laryng/o   _____

(i) pharyng/o   _____

(j) rhin/o   _____

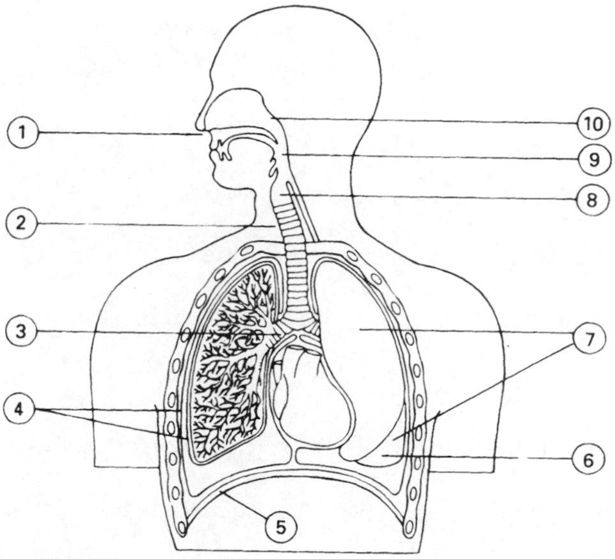

Figure 19   The breathing system

Score

[   ]
10

> **NOW TRY THE SELF-ASSESSMENT** <

SELF-ASSESSMENT

Test 3A

Below are some combining forms that refer to the anatomy of the breathing system. Indicate which part of the system they refer to by putting a number from the diagram (Fig. 19) next to each word. The numbers may be used more than once.

(a) bronch/o   _____

(b) nasopharyng/o   _____

(c) phren/o   _____

(d) lob/o   _____

Test 3B

Prefixes and Suffixes

Match each prefix and suffix in Column A with a meaning in Column C by inserting the appropriate number in Column B.

Column A	Column B	Column C
(a) -centesis	_____	1. measuring instrument
(b) -desis	_____	2. pertaining to originating in/formation
(c) -dynia	_____	3. opening into/ connection between two parts

Column A	Column B	Column C
(d) dys-	_____	4. between
(e) -ectomy	_____	5. abnormal condition/disease of
(f) -genic	_____	6. fixation (by surgery)
(g) hyper-	_____	7. condition of pain
(h) hypo-	_____	8. removal of
(i) inter-	_____	9. excessive flow/discharge
(j) -meter	_____	10. fast
(k) -metry	_____	11. above
(l) -osis	_____	12. difficult/painful
(m) -pexy	_____	13. surgical repair
(n) -plasty	_____	14. puncture
(o) -plegia	_____	15. condition of paralysis
(p) -rrhaphy	_____	16. to bind together
(q) -rrhoea (Am. rrhea)	_____	17. incision into
(r) -stomy	_____	18. below
(s) -tachy	_____	19. technique of measuring
(t) -tomy	_____	20. suturing/stitching

Score

20

Test 3C

Combining forms of word roots

Match each combining form in Column A with a meaning in Column C by inserting the appropriate number in Column B.

Column A	Column B	Column C
(a) bronch/o	_____	1. larynx
(b) cost/o	_____	2. diaphragm
(c) enter/o	_____	3. bronchus

Column A	Column B	Column C
(d) epiglott/o	_____	4. thorax
(e) gastr/o	_____	5. intestine
(f) hepat/o	_____	6. pleural membranes
(g) laryng/o	_____	7. stomach
(h) lob/o	_____	8. trachea
(i) myc/o	_____	9. breathing (wind)
(j) nas/o	_____	10. nose (i)
(k) pharyng/o	_____	11. nose (ii)
(l) phren/o	_____	12. fungus
(m) pleur/o	_____	13. lobe
(n) pneum/o	_____	14. pharynx
(o) pneumon/o	_____	15. liver
(p) pnoea (Am. pnea)	_____	16. gas/air/wind
(q) rhin/o	_____	17. lung
(r) sten/o	_____	18. epiglottis
(s) thorac/o	_____	19. rib
(t) trache/o	_____	20. narrowing

Score

20

Test 3D

Write the meaning of:

(a) bronchogenic _____

(b) tracheostenosis _____

(c) pulmonologist _____

(d) phrenograph _____

(e) laryngoplegia _____

Score

5

Test 3E

Build words that mean:

(a) surgical repair of the bronchus   _____

(b) technique of visually examining _____
    bronchi

(c) suturing of the trachea   _____

(d) study of the nose (use rhin/o)   _____

(e) pertaining to the diaphragm   _____
    and ribs

Score

5

Check answers to Self-Assessment Tests on page 299.

4 The cardiovascular system

Objectives

Once you have completed Unit 4 you should be able to:

- understand the meaning of medical words relating to the cardiovascular system

- build medical words relating to the cardiovascular system

- associate medical terms with their anatomical position

- understand medical abbreviations relating to the cardiovascular system.

Exercise Guide

Use this list of word components and their meanings to complete the word exercises in this unit.

Prefixes

a-	without
brady-	slow
dextro-	right
endo-	within/inside
pan-	all
peri-	around
tachy-	fast

Roots/Combining forms

dynam/o	force
ech/o	echo/reflected sound
electr/o	electrical
lith/o	stone
man/o	pressure
my/o	muscle
necr/o	death, dead
phon/o	sound/voice

Suffixes

-ac	pertaining to
-algia	condition of pain
-ar	pertaining to
-centesis	surgical puncture to remove fluid
-clysis	infusion/injection/irrigation
-ectasis	dilatation/stretching
-ectomy	removal of
-genesis	capable of causing/pertaining to formation
-gram	X-ray/tracing/recording
-graph	usually an instrument that records
-graphy	technique of recording/making X-ray
-ia	condition of
-ic	pertaining to
-itis	inflammation of
-logy	study of
-lysis	breakdown/disintegration
-megaly	enlargement
-meter	measuring instrument
-metry	process of measuring
-oma	tumour/swelling
-osis	abnormal condition/disease of
-ous	pertaining to/of the nature of
-pathy	disease of
-plasty	surgical repair/reconstruction
-pexy	surgical fixation/fix in place
-plegia	condition of paralysis
-poiesis	formation
-rrhaphy	stitching/suturing
-sclerosis	abnormal condition of hardening
-scope	an instrument to view/examine
-spasm	involuntary contraction of muscle
-stasis	stopping/controlling/cessation of movement
-stenosis	abnormal condition of narrowing
-tome	cutting instrument
-tomy	incision into
-um	thing/a structure/anatomical part
-us	thing/a structure/anatomical part

Heart

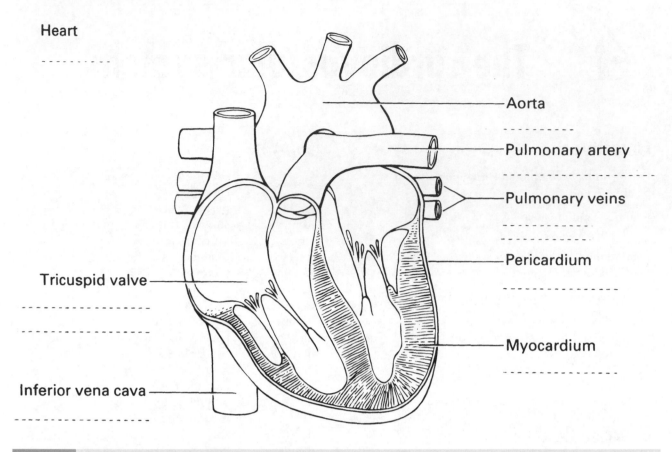

Aorta

Pulmonary artery

Pulmonary veins

Pericardium

Tricuspid valve

Myocardium

Inferior vena cava

Figure 20   The heart

ANATOMY EXERCISE

When you have finished Word Exercises 1–16, look at the word components listed below. Complete Figure 20 by writing the appropriate combining form on each dotted line – more than one component may relate to the same position. (You can check their meanings in the Quick Reference box on p. 50.)

Aort/o	Pericardi/o	Venacav/o
Arteri/o	Phleb/o	Ven/o
Cardi/o	Valv/o	
Myocardi/o	Valvul/o	

The cardiovascular system

In order to remain alive, cells within the body need a continuous supply of oxygen and nutrients for their metabolism. Any metabolic wastes excreted by these cells must be transported to the excretory organs where they can be removed from the body. The cardiovascular system provides a transport system for supply and removal of materials to and from the tissue cells; it consists of the heart and blood vessels.

The heart

The heart is a four chambered muscular pump that continuously pushes blood into arteries. The right and left atria (singular – atrium) form the top chambers and the right and left ventricles the lower chambers.

The atria receive blood from veins and push it into the ventricles. The right ventricle then forces blood through the pulmonary artery to the lungs where it is oxygenated. Simultaneously oxygenated blood that has returned to the left side of the heart is forced by the left ventricle through the aorta into the systemic circulation.

The heart muscle (myocardium) that forms the walls of the chambers, is stimulated to contract rhythmically by a special patch of tissue called the sino-atrial (SA) node or 'pacemaker'. Although the SA node gives the heart the ability to contract by itself, its rate of contraction is determined by nerve impulses from centres in the brain.

The heart muscle receives a supply of fully oxygenated blood from branches of the aorta known as the coronary arteries. If coronary arteries become blocked, the muscle dies triggering a heart attack. Another common cause of death is **heart failure**, defined as the inability of the heart to maintain a flow of blood sufficient to meet the body's needs; the term is most often applied to the heart muscle of either the left or right ventricle. If both ventricles are affected, it is known as **biventricular** heart failure (bi – meaning two).

(The term **atrial** means pertaining to an atrium and **ventricular** means pertaining to a ventricle (-al and -ar both mean pertaining to.)

Use the Exercise Guide at the beginning of this unit to complete Word Exercises 1–16 unless you are asked to work without it.

Root	Card
	(From a Greek word **kardia**, meaning heart.)
Combining forms	**Card/i/o**

WORD EXERCISE 1

Using your Exercise Guide, find the meaning of:

(a) **cardi**/ac

(b) **cardi**/algia

(c) **cardio**/scope

(d) **cardio**/graph

(e) **cardio**/gram

(f) tachy/**card**/ia

Using your Exercise Guide, build words using cardi/o that mean:

(g) enlargement of the heart

(h) surgical repair of the heart

(i) disease of the heart

(j) study of the heart

Using your Exercise Guide, find the meaning of:

(k) myo/**cardi**/um

(l) **cardio**/myo/pathy

(m) **cardio**/rrhaphy

(n) electro/**cardio**/graph

(o) endo/**card**/itis

(p) pan/**card**/itis

(q) brady/**card**/ia

(r) dextro/**card**/ia

(s) phono/**cardio**/graphy

(t) echo/**cardio**/graphy

(u) electro/**cardio**/gram

To make an electrocardiogram (ECG; Fig. 21) electrodes are attached to the skin at various sites on the body. The heart muscle generates electrical impulses that can be detected at the surface of the body, amplified and converted into a trace on a screen or paper. The P wave appears when the atria are stimulated, the QRS complex when the impulse passes to the ventricles and the T wave is generated when the ventricles contract. Abnormal electrical activity and changes in heart rate seen in coronary heart disease can be detected from the ECG.

The heart is continuously supplied with blood through coronary arteries. Narrowing of these vessels results in **ischaemia**, a deficient blood supply (isch- meaning to check) that produces the chest pain known as **angina**

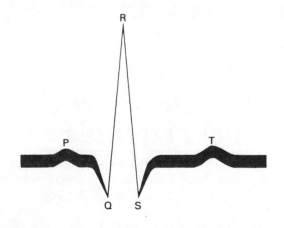

Figure 21   Electrocardiogram

pectoris. If the flow of blood to the heart muscle is interrupted, the muscle dies; this is a **myocardial infarction** or heart attack. Heart muscle deprived of oxygen produces a rapid, uncoordinated, quivering contraction known as **fibrillation**. Normal rhythm can sometimes be restored by applying an electric shock with an instrument known as a **defibrillator**.

Around the heart there is a double membranous sac known as the **pericardium** (peri-, prefix meaning around). Between the membranes is the pericardial cavity containing a small amount of fluid. The combining forms of pericardium are **pericard/o** and **pericardi/o**.

WORD EXERCISE 2

Without using your Exercise Guide, build a word that means:

(a) inflammation of the pericardium _____

Using your Exercise Guide, find the meaning of:

(b) cardio/**pericardio**/pexy _____

(c) **pericardio**/centesis _____

(d) **pericardi**/ectomy _____

Blood flow through the heart is controlled by **valves**. Between the right atrium and the right ventricle there is a **tricuspid valve** (with three flaps or cusps) that allows blood to flow from the right atrium to the right ventricle but not in the opposite direction. Similarly there is a valve on the left side of the heart that allows blood to flow from the left atrium to the left ventricle. This is known as the **bicuspid valve** or the **mitral valve** (with two flaps or cusps).

Root	**Valv**
	*(From Latin **valva**, meaning fold. In medicine it refers to a valve, i.e. a fold or membrane in a tube or passage permitting flow in one direction only.)*
Combining forms	**Valv/o**

WORD EXERCISE 3

Without using your Exercise Guide, build words that mean:

(a) surgical repair of a heart valve _____

(b) removal of a heart valve _____

Valvul/o is a New Latin combining form also derived from *valva*; using your Exercise Guide, find the meaning of:

(c) cardio/**valvulo**/tome _____

Note. -tome comes from *tomon*, meaning cutter.

(d) **valvul**/ar _____

(e) **valv**/o/tomy _____

The blood vessels

Blood circulates through a closed system of blood vessels throughout the body. It flows away from the heart in arteries that divide into smaller arterioles and then into capillaries. Blood flows back to the heart through venules and then into larger vessels known as veins. The system that supplies blood to the tissues is known as the **arterial system** and that which takes it away the **venous system**. Now we will look at some of the terms concerned with blood vessels.

Root	**Vas**
	*(A Latin word, meaning **vessel**. Here it refers to blood vessels of any type.)*
Combining forms	**Vas/o**
	Vascul/o, *also derived from vas, has the same meaning.*

WORD EXERCISE 4

Using your Exercise Guide, find the meaning of:

(a) **vaso**/spasm _____

Blood vessels can widen (**vaso**dilatation) and they can narrow (**vaso**constriction) because of the activity of smooth muscle in their walls. If a vessel widens then the blood pressure within it falls. Some drugs are designed to stimulate this action, i.e. reducing blood pressure, and are known as **vasodilators** and antihypertensives.

(b) a/**vascul**/ar _____

Without using your Exercise Guide, build words using vascul/o that mean:

(c) inflammation of blood vessels _____

(d) disease of blood vessels _____

Root

Angi
*(From a Greek word **angeion**, meaning vessel, in this case a blood vessel.)*

Combining forms   **Angi/o**

WORD EXERCISE 5

Without using your Exercise Guide, write the meaning of:

(a) **angio**/gram _____

(b) **angio**/cardio/gram _____

(c) **angio**/cardio/graphy _____

Digital subtraction angiography

Angiography is the technique of making X-rays or images of blood vessels. Both arteries and veins can be made visible on radiographic film following the injection of a contrast medium. This results in an X-ray film on which the injected vessels cast a shadow showing their size, shape and location.

Digital subtraction angiography (DSA) is very similar, except, instead of having an X-ray film, the X-rays are detected electronically and a computer builds an image of the blood vessels on a monitor.

One problem in visualizing blood vessels is that over-lying tissues cast an image on the picture. To eliminate these unwanted images, an X-ray is taken before and after dye is injected. A computer then subtracts the first image from the second, removing the interfering image. The picture produced by DSA is superior to a film-based angiogram.

Without using your Exercise Guide, build words that mean:

(d) study of blood vessels _____

(e) surgical repair of blood vessels _____

A common surgical repair is a balloon angioplasty. In this procedure a catheter containing an inflatable balloon is inserted into a narrowed vessel (see Fig. 22). When the balloon is inflated and moved along the lining any fatty plaques are displaced and the flow of blood through the vessel is restored.

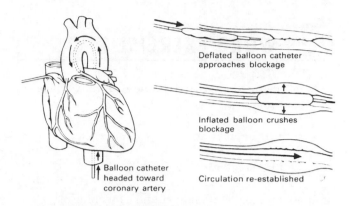

Deflated balloon catheter approaches blockage

Inflated balloon crushes blockage

Circulation re-established

Balloon catheter headed toward coronary artery

Figure 22   Balloon angioplasty

Using your Exercise Guide, find the meaning of:

(f) **angi**/oma _____

(g) **angi**/ectasis _____

(h) **angio**/poiesis _____

(i) **angio**/sclerosis _____

The above roots refer generally to blood vessels. Now we will look at roots that refer to specific types of vessel.

Root

Aort
*(From Greek **aorte**, meaning great vessel. It refers to the largest artery in the body, the aorta. This leaves the left ventricle of the heart and divides into smaller arteries that supply all body systems with oxygenated blood.)*

Combining forms   **Aort/o**

WORD EXERCISE 6

Without using your Exercise Guide, build words that mean:

(a) any disease of the aorta _____

(b) technique of X-raying the aorta _____

Root

Arter
*(From a Greek word **arteria**, meaning artery. The function of arteries is to move blood away from the heart. They divide into smaller arterioles and then into capillaries that exchange materials with the tissue cells.)*

Combining forms   **Arter/i/o**

WORD EXERCISE 7

Without using your Exercise Guide, build words using arteri/o that mean:

(a) suturing of an artery _____

(b) condition of hardening of arteries _____

Using your Exercise Guide, find the meaning of:

(c) end/**arter**/ectomy _____
(In this procedure fatty deposits are removed from the lining of the artery.)

(d) **arterio**/necr/osis _____

(e) **arterio**/stenosis _____

Root	Vena cav
	*(From Latin **vena cavum**, meaning hollow vein, it is used to mean venae cavae.)*

Combining forms **Venacav/o**

Venae cavae are the great veins of the body; the **superior vena cava** drains blood from the head and the **inferior vena cava** drains blood from the lower parts of the body. They pass their blood into the right atrium of the heart.

WORD EXERCISE 8

Without using your Exercise Guide, write the meaning of:

(a) **venacavo**/gram _____

(b) **venacavo**/graphy _____

Root	Ven
	*(From a Latin word **vena**, meaning vein. The function of veins is to transfer blood back to the heart. Capillaries are drained by small vessels called venules, these join and form larger veins. Unlike arteries, veins contain valves that prevent the backflow of blood.)*

Combining forms **Ven/o**

WORD EXERCISE 9

Using your Exercise Guide, find the meaning of:

(a) **ven**/ectasis _____

(b) **veno**/clysis _____

(c) **ven**/ous _____

Without using your Exercise Guide, build words that mean:

(d) X-ray picture of a vein _____
(after injection of opaque dye)

(e) technique of making an _____
X-ray of a vein/venous system

Root	Phleb
	*(From a Greek word **phlebos**, meaning vein.)*

Combining forms **Phleb/o**

WORD EXERCISE 10

Without using your Exercise Guide, write the meaning of:

(a) **phleb**/arteri/ectasis _____

(b) **phlebo**/clysis _____

(c) **phlebo**/tomy _____

Using your Exercise Guide, find the meaning of:

(d) **phlebo**/stasis _____

(e) **phlebo**/mano/meter _____

(f) **phlebo**/lith _____

Root	Thromb
	*(From a Greek word **thrombos**, meaning a clot. Clots are formed mainly of platelets, fibrin and blood cells. They can block blood vessels, restricting or stopping the flow of blood.)*

Combining forms **Thromb/o**

WORD EXERCISE 11

Without using your Exercise Guide, write the meaning of:

(a) **thrombo**/poiesis _____

(b) **thrombo**/phleb/itis _____

(c) **thrombo**/end/arter/ectomy _____

Without using your Exercise Guide, build words that mean:

(d) abnormal condition of having _____ a clot

(e) removal of a clot _____

Using your Exercise Guide, find the meaning of:

(f) **thrombo**/genesis _____

(g) **thrombo**/lysis _____

The sudden blocking of an artery by a clot is referred to as an **embolism**. Emboli can be caused by thrombi as well as other foreign materials, such as fat, air and infective material. The combining form **embol/o** is used when referring to an **embolus**, e.g. as in **embol**ectomy.

Thrombolytic therapy

Recently developed enzymes are being used to dissolve blood clots in situ. The drug streptokinase, extracted from bacteria, can be injected into the coronary vessels to lyse a clot and thereby restore blood in the coronary system. The thrombolytic drugs streptokinase, altepase and anistreplase have been shown to reduce mortality when given by the intravenous route following a heart attack (acute myocardial infarction).

Root	Ather
	*(From a Greek word **athere**, meaning porridge. Used to mean fatty plaques on walls of vessels.)*
Combining forms	**Ather/o**

Atheroma is used to refer to another very common disorder of the blood vessels. The meaning of this word is a porridge-like tumour but it is used to describe the yellow plaques of fatty material which are deposited in the lining of the arteries. The presence of such deposits is believed to be partly related to diets rich in certain types of fat. Atheroma in coronary arteries increases the chance of their becoming blocked, thus predisposing the heart to myocardial infarction (death of heart muscle due to lack of oxygen, i.e. a heart attack).

WORD EXERCISE 12

Without using your Exercise Guide, write the meaning of:

(a) **athero**/genesis _____

(b) **athero**/embolus _____

Atherosclerosis refers to the hardening of arteries and to the presence of atheroma.

Root	Aneurysm
	*(From Greek **aneurysma**, meaning a dilatation. Here it is used to refer to a dilated vessel, usually an artery. It is due to a local fault in the wall through defect, disease or injury. An aneurysm appears as a pulsating swelling that can rupture.)*
Combining forms	**Aneurysm/o**

WORD EXERCISE 13

Without using your Exercise Guide, write the meaning of:

(a) **aneurysmo**/plasty _____

(b) **aneurysmo**/rrhaphy _____

Root	Sphygm
	*(From a Greek word **sphygmos**, meaning pulsation. We use it to refer to the pulse that can be felt wherever an artery is near to the surface of the body. The pulsation is due to the heart forcing blood into the arterial system at ventricular systole (contraction). Pulse rate is therefore a measure of heart rate.)*
Combining forms	**Sphygm/o**

WORD EXERCISE 14

Using your Exercise Guide, find the meaning of:

(a) **sphygmo**/dynamo/meter _____

(b) **sphygmo**/mano/meter _____

(c) **sphygmo**/metry _____

Without using your Exercise Guide, write the meaning of:

(d) **sphygmo**/graph _____

(e) **sphygmo**/gram _____
    (refers to movements created
    by arterial pulse)

(f) **sphygmo**/cardio/graph _____

Note. Mano comes from Greek *manos*, meaning rare. Manometers were first used for measuring rarefied air, i.e. gases. The combining form **man/o** is now used to mean pressure.

Figure 23 is a drawing of an instrument that uses a manometer to measure blood pressure. Two pressures are measured: the **systolic** pressure when the ventricles of the heart are forcing blood into the circulation, and

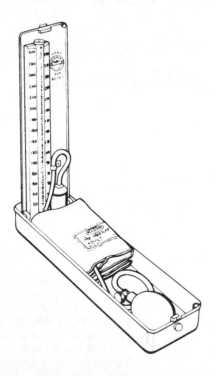

Figure 23   Sphygmomanometer

the **diastolic** pressure which is the pressure within the vessels when the heart is dilating and refilling.

The sphygmomanometer can be used to detect **hypertension**, i.e. a persistently high arterial blood pressure, or **hypo**tension, an abnormally low blood pressure. Both of these conditions have a variety of causes.

The **stethoscope** (Fig. 24) is used in conjunction with the sphygmomanometer to listen to the sounds made by blood flowing through the brachial artery when recording the blood pressure.

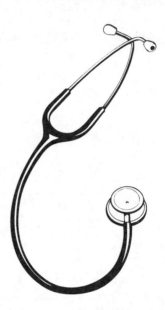

Figure 24   Stethoscope

Note. In medicine the suffix -scope usually refers to an instrument for visual examination. Here we are using it in stethoscope, an instrument used for listening to body sounds. We can use it in this way because scope comes from the Greek word *skopein* which also means to examine. **Steth/o** means breast, therefore stethoscope means an instrument to examine the breast.

Medical equipment and clinical procedures

In this unit we have named many instruments used for examining the cardiovascular system. Two new combining forms have been used with them and we will revise them before completing the next exercise.

---

mano
    means pressure. In sphygmo**mano**meter it refers to the pressure of the pulse, i.e. arterial blood pressure.

dynam
    means power. In sphygmo**dynamo**meter it refers to the force of the pulse (volume and pressure).

Note. Words ending in **-graph** usually refer to a recording instrument and those ending in **-scope** to a viewing instrument (except for the stethoscope which is used for listening).

Revise the names of all instruments mentioned in this unit and then complete Exercises 15 and 16.

WORD EXERCISE 15

Match each term in Column A with a description from Column C by placing an appropriate number in Column B.

Column A	Column B	Column C
(a) cardioscope	_____	1. instrument that measures arterial blood pressure (pressure of the pulse)
(b) cardiograph	_____	2. instrument used to cut a heart valve
(c) electro-cardiograph	_____	3. technique of X-raying heart and blood vessels after injection of radio-opaque dye
(d) cardioval-votome	_____	4. instrument that records heart (beat)
(e) angiocardio-graphy	_____	5. instrument that records the electrical activity of the heart
(f) sphygmo-manometer	_____	6. instrument to view the heart

WORD EXERCISE 16

Match each term in Column A with a description from Column C by placing an appropriate number in Column B.

Column A	Column B	Column C
(a) echocardio-graphy	_____	1. recording of heart sounds
(b) sphygmocar-diograph	_____	2. instrument used to listen to sounds within the chest
(c) stethoscope	_____	3. tracing or recording of the electrical activity of the heart

Column A	Column B	Column C
(d) phonocardio-gram	_____	4. instrument that measures the pressure within a vein
(e) electrocardio-gram	_____	5. instrument that records pulse and heart beat
(f) phlebomano-meter	_____	6. technique of recording heart using reflected ultrasound

ANATOMY EXERCISE

Now complete the Anatomy Exercise on page 42.

CASE HISTORY 4

The object of this exercise is to understand words associated with a patient's medical history.
To complete the exercise:

• read through the passage on cardiac failure; unfamiliar words are underlined and you can find their meaning using the Word Help

• write the meaning of the medical terms shown in bold print.

Cardiac failure

Mr D, a 65-year-old male builder, was referred by his GP to the **Cardiology** Unit. He had been healthy until 8 months previously but since then he has developed fatigue, exertion dyspnoea and paroxysmal nocturnal dyspnoea. He also described discomfort in his chest and felt his heart was 'thumping'.

On the morning of admission he had become unwell and was pale, cold and sweating and seemed confused. Initial examination revealed tender, smooth hepatic enlargement and the presence of ascites. His jugular **venous** pulse was raised and pitting oedema (Am. edema) was present in his ankles. Auscultation revealed a left ventricular third sound with **tachycardia** (a gallop rhythm) and crepitations were heard at the lung bases. Mr D was connected to a 12 lead **electrocardiograph** to monitor his heart rate and rhythm. A posteroanterior chest X-ray revealed **cardiomegaly** and pulmonary oedema and he was diagnosed as having acute **biventricular** heart failure.

Mr D was treated with furosemide (frusemide) a underline{diuretic} to promote renal excretion of fluid. The loss of fluid provided symptomatic and underline{haemodynamic} (Am. hemodynamic) benefits relieving his dyspnoea and reducing ventricular filling pressure. **Cardiac** output was improved by **vasodilator** therapy with underline{ACE inhibitors} in combination with positive underline{inotropic} agents.

WORD HELP

ACE inhibitor angiotensin-converting enzyme (drug used to reduce blood pressure)

ascites free fluid in the abdominal cavity

auscultation a method of listening to body sounds for diagnostic purposes

crepitations rattling or crackling sounds

diuretic agent that increases the flow of urine

dyspnoea difficult/laboured breathing

GP general practitioner (family doctor)

haemodynamic pertaining to the force of blood

inotropic pertaining to affecting the contraction of (heart) muscle increasing or decreasing the force of contraction

jugular pertaining to the neck/throat

nocturnal pertaining to during the night

oedema (Am. edema) accumulation of fluid in a tissue

paroxysmal intensification of symptoms / an attack

posteroanterior from the back/posterior to the front

pitting when pressure on a tissue leaves a mark

Now write the meaning of the following words from the case history without using your dictionary lists:

(a) cardiology

(b) venous

(c) tachycardia

(d) electrocardiograph

(e) cardiomegaly

(f) biventricular

(g) cardiac

(h) vasodilator

(Answers to the case history exercise are given in the Answers to Word Exercises beginning on page 275.)

Quick Reference

Combining forms relating to the cardiovascular system:

Aneurysm/o	aneurysm
Angi/o	vessel
Aort/o	aorta
Arteri/o	artery
Ather/o	atheroma
Atri/o	atrium
Cardi/o	heart
Embol/o	embolism
My/o	muscle
Myocardi/o	myocardium
Pericardi/o	pericardium
Phleb/o	vein
Sphygm/o	pulse
Steth/o	breast
Thromb/o	thrombus/clot
Valv/o	valve
Valvul/o	valve
Vas/o	vessel
Vascul/o	vessel
Venacav/o	vena cava
Ven/o	vein
Ventricul/o	ventricle

Abbreviations

Some common abbreviations related to the cardiovascular system are listed below. Note, some are not standard and their meaning may vary from one health care setting to another. There is a more extensive list for reference on page 307.

AAA	abdominal aortic aneurysm
AF	atrial fibrillation
AMI	acute myocardial infarction
CABG	coronary artery bypass grafting
CAD	coronary artery disease
CCU	coronary care unit
CPR	cardiopulmonary resuscitation
CT	coronary thrombosis
ECG	electrocardiogram
iv	intravenous
MI	myocardial infarction
MS	mitral stenosis

 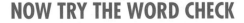 **NOW TRY THE WORD CHECK**

WORD CHECK

This self-check exercise lists all word components used in this unit. First write down the meaning of as many word components as you can. Then check your answers using the Exercise Guide and Quick Reference box or the Glossary of Word Components (pp. 319–341).

Prefixes

a-	without
bi-	two
brady-	slow
dextro-	right
electro-	electrical
endo-	within / inside
hyper-	above
hypo-	below
pan-	all
peri-	around
tachy-	fast
tri-	three

Combining forms of word roots

aneurysm/o	aneurysm
angi/o	vessel
aort/o	aorta
arteri/o	artery
ather/o	atheroma
atri/o	atrium
cardi/o	heart
ech/o	echo
embol/o	embolus
dynam/o	force
man/o	pressure

my/o	muscle
necr/o	death / dead
pericardi/o	around the heart
phleb/o	vein
phon/o	sound
sphygm/o	pulse
sten/o	narrowing
steth/o	chest
thromb/o	clot
valv/o	valve
valvul/o	valve
vas/o	vessel
vascul/o	vessel
venacav/o	venacava
ven/o	vein
ventricul/o	ventricle

Suffixes

-algia	condition of pain
-ar	pertaining to
-centesis	surgical puncture to remove fluid
-clysis	injection
-ectasis	dilation / stretching
-ectomy	removal of
-genesis	formation
-gram	x-ray / recording
-graph	instrument that records
-graphy	technique of recording
-ia	condition of
-ic	pertaining to
-itis	inflammation of
-ium	thing / anatomical structure

-lith _____ stone _____
-logy _____ study of. _____
-lysis _____ breakdown _____
-megaly _____ enlargement of _____
-meter _____ instrument that measures _____
-metry _____ technique of measuring. _____
-oma _____ tumour/swelling. _____
-osis _____ abnormal condition of. _____
-ous _____ pertaining to _____
-pathy _____ disease of. _____
-pexy _____ surgical fixation _____
-plasty _____ surgical repair _____
-poiesis _____ fixation _____
-rrhage _____ bursting forth of blood. _____
-rrhaphy _____ suturing _____
-sclerosis _____ abnormal hardening _____
-scope _____ instrument to view. _____
-stasis _____ stopping/controlling. _____
-tome _____ cutting instrument _____
-tomy _____ incision into _____
-um _____ thing _____

> **NOW TRY THE SELF-ASSESSMENT** <

SELF-ASSESSMENT

Test 4A

Below are some combining forms that refer to the anatomy of the cardiovascular system. Indicate which part of the system they refer to by putting a number from the diagram (Fig. 25) next to each word.

(a) aort/o _____ aorta (6) _____

(b) venacav/o _____ vena cava (1) _____

(c) endocardi/o _____ inside the heart (4) _____

(d) valv/o _____ valve (5) _____

(e) pericardi/o _____ pericardium (2) _____

(f) myocardi/o _____ myocardium (3) _____

Score

6

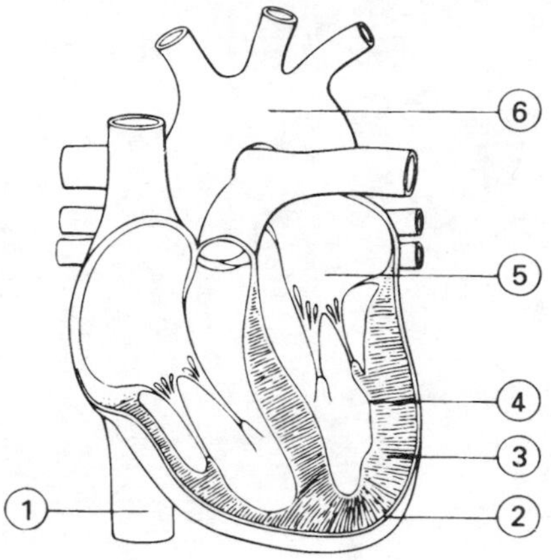

Figure 25   The heart

Test 4B

Prefixes and suffixes

Match each prefix or suffix in Column A with a meaning in Column C by inserting the appropriate number in Column B.

Column A	Column B	Column C
(a) a-	8	1. to hold back/check
(b) bi-	5	2. formation (i)
(c) brady-	15	3. formation (ii)
(d) -clysis	4	4. infusion/injection
(e) dextro-	10	5. two
(f) -ectasis	7	6. fast
(g) electro-	12	7. dilatation
(h) endo-	20	8. without

Column A	Column B	Column C
(i) -genesis	2/3	9. fixation
(j) isch-	1	10. right
(k) -megaly	19	11. around
(l) pan-	18	12. electrical
(m) peri-	11	13. stopping/cessation
(n) -pexy	9	14. hardening
(o) -poiesis	3/2	15. slow
(p) -sclerosis	14	16. tissue/thing
(q) -stasis	13	17. three
(r) tachy-	6	18. all
(s) tri-	17	19. enlargement
(t) -um	16	20. inside

Score

20

Column A	Column B	Column C
(h) ech/o	1	8. heart
(i) man/o	13	9. vessel (i)
(j) my/o	14	10. vessel (ii)
(k) necr/o	3	11. force
(l) phleb/o	15/16	12. aneurysm (swelling)
(m) phon/o	4	13. pressure/rare
(n) sphygm/o	19	14. muscle
(o) sten/o	18	15. vein (i)
(p) steth/o	20	16. vein (ii)
(q) thromb/o	17	17. clot
(r) valv/o	5	18. narrowing
(s) vas/o	10/9	19. pulse
(t) ven/o	16/15	20. breast

Score

20

Test 4C

Combining forms of word roots

Match each combining form in Column A with a meaning in Column C by inserting the appropriate number in Column B.

Column A	Column B	Column C
(a) aneurysm/o	12	1. echo/reflected sound
(b) angi/o	9/10	2. artery
(c) aort/o	6	3. death/corpse
(d) arteri/o	2	4. sound
(e) ather/o	7	5. valve
(f) cardi/o	8	6. aorta
(g) dynam/o	11	7. porridge (yellow plaque on wall of blood vessel)

Test 4D

Write the meaning of:

(a) cardiovalvulitis — inflammation of heart valves

(b) aortorrhaphy — suturing of the aorta

(c) angioscope — instrument view vessels

(d) phlebostenosis — abnormal condition of narrowing of veins

(e) thromboendarteritis — inflammation of lining of an artery caused by a thrombus (clot)

Score

5

Test 4E

Build words that mean:

(a) Inflammation of an artery associated with a thrombosis

thromboarteritis

(b) Puncture of the heart

cardiocentesis

(c) Disease of an artery

arteriopathy

(d) Removal of a vein

phlebectomy

(e) Study of heart and blood vessels (use angi/o)

angiocardiology

Score

5

Check answers to Self-Assessment Tests on page 299.

5 The blood

Objectives

Once you have completed Unit 5 you should be able to:

- understand the meaning of medical words relating to the blood

- build medical words relating to blood

- associate medical terms with the components of blood

- understand medical abbreviations relating to the blood.

Exercise guide

Use this list of word components and their meanings to complete the word exercises in this unit.

Prefixes

a-	without
an-	without/not
ellipto-	shaped like an ellipse
hyper-	above/abnormal increase
hypo-	below/abnormal decrease
macro-	large
micro-	small
normo-	normal/rule
peri-	around
poikil/o	varied/irregular
poly-	many

Roots/Combining forms

cyt/e/o	cell
dynam/o	force/movement
fibr/o	fibre
is/o	equal/same
path/o	disease
pericardi/o	pericardium
septic/o	sepsis/infection/putrefaction

Suffixes

-aemia	condition of blood
-apheresis	removal
-blast	germ cell/embryonic/immature
-chromia	condition of colour/haemoglobin
-crit	separate/device for measuring cells
-cytosis	increased number of cells
-emia (Am.)	condition of blood
-genesis	capable of causing/pertaining to formation
-globin	protein
-ia	condition of
-ic	pertaining to
-ium	structure/anatomical part
-logy	study of
-lysis	breakdown/disintegration
-meter	measuring instrument
-oma	tumour/swelling
-osis	abnormal condition/disease of
-penia	condition of lack of/deficiency
-poiesis	formation
-ptysis	spitting up
-rrhage	bursting forth (of blood/bleeding)
-stasis	stopping/controlling/cessation of movement
-toxic	pertaining to poisoning
-um	thing/structure/anatomical part
-uria	condition of urine

Blood (a stained smear)

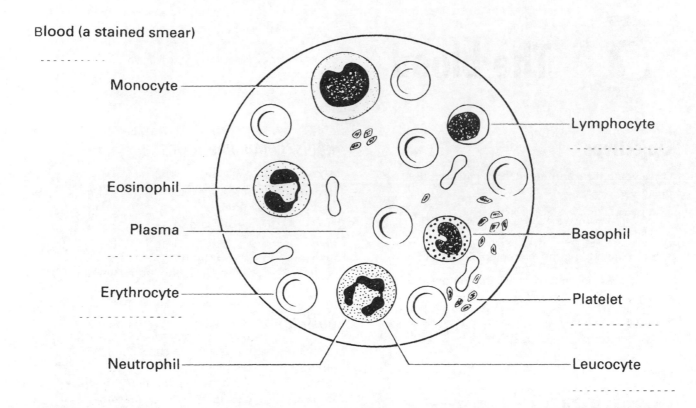

Monocyte

Lymphocyte

Eosinophil

Plasma

Basophil

Erythrocyte

Platelet

Neutrophil

Leucocyte

| Figure 26 | Blood |

ANATOMY EXERCISE

When you have finished Word Exercises 1–7, look at the word components listed below. Complete Figure 26 by writing the appropriate combining form on each dotted line – more than one component may relate to the same position. (You can check their meanings in the Quick Reference box on p. 61.)

Erythrocyt/o	Leucocyt/o	Plasma-
Haem/o	Lymphocyt/o	Thrombocyt/o

The blood

Blood is a complex fluid classified as a connective tissue because it contains cells, plus an intercellular matrix known as plasma. Here we can see the main components of whole blood:

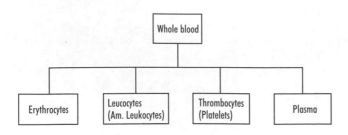

The blood cells carry out a variety of functions: erythrocytes (red blood cells) transport gases whilst leucocytes (white blood cells) defend the body against invasion by microorganisms and foreign antigens. Thrombocytes, or platelets, are actually fragments of larger cells concerned with the formation of blood clots following injury.

The plasma carries nutrients, wastes, hormones, antibodies and blood-clotting proteins. The study of blood is very important in medicine for the diagnosis of disease.

Use the Exercise Guide at the beginning of the unit to complete Word Exercises 1–7 unless you are asked to work without it.

Root   Haem
(From a Greek word **haima**, *meaning blood.)*

Combining forms   **Haem/o, haemat/o, -aem-**
(Am. **Hem/o, hemat/o, -em-***)*

WORD EXERCISE 1

Using your Exercise Guide, find the meaning of:

(a) **haemato**/logy
(Am. hemato/logy)

(b) **haemo**/patho/logy
(Am. hemo/patho/logy)

(c) **haemo**/dynam/ics
(Am. hemo/dynam/ics)

(d) **haemo**/poiesis
(Am. hemo/poiesis)

(e) **haemo**/stasis
(Am. hemo/stasis)

(f) **haemo**/pericardi/um (Fig. 27)
(Am. hemo/pericardi/um)

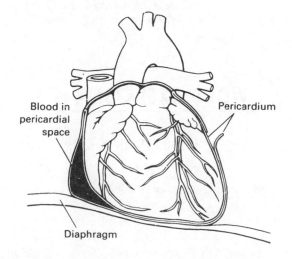

Blood in
pericardial
space

Pericardium

Diaphragm

Figure 27   Haemopericardium (Am. hemopericardium)

(g) **haemo**/ptysis
(Am. **hemo**/ptysis)

Using your Exercise Guide, build words that mean:

(h) Tumour/swelling containing blood

(i) Breakdown/disintegration of blood

(j) Condition of blood in the urine

(k) Bursting forth of blood

Using your Exercise Guide, find the meaning of:

(l) poly/cyt/**haem**/ia
(Am. poly/cyt/hem/ia)

(m) an/**aem**/ia
(Am. an/em/ia)

(n) septic/**aem**/ia
(Am. septic/em/ia)

Haemoglobin is a red pigment (globular protein) found inside red blood cells, it functions to transport oxygen and carbon dioxide. The haemoglobin present in the blood is of great importance to the efficiency of gaseous transport and several types of investigation are performed to estimate its concentration.

The three medical terms that follow use the combining form **haemoglobin/o** meaning haemoglobin.

Using your Exercise Guide, find the meaning of:

(o) **haemo/globino**/meter
(Am. hemo/globino/meter)

Without using your Exercise Guide, write the meaning of:

(p) **haemo/globin**
(Am. hemo/globin)

(q) **haemoglobin**/uria
(Am. hemoglobin/uria)

The amount of haemoglobin within red blood cells can be estimated and abnormal levels are found in some patients. Terms describing these conditions have been formed from the suffix **-chromia** (from Greek *chromos*, meaning colour). Here the colour refers to the red pigment haemoglobin.

Using your Exercise Guide, find the meaning of:

(r) hypo/**chrom**/ia

(s) hyper/**chrom**/ia

(t) normo/**chrom**/ic

Another common term relating to the colour of haemoglobin is **cyanosis**. **Cyan/o** means blue. In the absence of oxygen, haemoglobin develops a bluish tinge. Nailbeds, lips and skin show signs of cyanosis (i.e. look blue) when oxygenation of the blood is deficient. Tissues deprived of oxygen can also be described as **anoxic**.

Now we will examine word roots which refer to the different types of blood cells. All of these cells are suspended in the liquid matrix of the blood known as plasma.

Root	**Erythr** *(From a Greek word **erythros**, meaning red. Here it is used to refer to red blood cells, i.e. erythrocytes.)*

Combining forms   **Erythr/o**

 WORD EXERCISE 2

Using your Exercise Guide, find the meaning of:

(a) **erythro**/penia _____

(b) **erythro**/genesis _____

(c) **erythro**/blast _____
(This refers to the cell which eventually forms the mature erythrocyte.)

Without using your Exercise Guide, write the meaning of:

(d) **erythro**/poiesis _____

(e) **erythrocyto**/lysis _____

(f) **erythrocyt**/haem/ia _____
(Am. erythrocyt/hem/ia)

This last condition is synonymous with **erythrocytosis** meaning an abnormal condition of red cells, i.e. too many red cells. This condition is usually a physiological response to low levels of oxygen circulating in the blood. Besides changes in number, individual erythrocytes can suffer from various abnormalities, some of which are listed below.

Using your Exercise Guide, find the meaning of:

(g) micro/**cytosis** _____
(NB: Cytosis is used in (g) to (k) to mean too many red blood cells.)

(h) macro/**cytosis** _____

(i) ellipto/**cytosis** _____

(j) an/iso/**cytosis** _____

(k) poikilo/**cytosis** _____

(l) normo/**cyt**/ic _____

Root	**Reticul** *(From a Latin word **reticulum**, meaning small net. Here, it refers to a very young erythrocyte lacking a nucleus called a reticulocyte; its cytoplasm gives it a net-like appearance with basic dyes.)*

Combining forms   **Reticul/o**

 WORD EXERCISE 3

Without using your Exercise Guide, build words that mean:

(a) an immature erythrocyte _____

(b) condition of too many immature erythrocytes _____

(c) condition of deficiency of reticulocytes _____

Root	**Leuc** *(From a Greek word **leukos**, meaning white. Here it is referring to white blood cells, i.e. leucocytes.)*

Combining forms   **Leuc/o, leuk/o**
*(**Leuc/o** is more commonly used in the UK, **leuk/o** in America.)*

 WORD EXERCISE 4

Without using your Exercise Guide, build words that mean:

(a) condition of deficiency of white cells _____

(b) the formation of white blood cells _____

Without using your Exercise Guide, write the meaning of:

(c) **leuco**/cyto/genesis _____
(Am. leuko/cyto/genesis)

(d) **leuk**/aem/ia _____
(Am. leuk/em/ia. This is a malignant condition, i.e. a type of cancer.)

(e) **leuco**/cytosis _____
(Am. leuko/cytosis. This refers to an excess of white cells as seen during infection.)

(f) **leuco**/cyt/oma
(Am. leuko/cyt/oma) _____

(g) **leuco**/blast
(Am. leuko/blast) _____

(h) **leuco**/blast/osis
(Am. leuko/blast/osis) _____

Using your Exercise Guide, find the meaning of:

(i) **leuco**/toxic
(Am. leuko/toxic) _____

Leucocyte is a general term meaning white cell but there are many types of white cell. Some leucocytes contain granules and are known as **granulocytes**, those without granules are called **agranulocytes** (*a-* meaning without, *granul/o-* granule and *-cyte* cell).

Among the commonest granulocytes are polymorphonuclear granulocytes or polymorphs. These all have nuclei which show many shapes (*poly* – many, *morpho* – shape). There are three types of polymorph:

Neutrophils
From *neutro*, meaning neither, and *philein*, meaning to love. These cells stain well with (love) **neutral** dyes. Neutrophils engulf microorganisms that have entered the blood and destroy them. These cells are sometimes referred to as phagocytes (*phago* means eat, i.e. cells that eat). The process of engulfing particles is known as phagocytosis.

Basophils
These cells stain well with **basic** (alkaline) dyes.

Eosinophils
These cells stain well with acid dyes like **eosin**, a red dye.

Among the agranular leucocytes are lymphocytes and large monocytes (*mono* means single). The latter can leave the blood and wander to the site of infections. Lymphocytes will be studied in Unit 6.

Note. The condition **pancytopenia** refers to an abnormal depression of all the cellular components of the blood (*pan-* meaning all, *cyt/o-* cell and *-penia* condition of deficiency).

Root   **Myel**
(*From a Greek word* **myelos**, *meaning marrow. Here it is used to refer to the bone marrow which gives rise to the granulocyte, a type of white blood cell.*)

Combining forms   **Myel/o**

WORD EXERCISE 5

Without using your Exercise Guide, write the meaning of:

(a) **myelo**/cyte _____

(b) **myelo**/fibr/osis _____

Without using your Exercise Guide, build words that mean:

(c) germ cell of the marrow _____

(d) tumour of myeloid tissue _____

WORD EXERCISE 6

We have already used the combining form **thromb/o** meaning clot; here it is combined with cyte to make **thrombocyte**. Thrombocytes or **platelets** are fragments of cells that circulate in the blood. They play a major role in the clotting of blood.

Without using your Exercise Guide, write the meaning of:

(a) **thrombocyto**/penia _____

(b) **thrombocyto**/poiesis _____

(c) **thrombocyto**/lysis _____

(d) **thrombocyto**/pathy _____

The numbers and proportions of blood cells found in whole blood are important in the diagnosis of disease. The percentage volume of erythrocytes is known as the **haematocrit** (Am. hematocrit) (from Greek *krites*, meaning separate/judge/discern). The word haematocrit is also used for the apparatus that measures the volume of erythrocytes in a blood sample.

Now write down what is meant by:

(e) **thrombocyto**/crit _____

The number of blood cells can be counted using a device known as a **haemocytometer**. The simplest type of counter consists of a specially designed microscope slide that holds a precise volume of blood and a grid for the manual counting of cells. Today, the process of counting cells is performed automatically in a Coulter counter. A doctor may request particular types of cell count to aid diagnosis, for example:

Blood count
A count of the number of red cells and/or white cells in a sample of blood. Reference intervals for the number of cells in a sample from a healthy person are:
Red blood cells 4.5–6.5 $\times$ 10^{12}/l in males, 4.0–6.0 $\times$ 10^{12}/l in females
White cells 3.5–11.0 $\times$ 10^{9}/l.

Differential count
A count of the proportions of different types of cells in stained smears. Examples of reference intervals for the number of cells in a sample from a healthy person are:
Neutrophils (30–75%) 1.5–7.5 $\times$ 10^{9}/l
Basophils (<1%) <0.1 $\times$ 10^{9}/l
Eosinophils (1–6%) 0.04–0.4 $\times$ 10^{9}/l.

Platelet count
A count of the number of platelets in a sample of blood. The reference interval for the number of platelets in a sample from a healthy person is: 150–400 $\times$ 10^{9}/l.

Techniques have been developed to take blood from a donor, remove wanted or unwanted components from it and return the cells in fresh or frozen plasma back into the body. When plasma is removed the technique is known as **plasmapheresis**. Plasma refers to the liquid matrix of the blood in which cells are suspended and nutrients and wastes dissolved. Apheresis is from the Greek *hairein*, meaning take/remove.

Without using your Exercise Guide, write the meaning of:

(f) erythrocyt/**apheresis** _____

(g) thrombocyt/**apheresis** _____

(h) leuc/**apheresis** _____

Medical equipment and clinical procedures

Revise the names of all instruments and procedures mentioned in this unit and then complete Exercise 7.

WORD EXERCISE 7

Match each term in Column A with a description from Column C by placing an appropriate number in Column B.

Column A	Column B	Column C
(a) plasmapheresis	_____	1. count of numbers of blood cells/Litre of blood
(b) differential count	_____	2. instrument that estimates the percentage volume of red cells in blood, or the actual value (as a percentage of the volume) of red cells in blood
(c) haematocrit	_____	3. estimate of proportions/ numbers of white cells in a stained smear
(d) haemoglo-binometer	_____	4. continuous removal of plasma from blood and retransfusion of cells
(e) blood count	_____	5. instrument which measures amount of haemoglobin in a sample

ANATOMY EXERCISE

Now complete the Anatomy Exercise on page 56.

CASE HISTORY 5

The object of this exercise is to understand words associated with a patient's medical history.

To complete the exercise:

- read through the passage on aplastic anaemia (Am. anemia); unfamiliar words are underlined and you can find their meaning using the Word Help

- write the meaning of the medical terms shown in bold print.

Aplastic anaemia (Am. anemia)

Mr E, a 44-year-old chemistry teacher and former industrial chemist, had been unwell for many weeks before seeking advice from his GP. He complained of headache, breathlessness, fatigue and palpitation; the previous day he had become concerned about his condition following a severe epistaxis and **haemoptysis** (Am. hemoptysis). On examination he appeared to have a lower respiratory tract infection and oral thrush. Initial blood investigation revealed a **pancytopenia,** and he was referred to the Haematology (Am. Hematology) Department.

Mr E looked pale and was troubled by ulcerative lesions in his mouth and pharynx. There was no lymphadenopathy or hepatosplenomegaly. A bone marrow trephine biopsy and smear confirmed a hypocellularity with the virtual absence of reticulocytes; no **leukaemic** or neoplastic cells were observed. Detailed haematological (Am. hematological) examination revealed a **normochromic**, **normocytic** anaemia with **granulocytopenia** and **thrombocytopenia.**

Mr E was diagnosed with a severe, secondary aplastic **anaemia** (Am. anemia) and was advised of its serious prognosis. He resigned from his post as a teacher and a programme of supportive care aimed at treating his respiratory tract infection was established. He is currently being assessed for bone marrow transplantation by his HLA identical brother.

(c) leukaemic
    (Am. leukemic) _____

(d) normochromic _____

(e) normocytic _____

(f) granulocytopenia _____

(g) thrombocytopenia _____

(h) anaemia
    (Am. anemia) _____

(Answers to the case history exercise are given in the Answers to Word Exercises beginning on page 275.)

WORD HELP

aplastic pertaining to without growth/unable to form new cells

epistaxis a nose bleed

GP general practitioner (family doctor)

haematological pertaining to study of blood (Am. hematological)

hepatosplenomegaly enlargement of the spleen and liver

HLA identical human leucocyte (Am. leukocyte) antigen, important for cross-matching of donor and recipient

hypocellularity condition of below normal number of cells

lesion pathological change in a tissue

lymphadenopathy disease of lymph nodes

neoplastic pertaining to new, abnormal growth of cells (cancer cells)

oral thrush fungal infection in the mouth (with *Candida albicans*)

palpitation unusual awareness of one's heartbeat

prognosis a forecast of the probable course and outcome of a disease

reticulocyte an immature erythrocyte

secondary here refers to a second type of aplastic anaemia caused by direct damage of the bone marrow by chemicals, radiation or infection

smear spreading material across a slide for microscopic examination

trephine biopsy using a trephine (device that removes a circular disc of bone) to take a sample of bone marrow

ulcerative having the form of an ulcer

Now write the meaning of the following words from the case history without using your dictionary lists:

(a) haemoptysis
    (Am. hemoptysis) _____

(b) pancytopenia _____

Quick Reference

Combining forms relating to the blood:

Cyt/o	cell
Erythr/o	red
Erythrocyt/o	erythrocyte/red cell
Fibr/o	fibre
Globin/o	protein
Granul/o	granule
Haem/o	blood
Hem/o (Am.)	blood
Leuc/o	white
Leucocyt/o	leucocyte/white cell
Leuk/o (Am.)	white
Leukocyt/o (Am.)	leukocyte/white cell
Lymphocyt/o	lymph cell
Morph/o	shape/form
Myel/o	marrow/myelocyte
Phag/o	eating/consuming
Reticul/o	immature erythrocyte
Thromb/o	clot
Thrombocyt/o	platelet

Abbreviations

Some common abbreviations related to the blood are listed below. Note, some are not standard and their meaning may vary from one health care setting to another. There is a more extensive list for reference on page 307.

ALL	acute lymphocytic leukaemia
AML	acute myeloid leukaemia
Diff	differential blood count (of cell types)

Abbreviations (contd.)

ESR	erythrocyte sedimentation rate
FBC	full blood count
Hb	haemoglobin (Am. hemoglobin)
Hct	haematocrit (Am. hematocrit)
MCH	mean corpuscular haemoglobin
MCHC	mean corpuscular haemoglobin concentration
PCV	peaked cell volume
RBC	red blood cell/count
WBC	white blood cell/count

> ## NOW TRY THE WORD CHECK <

WORD CHECK

This self-check exercise lists all the word components used in this unit. First write down the meaning of as many word components as you can. Then check your answers using the Exercise Guide and Quick Reference box or the Glossary of Word Components (pp. 319–341).

Prefixes

a-	without
an-	without
basi-	base / basic
ellipto-	shaped like an ellipse
eosino-	red dye
hyper-	above / abnormal increase
hypo-	below / abnormal decrease
macro-	large
micro-	small
neutro-	neutral
normo-	normal
pan-	all

peri-	around
poikil/o	varied
poly-	many

Combining forms of word roots

cardi/o	heart
cyan/o	blue
cyt/o	cell
dynam/o	force
erythr/o	red
fibr/o	fibre
globin/o	protein
granul/o	granule
haem/o (Am. hem/o)	blood
is/o	equal / same
leuc/o (Am. leuk/o)	white
morph/o	shape / form
myel/o	marrow
norm/o	normal
ox/y	oxygen
path/o	disease
phag/o	eating / consuming
reticul/o	immature erythrocyte
sept/i	poison
thromb/o	clot
thrombocyt/o	platelet

Suffixes

-aemia (Am. -emia)	condition - of blood
-apheresis	removal of

-blast	*immature germ cell*	(c) haemoglobin/o (Am. hemoglobin/o)	*1/3*
-chromia	*condition of colour*	(d) leucocyt/o (Am. leukocyt/o)	*2*
-crit	*instrument for measuring volume*	(e) thrombocyt/o	*4*
-genesis	*formation*		
-ic	*pertaining to*		
-ium	*structure*		
-logy	*study of*		
-lysis	*breakdown*		
-meter	*instrument for measuring*		
-oma	*tumour/swelling*		
-osis	*abnormal condition of*		
-penia	*condition of deficiency*		
-phil	*love*		
-poiesis	*formation*		
-rrhage	*bursting forth of blood*		
-stasis	*stopping/controlling*		
-toxic	*pertaining to poisoning*		
-um	*structure*		
-uria	*condition of urine*		

Score

5

> **NOW TRY THE SELF-ASSESSMENT** <

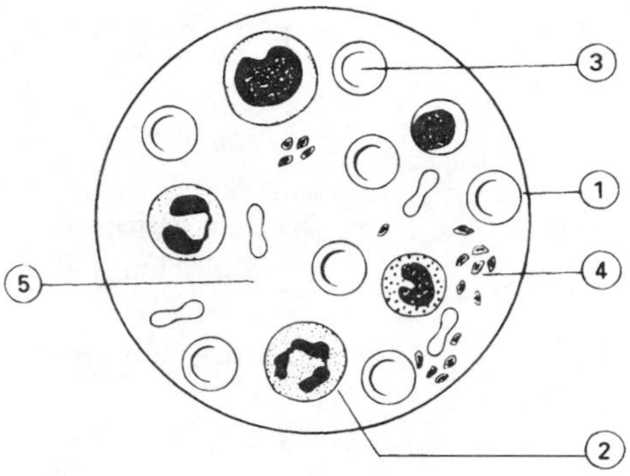

Figure 28 Blood

Test 5B

Prefixes, suffixes and combining forms of word roots

Match each word component in Column A with a meaning in Column C by inserting the appropriate number in Column B.

SELF-ASSESSMENT

Test 5A

Below are some combining forms that relate to the components of blood. Indicate which part of the blood they refer to by putting a number from the diagram (Fig. 28) next to each word. You may use a number more than once.

(a) plasma _____5_____

(b) erythr/o _____3/1_____

Column A	Column B	Column C
(a) -aemia (Am. -emia)	*10*	1. condition of urine
(b) an-	*17*	2. disintegration/ breakdown
(c) is/o	*9*	3. red
(d) baso-	*6*	4. measuring instrument
(e) -blast	*13*	5. abnormal condition/ disease of
(f) -chromia	*19*	6. basic/alkaline
(g) ellipt/o	*20*	7. white

Column A	Column B	Column C
(h) eosin/o	22	8. clot
(i) erythr/o	3	9. equal/same
(j) granul/o	12	10. condition of blood
(k) leuc/o (Am. leuk/o)	7	11. disease
(l) -lysis	2	12. granule
(m) macro-	21	13. germ cell
(n) -meter	4	14. cessation of flow
(o) micro-	18	15. affinity for/loving
(p) neutr/o	23	16. condition of deficiency/lack of
(q) -osis	5	17. not/without
(r) -pathy	11	18. small
(s) -penia	16	19. condition of colour/haemoglobin
(t) -phil	15	20. oval/elliptoid
(u) sept/i	24	21. large
(v) -stasis	14	22. eosin (acid dye)
(w) thromb/o	8	23. neutral
(x) -uria	1	24. decay/sepsis/infection

Score

24

(c) erythrocyturia — condition of red blood cells in urine

(d) thrombocythaemia (Am. thrombocythemia) — condition of blood with platelets

(e) phagocytolysis — breakdown of phagocytes

Score

5

Test 5D

Build words that mean:

(a) any disease of blood (use haem/o, Am. hem/o) — haemopathy

(b) condition of deficiency in the number of red cells — erythrocytopenia

(c) a physician who specializes in the study of blood (use haemat/o, Am. hemat/o) — haematologist

(d) pertaining to the poisoning of blood — haemotoxic

(e) condition of deficiency in the number of neutrophils — neutropenia

Score

5

Check answers to Self-Assessment Tests on page 299.

Test 5C

Write the meaning of:

(a) leucocyturia (Am. leukocyturia) — condition of white blood cells in urine

(b) myelocytosis — abnormal condition of too many marrow cells.

The lymphatic system and immunology

Objectives

Once you have completed Unit 6 you should be able to:

- understand the meaning of medical words relating to the lymphatic system and immunology

- build medical words relating to the lymphatic system and immunology

- associate medical terms with their anatomical position

- understand medical abbreviations relating to the lymphatic system and immunology.

Exercise Guide

Use this list of word components and their meanings to complete the word exercises in this unit.

Prefixes

auto-	self

Roots/Combining forms

aden/o	gland
angi/o	vessel
cyt/o – cyte	cell
helc/o	ulcer
hepat/o	liver
path/o	disease
pharyng/o	pharynx
port/o	portal vein

Suffixes

-aemia	condition of blood
-cele	swelling/protrusion/hernia
-cytosis	abnormal increase in cells
-eal	pertaining to
-ectasis	dilatation/stretching
-ectomy	removal of
-emia (Am.)	condition of blood
-genesis	pertaining to formation
-genic	pertaining to formation/ originating in
-globulin	protein
-gram	X-ray/tracing/recording
-graphy	technique of recording/making X-ray
-ic	pertaining to
-itis	inflammation of
-ity	state/condition
-logy	study of
-lysis	breakdown/disintegration
-malacia	condition of softening
-megaly	enlargement
-oma	tumour/swelling
-osis	abnormal condition/disease of
-pathy	disease of
-pexy	surgical fixation/fix in place
-poiesis	formation
-rrhagia	condition of bursting forth
-rrhea (Am.)	excessive discharge/flow
-rrhoea	excessive discharge/flow
-tic	pertaining to
-tome	cutting instrument

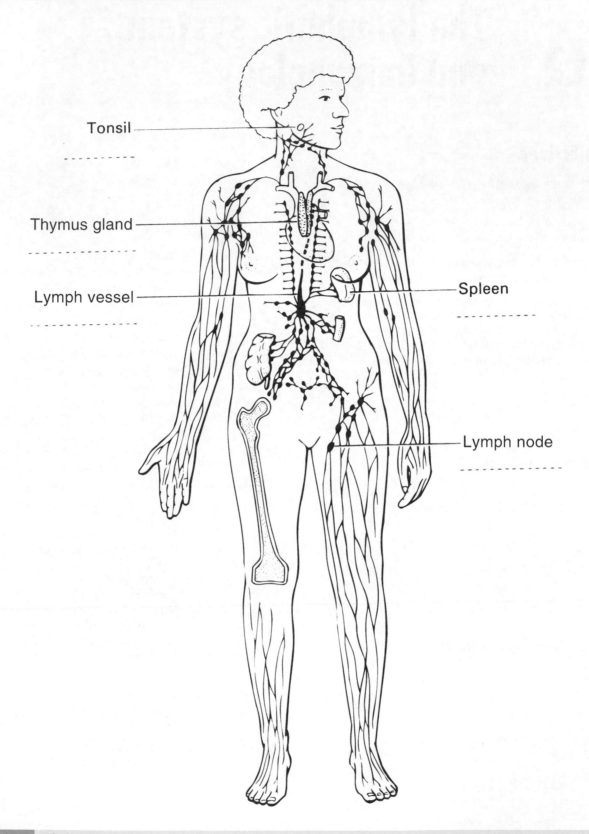

Tonsil

Thymus gland

Lymph vessel

Spleen

Lymph node

Figure 29   The lymphatic system

ANATOMY EXERCISE

When you have finished Word Exercises 1–8, look at the word components listed below. Complete Figure 29 by placing the appropriate combining form on each dotted line. (You can check their meanings in the Quick Reference box on p. 72.)

Lymphaden/o   Splen/o   Tonsill/o
Lymphangi/o   Thym/o

The lymphatic system

The lymphatic system consists of capillaries, vessels, ducts and nodes that transport a fluid known as lymph. Lymph is formed from the tissue fluid that surrounds all tissue cells. It performs three important functions: (i) transportation of lymphocytes that defend the body against infection and foreign antigens, (ii) transportation of lipids and (iii) by its formation, the drainage of excess fluid from the tissues.

Let us begin by examining the terms associated with the cells and components of the system. Use the Exercise Guide at the beginning of this unit to complete Word Exercises 1–8 unless you are asked to work without it.

Root	Lymph
	*(From Greek **lympha**, meaning water. It is used to mean the fluid lymph or lymphatic tissue.)*
Combining forms	**Lymph/a/o**

WORD EXERCISE 1

Using your Exercise Guide, find the meaning of:

(a) **lympho**/cyt/osis _____

(b) **lympho**/rrhagia _____

(c) **lymph**/angio/graphy _____

(d) **lymph**/angio/gram _____

(e) **lymph**/angi/ectasis _____

Note.   The next four words use the combining form **lymphaden/o** meaning lymph gland. The structures referred to by this combining form are no longer called glands because unlike true glands, they do not produce secretions. Lymphaden/o is now used to mean **lymph node**. A node is a mass of lymphoid tissue containing cells that defend the body against noxious agents such as microorganisms and toxins.

(f) **lymphaden**/oma _____

(g) **lymphaden**/ectomy _____

(h) **lymphadeno**/pathy _____

(i) **lymphaden**/itis _____

Lymph nodes consist of lymphatic channels held in place by fibrous connective tissue that forms a capsule. The nodes contain **lymphocytes** (lymph cells, *-cyte* meaning cell), and special cells called **macrophages** (large-eaters) which, like neutrophils, can engulf foreign substances and microorganisms (by phagocytosis). Lymph nodes often trap and destroy malignant cells as well as microorganisms. During infection lymphocytes and macrophages multiply rapidly, causing the nodes to swell; they may become inflamed and sore. Lymphocytes and macrophages leave the nodes in lymph (a clear fluid) that eventually drains through ducts into blood vessels near the heart. These cells then circulate in the blood and form a proportion of the white blood cell population.

If disease in the lymphatic system is suspected, a **nodal** (*-al* meaning pertaining to) **biopsy** may be performed; in this procedure a node is removed for examination by a histopathologist (*hist/o* meaning tissue, *path/o* disease and *-logist* a specialist who studies).

The macrophages that line the lymph organs are part of a large system of cells known as the **reticuloendothelial system** or macrophage system. Cells that form this network have a common ancestry and carry out phagocytosis (Fig. 30) in the liver, bone marrow, lymph nodes,

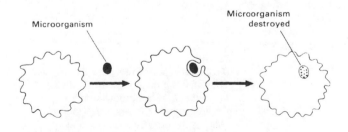

Figure 30   Phagocytosis

spleen, nervous system, blood and connective tissues. Macrophages found in connective tissues are known as **histiocytes** (i.e. tissue cells). If there is an increase in the number of histiocytes without infection this is known as a **histiocytosis**.

Distinct patches of lymphatic tissue have been given specific names; the familiar ones mentioned here include the spleen, tonsils, adenoids and thymus.

Root	Splen
	(A Greek word, meaning spleen. This organ has four main functions: destruction of old blood cells, blood storage, blood filtration and participation in the immune response.)

Combining forms **Splen/o**

WORD EXERCISE 2

Using your Exercise Guide, find the meaning of:

(a) **spleno**/megaly _____

(b) **spleno**/hepato/megaly _____

(c) **spleno**/pexy _____

(d) **spleno**/cele _____

(e) **spleno**/malacia _____

(f) **spleno**/lysis _____

Without using your Exercise Guide, write the meaning of:

(g) **spleno**/gram _____

(h) **spleno**/porto/gram _____

(**Port/o** refers to the portal vein which drains blood from the intestines, stomach, pancreas and spleen into the liver.)

Root	Tonsill
	*(From Latin **tonsillae**, meaning tonsils. These form a ring of lymphoid tissue at the back of the mouth and nasopharynx. They are important in the formation of antibodies and lymphocytes.)*

Combining forms **Tonsill/o**

WORD EXERCISE 3

Without using your Exercise Guide, build words that mean:

(a) inflammation of the tonsils _____

(b) removal of the tonsils _____

Using your Exercise Guide, find the meaning of:

(c) **tonsillo**/pharyng/eal _____

(d) **tonsillo**/tome _____

Note. The enlarged nasopharyngeal tonsil is known as the **adenoids**. Sometimes this obstructs the passage of air or interferes with hearing when it blocks the entrance to the auditory tube. Removal of the adenoids is known as an **adenoid**ectomy.

Root	Thym
	*(From a Greek word **thymos**, meaning soul/emotion. It is used to mean the thymus gland which lies high in the chest above the aorta. It controls the development of the immune system in early life.)*

Combining forms **Thym/o, thymic/o**

WORD EXERCISE 4

Without using your Exercise Guide, build words using thym/o that mean:

(a) a cell of the thymus _____

(b) disease of the thymus _____

(c) protrusion/swelling of the thymus _____

Using your Exercise Guide, find the meaning of:

(d) **thym**/elc/osis (Look up helc.) _____

(e) **thymico**/lympha/tic _____

Immunology

Immunology is the scientific study of immunity and related disciplines such as immunotherapy and immunochemistry. Immunological research has intensified recently because of the spread of the immuno-deficiency virus (HIV) that causes AIDS. Many pharmaceutical companies are actively engaged in the search for vaccines and new treatments based on our increased knowledge of the immune process.

Immunity is the condition of being immune to infectious disease and antigenic substances that might damage the body. It is brought about by the production of antibodies and cells that destroy invading pathogens before they can do us harm. During our lifetime we acquire an immunity to common disease-producing organisms, such as viruses that cause colds and influenza. We can also acquire an immunity to more serious diseases by vaccination.

Understanding the meaning of the following terms will help you understand the basis of the immune process.

Antigen
An antigen is any foreign substance that enters the body and stimulates antibody production or a response associated with sensitized T-cells. Note, antigens will be present on the surface of any foreign cell that enters the body and these will provoke a response from the immune system.

Antibody
An antibody is a chemical that circulates in the blood destroying or precipitating specific foreign substances (antigens) that have entered the body. (*Anti-* means against, *-body* is an Anglo-Saxon word, in this case referring to a foreign body.)

Root	Immun
	*(From Latin **immunis**, meaning exempt from public burden. In medicine it means exemption from disease, i.e. immunity.)*

Combining forms   **Immun/o**

WORD EXERCISE 5

Using your Exercise Guide, build words that mean:

(a) the study of immunity   _____

(b) branch of medicine concerned with the study of immune reactions associated with disease   _____

Using your Exercise Guide, find the meaning of:

(c) **immuno**/genesis   _____

(d) auto/**immun**/ity   _____

(e) **immuno**/globulin   _____

Immunity is brought about by two basic types of cell.

T-cells (thymic cells)

T-cells are types of lymphocyte formed in the bone marrow of the embryo that move to the thymus to be processed into T-cells (hence the name T-cell). The T-cells then move to other parts of the lymphatic system where they are responsible for the **cell-mediated response**. Once sensitized to a specific antigen, these cells multiply rapidly, producing various cell types all of which play a role in the immune response. One type of cell that forms is the cytotoxic (killer) T-cell, this attacks and kills infectious microorganisms containing the specific antigen. These cells are particularly effective against slowly growing bacteria and fungi, cancer cells and skin grafts.

B-cells

B-cells are types of lymphocyte named for historical reasons after the site where they were first seen in birds, the Bursa of Fabricius. In humans, B-cells first differentiate in the fetal liver and transform into large **plasma cells** when confronted with specific antigens. Once sensitized by an antigen, the plasma cell multiplies to form a large clone of similar cells (**plasmacytosis**). Each cell in the clone secretes the same antibody to the sensitizing antigen; this is known as the **humoral response**. Some antibodies activate a protein in the blood known as **complement**, which aids the antibody in destroying antigen. (Note, plasmacytosis means an excess of plasma cells in the blood).

Root	Ser
	*(From a Latin word **serum**, meaning whey. It is used in medicine to mean the clear portion of any liquid separated from its more solid elements. Blood serum is the supernatant liquid formed when blood clots. It can be used as a source of antibodies.)*

Combining forms   **Ser/o**

WORD EXERCISE 6

Without using your Exercise Guide, build a word that means:

(a) the scientific study of sera   _____

Serum investigations can lead to a patient being sero-negative or seropositive for the presence of a particular antibody. For example people assessed as HIV positive have antibodies in their blood to the human immuno-deficiency virus. This means that the virus has entered their bodies and stimulated the immune system to make antibodies. If the virus is not destroyed by the immune system or inhibited by drug therapy it will continue to replicate and lead to the development of AIDS.

Seronegative
means showing a lack of antibody.

Seropositive
means showing the presence of a high level of antibody.

Root   **Py**
(From a Greek word **pyon***, meaning pus.)*

Combining forms   **Py/o**

Pus is a yellow, protein-rich liquid, composed of tissue fluids containing bacteria and leucocytes. When a wound is forming or discharging pus it is said to be **suppurating**. Pus is formed in response to certain types of infection.

WORD EXERCISE 7

Using your Exercise Guide, find the meaning of:

(a) **py**/aemia
    (Am. py/emia)   _____

(b) **pyo**/genic   _____

(c) **pyo**/rrhoea
    (Am. pyo/rrhea)   _____

(d) **pyo**/poiesis   _____

The immune response of the lymphatic system not only resists invasion by infective organisms but also functions to identify and destroy everything described as 'non-self', i.e. foreign antigens that have entered the body, such as in transplanted organs or body cells that have changed their form, such as malignant cells.

Patients infected with microorganisms, for example those who present with tonsillitis, experience swollen lymph nodes and their blood counts indicate an increase in circulating white blood cells. The nodes swell because they contain plasma cells and T-cells forming clones of cells to 'fight' the infection. Once the foreign cells have been destroyed, the nodes return to their normal size. The response of the body to the initial sensitization with the antigen is called the *primary response*.

An important feature of the immune response is that some activated B-cells develop into **memory B-cells** rather than plasma cells. These remain in the nodes and other lymphoid tissue ready to respond should the same antigen enter the body again. If the same antigen is contacted the memory B-cells divide rapidly to produce plasma cells. These release large amounts of antibody, destroying the antigen before symptoms appear.

In a similar way some **memory T-cells** remain in the lymphoid tissue, and can be rapidly activated in response to another contact with the same antigen. The accelerated and increased response of the memory cells is called the *secondary response*, and it endows us with immunity.

Medical equipment and clinical procedure

The lymphatic system is investigated by radiological examination and few specific instruments are used to examine it. Revise the meaning of **-gram** and **-graphy** and then try Exercise 8.

WORD EXERCISE 8

Match each term in Column A with a description from Column C by placing an appropriate number in Column B.

Column A	Column B	Column C
(a) tonsillotome	_____	1. X-ray picture of portal veins and spleen
(b) lymphangio-graphy	_____	2. X-ray picture of lymphatic system
(c) lymphadeno-graphy	_____	3. instrument for cutting tonsils
(d) lymphogram	_____	4. technique of making an X-ray of lymph vessels
(e) splenoporto-gram	_____	5. the technique of making an X-ray of the lymphatic system
(f) lymphography	_____	6. technique of making an X-ray of lymph nodes

ANATOMY EXERCISE

Now complete the Anatomy Exercise on page 67.

CASE HISTORY 6

The object of this exercise is to understand words associated with a patient's medical history.

To complete the exercise:

- read through the passage on non-Hodgkin's lymphoma; unfamiliar words are underlined and you can find their meaning using the Word Help

- write the meaning of the medical terms shown in bold print.

Non-Hodgkin's Lymphoma

Mr F, a 48-year-old male, presented to his GP with a painless swelling in the right axilla. The lump had been present for at least two months before his consultation and he had not been unduly concerned until he noticed a similar lump in his left axilla that appeared to be increasing in size. The patient indicated he had a good appetite and denied weight loss. There had been no change to his bowel and bladder habits and apart from a recent cold and **tonsillitis** he had not suffered any infection. He had smoked for 32 years and admitted moderate drinking. The only problem he mentioned was difficulty in sleeping; sometimes he would wake sweating copiously.

Examination revealed prominent lymph node enlargement in the right and left axillae and inguinal areas. The largest node was located in the right axilla, approximately 2 cm across. Examination of the head and neck also revealed enlarged cervical nodes, the largest approximately 1.5 cm across. The nodes were firm, tender and rubbery on palpation.

Cardiovascular and pulmonary examination was normal. He had **splenomegaly** that was palpable 3 cm below the left costal margin. His tonsils appeared swollen. It was evident from initial examination that Mr F was suffering from a generalized **lymphadenopathy** that did not appear to be associated with infection.

Mr F underwent axillary **nodal** biopsy and his specimen was sent to **histopathology**. Examination of the tissue revealed a follicular, small, cleaved cell non-Hodgkin's **lymphoma** (NHL). This was followed by a bilateral bone marrow trephine biopsy that demonstrated cells suspicious for lymphoma similar to those found in the nodes. The **lymphocytes** forming the

tumour were classified as being of **B-cell** origin. Computerized tomography (CT) was used to assess nodal enlargement and he was referred to the oncology department for staging.

Mr F underwent four cycles of chemotherapy (CHOPS) and since then no disease is evident in his bone marrow and his lymphadenopathy has regressed.

WORD HELP

axilla the armpit (Pl. axillae)

bilateral pertaining to two sides

biopsy removal and examination of living tissue

cervical pertaining to the neck

chemotherapy treatment with chemicals i.e. cytotoxic drugs that kill cancer cells

CHOPS type of chemotherapy regimen (Using **c**yclophosphamide, **h**ydroxydaunorubicin, **o**ncovin and **p**rednisolone)

cleaved cut/separated (here refers to indentations in the nucleus of a lymph cell)

costal pertaining to the ribs

follicular pertaining to a follicle (here a well-defined collection of multiplying lymph cells)

GP general practitioner (family doctor)

inguinal pertaining to the groin

non-Hodgkin's not Hodgkin's disease (a type of lymphoma)

oncology study of tumours/cancers

palpation act of feeling with the fingers using light pressure

regressed reverted (towards former condition)

staging system of classifying malignant disease that will influence its treatment

tomography technique of using X-rays to image a section through the body

trephine instrument with a circular cutting edge that removes a disc of tissue

Now write the meaning of the following words from the case history without using your dictionary lists:

(a) tonsillitis   _____

(b) splenomegaly   _____

(c) lymphadenopathy   _____

(d) nodal   _____

(e) histopathology   _____

(f) lymphoma   _____

(g) lymphocyte   _____

(h) B-cell   _____

(Answers to the case history exercise are given in the Answers to Word Exercises beginning on page 275.)

Quick Reference

Combining forms relating to the lymphatic system and immunology:

Aden/o	gland
Adenoid-	adenoids
Cyt/e/o	cell
-globulin	protein
Hist/i/o	tissue
Immun/o	immune
Lymph/o	lymph
Lymphaden/o	lymph node
Lymphangi/o	lymph vessel
Phag/o	eating/consuming
Plasma-	plasma cell
Py/o	pus
Ser/o	serum
Splen/o	spleen
Thym/o	thymus gland
Thymic/o	thymus gland
Tonsill/o	tonsil

Abbreviations

Some common abbreviations related to the lymphatic system are listed below. Note, some are not standard and their meaning may vary from one health care setting to another. There is a more extensive list for reference on page 307.

AIDS	acquired immune deficiency syndrome
ALL	acute lymphocytic leukaemia (Am. leukemia)
BM (T)	bone marrow (trephine)
CLL	chronic lymphocytic leukaemia (Am. leukemia)
HLA	human leucocyte antigen
Ig	immunoglobulin
LAS	lymphadenopathy syndrome
Lymphos	lymphocytes
T & A	tonsils and adenoids
TD	thymus-dependent cells
TI	thymus-independent cells
TLD	thoracic lymph duct

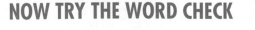 **NOW TRY THE WORD CHECK**

WORD CHECK

This self-check exercise lists all the word components used in this unit. First write down the meaning of as many word components as you can. Then check your answers using the Exercise Guide and Quick Reference box or the Glossary of Word Components (pp. 319–341).

Prefixes

anti-	*against*
auto-	*self*
macro-	*large*

Combining forms of word roots

aden/o	*node*
angi/o	*vessel*
cyt/o	*cell*
-globulin	*protein*
helc/o	*ulcer*
hepat/o	*liver*
hist/i/o	*tissue*
immun/o	*immune*
lymph/o	*lymph*
lymphaden/o	*lymph node*
lymphangi/o	*lymph vessel*
phag/o	*eating/consuming*
pharyng/o	*pharynx*
plasm/a	*plasma*
port/o	*portal vein*
py/o	*pus*
reticul/o	*immature erythrocyte*
ser/o	*serum*
splen/o	*spleen*

thym/o — *thymus gland*

tonsill/o — *tonsils*

-tic — *pertaining to*

-tome — *cutting instrument*

Suffixes

-aemia (Am. -emia) — *condition of blood*

-al — *pertaining to*

-cele — *hernia/swelling*

-eal — *pertaining to*

-ectasis — *dilation/stretching*

-ectomy — *removal of*

-genesis — *formation*

-genic — *pertaining to formation*

-gram — *x-ray/recording*

-graphy — *technique of taking x-ray*

-ia — *condition of*

-ic — *pertaining to*

-itis — *inflammation of*

-ity — *state/condition*

-logy — *study of*

-lysis — *breakdown/disintegration*

-malacia — *condition of softening*

-megaly — *enlargement of*

-oma — *tumour/swelling*

-osis — *abnormal condition of*

-pathy — *disease of*

-pexy — *surgical fixation*

-poiesis — *formation*

-rrhagia — *condition of bursting forth*

-rrhoea (Am. -rrhea) — *excessive flow/discharge*

> **NOW TRY THE SELF-ASSESSMENT** <

SELF-ASSESSMENT

Test 6A

Below are some medical terms that refer to the anatomy of the lymphatic system. Indicate which part of the system they refer to by putting a number from the diagram (Fig. 31) next to each word.

(a) lymphaden/o — 5

(b) splen/o — 3

(c) thym/o — 2

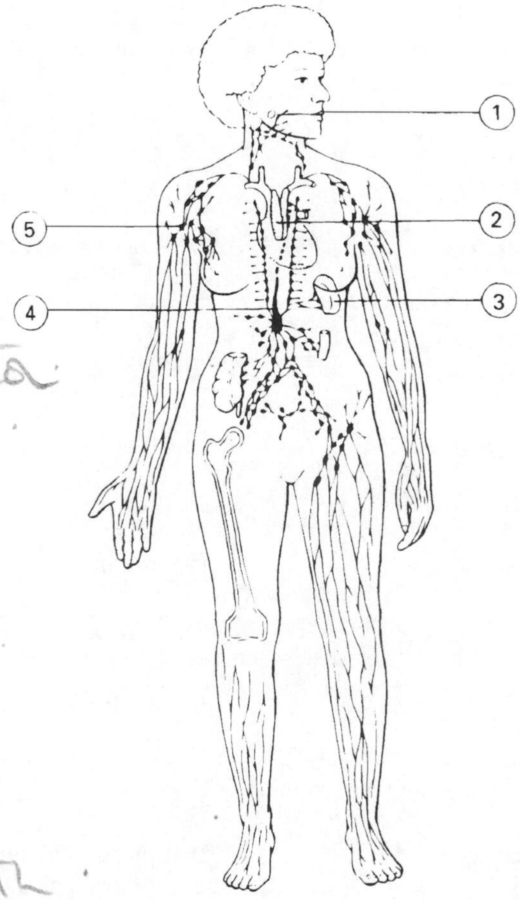

Figure 31 The lymphatic system

(d) tonsill/o _____ *1*

(e) lymphangi/o _____ *4*

Score

5

Column A	Column B	Column C
(r) thym/o	*20*	18. disintegration/breakdown
(s) -tome	*7*	19. portal vein
(t) tonsill/o	*12*	20. thymus gland

Score

20

Test 6B

Prefixes, suffixes and combining forms of word roots

Match each word component in Column A with a meaning in Column C by inserting the appropriate number in Column B.

Column A	Column B	Column C
(a) aden/o	*14*	1. protein/ball
(b) angi/o	*5*	2. swelling/hernia/protrusion
(c) anti-	*8*	3. immune
(d) auto-	*4*	4. self
(e) -cele	*2*	5. vessel
(f) -globin	*1*	6. pus
(g) -gram	*16*	7. cutting instrument
(h) helc/o	*10*	8. against
(i) immun/o	*3*	9. spleen
(j) lymph/o	*13*	10. ulcer
(k) -lysis	*18*	11. serum
(l) -malacia	*17*	12. tonsil
(m) port/o	*19*	13. lymph
(n) py/o	*6*	14. gland
(o) -rrhoea (Am. -rrhea)	*15*	15. excessive flow
(p) ser/o	*11*	16. picture/tracing/recording
(q) splen/o	*9*	17. condition of softening

Test 6C

Write the meaning of:

(a) lymphorrhoea (Am. lymphorrhea) — *excessive flow of lymph*

(b) splenic — *pertains to the spleen*

(c) lymphadenectasis — *dilation of lymph nodes*

(d) thymolysis — *breakdown of thymus*

(e) serologist — *specialist who studies sera*

Score

5

Test 6D

Build words that mean:

(a) tumour of lymph (tissue) — *lymphoma*

(b) X-ray examination of the lymph system — *lymphogram*

(c) removal of the spleen — *splenectomy*

(d) condition of bleeding/bursting forth of the spleen — *splenorrhagia*

(e) tumour of a lymph vessel — *lymphangioma*

Score

5

Check answers to Self-Assessment Tests on page 299.

The urinary system

Objectives

Once you have completed Unit 7 you should be able to:

- understand the meaning of medical words relating to the urinary system

- build medical words relating to the urinary system

- associate medical terms with their anatomical position

- understand medical abbreviations relating to the urinary system.

Exercise Guide

Use this list of word components and their meanings to complete the word exercises in this unit.

Prefixes

dys-	difficult/painful
hyper-	above normal/excessive
intra-	within/inside
oligo-	deficiency/few/little
poly-	many/much

Roots/Combining forms

albumin/o	albumin/albumen
azot/o	urea
calc/i	calcium
col/o	colon
enter/o	intestine
gastr/o	stomach
haemat/o	blood
hemat/o (Am.)	blood
hydr/o	water
lith/o	stone
metr/o	a measure
proct/o	anus/rectum
py/o	pus

sigmoid/o	sigmoid colon
trigon/o	trigone of the bladder

Suffixes

-al	pertaining to
-algia	condition of pain
-cele	swelling/protrusion/hernia
-clysis	infusion/injection/irrigation
-dynia	condition of pain
-ectasis	dilatation/stretching
-ectomy	removal of
-ferous	pertaining to carrying/bearing
-genesis	capable of causing/pertaining to formation
-gram	X-ray/tracing/recording
-graphy	technique of recording/making an X-ray
-ia	condition of
-iasis	abnormal condition
-ic	pertaining to
-itis	inflammation of
-lapaxy	empty/wash out/evacuate
-lithiasis	abnormal condition of stones
-logist	specialist who studies
-lysis	breakdown/disintegration
-meter	measuring instrument
-metry	process of measuring
-osis	abnormal condition/disease of
-ous	pertaining to/of the nature of
-pathy	disease of
-pexy	surgical fixation/fix in place
-phyma	tumour/boil
-plasty	surgical repair/reconstruction
-ptosis	falling/diplacement/prolapse
-rrhagia	condition of bursting forth of blood/bleeding
-rrhaphy	suture/stitch
-sclerosis	hardening
-scope	instrument to view
-scopy	visual examination
-stenosis	abnormal condition of narrowing
-stomy	to form a new opening or outlet
-tome	cutting instrument
-tomy	incision into
-tripsy	act of crushing
-triptor	instrument to crush/fragment (using shock waves)
-trite	instrument to crush/fragment
-uresis	excrete in urine/urinate

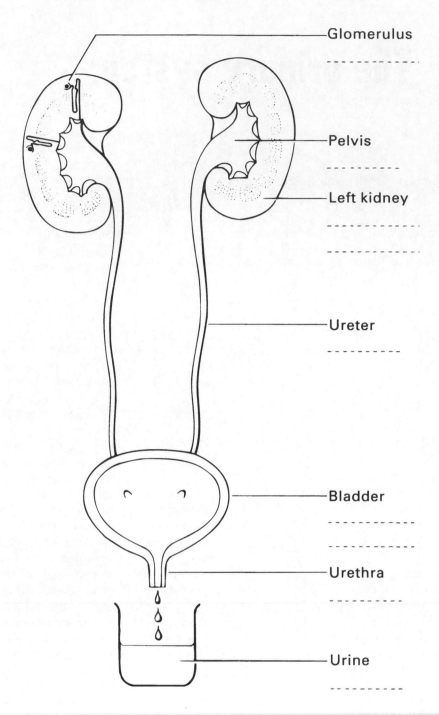

Glomerulus

- - - - - - - - - - - -

Pelvis

- - - - - - - - - -

Left kidney

- - - - - - - - - - - -

- - - - - - - - - - - -

Ureter

- - - - - - - - - -

Bladder

- - - - - - - - - - -

- - - - - - - - - - -

Urethra

- - - - - - - - - -

Urine

- - - - - - - - - -

Figure 32 The urinary system

ANATOMY EXERCISE

When you have finished Word Exercises 1–11, look at the word components listed below. Complete Figure 32 by writing the appropriate combining form on each dotted line – more than one component may relate to the same position. (You can check their meanings in the Quick Reference box on p. 83.)

Cyst/o	Ren/o	Urin/o
Glomerul/o	Ureter/o	Vesic/o
Nephr/o	Urethr/o	
Pyel/o		

The urinary system

The main components of the urinary system are the kidneys, that remove metabolic wastes from the blood by forming them into urine. This yellow liquid is passed from the kidneys through the ureters to the urinary bladder where it is stored. Periodically urine is passed out of the body through the urethra in the process of urination.

Besides removing waste substances that could be toxic to tissue cells, the kidneys maintain the volume of water in the blood and regulate its salt concentration and pH. The kidneys are therefore involved in homeostasis, i.e. maintaining constant conditions within the tissue fluids of the body. The continuous activity of the kidneys is required to maintain life.

Use the Exercise Guide at the beginning of this unit to complete Word Exercises 1–11 unless you are asked to work without it.

Root	Ren
	*(A Latin word **ren**, meaning kidney.)*
Combining forms	**Ren/o**

WORD EXERCISE 1

Using your Exercise Guide, find the meaning of:

(a) **reno**/gastr/ic _____

(b) **reno**/gram _____

(c) **reno**/graphy _____

Renography may show up a renal calculus (from Latin *calcis* – small stone), i.e. a kidney stone. The presence of a stone in a ureter leads to severe pain and is referred to as **renal colic**. Renal colic can also be caused by disorder and disease within a kidney.

Radioisotope renograms are useful in assessing kidney function. They are made following injection of radio-isotopes into the bloodstream. The technique of making this type of recording is discussed in more detail in Unit 18.

Root	Nephr
	*(From a Greek word **nephros**, meaning kidney.)*
Combining forms	**Nephr/o**

WORD EXERCISE 2

Using your Exercise Guide, find the meaning of:

(a) **nephro**/ptosis _____

(b) hydro/**nephr**/osis _____

(c) **nephro**/cele _____

(d) **nephr**/algia _____

Using your Exercise Guide, build words that mean:

(e) surgical fixation of a kidney (e.g. floating kidney) _____

(f) surgical repair of a kidney _____

(g) incision into a kidney _____

(h) condition of stones in the kidney _____

(i) removal of a kidney _____

Within each kidney there are approximately one million kidney tubules or nephrons that do the work of the kidney. At the beginning of each nephron is a **glomerulus**, a ball of capillaries surrounded by porous membranes that filter metabolic wastes from the blood. When glomeruli undergo pathological change the filtering mechanism of the kidneys is seriously affected, reducing their ability to maintain homeostasis.

Using your Exercise Guide, find the meaning of:

(j) **glomerul**/itis (suppurative) _____

(k) **glomerulo**/pathy _____

(l) **glomerulo**/sclerosis _____

Infections and disorders of the kidneys sometimes lead to kidney failure. This results in the waste products of metabolism increasing in concentration within the blood and a failure to regulate water, mineral metabolism and pH; these changes will lead to death. The patient with kidney failure can be kept alive if one of the following procedures is applied.

Haemodialysis (Am. hemodialysis)

This involves diverting the patient's blood through a dialyser, commonly called a kidney machine (Fig. 33). In the dialyser waste products are removed from the blood which is then returned to the body via another blood vessel. The patient must be connected to the dialyser for many hours per week and so cannot lead a normal life. (Dialysis means separating, i.e. separating wastes from the blood.)

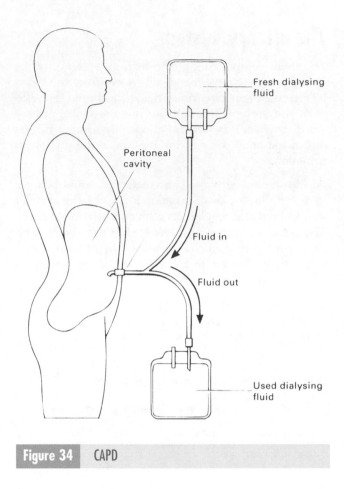

Figure 34   CAPD

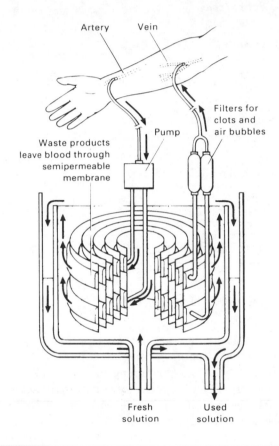

Figure 33   Haemodialysis (Am. hemodialysis)

CAPD (continuous ambulatory peritoneal dialysis)

The patient is fitted with a peritoneal catheter (tube) (Fig. 34). Every 6 hours approximately 2 litres of dialysing fluid is passed into the peritoneum. Toxic wastes diffuse into the dialysing fluid and are removed from the body when the fluid is changed. This procedure is repeated four times a day, 7 days a week. CAPD has been used on a long-term basis but there is danger from peritonitis caused by infection.

Kidney transplant

A kidney can be transplanted between two individuals of the same species, i.e. between two humans who are not closely related. This type of transplant or graft is known as a homotransplant or homograft (*homo* meaning the same, synonymous with allograft). The donor could be living, and survive with one remaining kidney, or a victim of a fatal accident. A transplant may keep a patient alive for many years and avoids the inconvenience and dangers associated with CAPD and dialysis. Transplants between genetically identical twins are more successful. These are known as isografts (*iso* means same/equal).

Root	**Pyel**
	*(From a Greek word **pyelos**, meaning trough. Here it refers to the space inside a kidney called the renal pelvis in which urine collects after its formation.)*
Combining forms	**Pyel/o**
	(Do not confuse this with pyo, meaning pus.)

WORD EXERCISE 3

Without using your Exercise Guide, write the meaning of:

(a) **pyelo**/nephr/itis _____

(This is often due to a bacterial infection.)

(b) **pyelo**/litho/tomy _____

(c) **pyelo**/nephr/osis _____

Without using your Exercise Guide, build words that mean:

(d) surgical repair of the renal pelvis _____

(e) X-ray picture of the renal pelvis _____

The technique of making an X-ray of the renal pelvis is known as **pyelo**graphy. It involves filling the pelvis with a radio-opaque dye. There are several ways of doing this:

> **Intravenous pyelography**
> Here the dye is injected into the bloodstream and it eventually passes through the kidney pelvis (**intra** – meaning inside, **ven/o** – meaning vein).
>
> **Antegrade pyelography**
> Here the dye is injected into the renal pelvis (**ante** – meaning before/in front; **grad** – meaning take steps/to go (Latin)). It refers to the fact that the dye goes into the pelvis before it leaves the kidney. The dye is injected through a percutaneous catheter, i.e. through the skin.
>
> **Retrograde (or ascending) pyelography**
> Here the dye is injected into the kidney via the ureter, so it is being forced backwards up the ureter into the urine within the pelvis (**retro** – Latin, means backwards).

Root   Ureter

*(From a Greek word **oureter**, meaning urinary canal. Now used to mean ureter, the narrow tube that connects each kidney to the bladder. Urine flows through the ureters assisted by the action of smooth muscle.)*

Combining forms   **Ureter/o**

WORD EXERCISE 4

Without using your Exercise Guide, write the meaning of:

(a) **uretero**/cele _____

(b) **uretero**/cel/ectomy _____

Using your Exercise Guide, find the meaning of:

(c) **uretero**/rrhagia _____

(d) **uretero**/rrhaphy _____

(e) **ureter**/ectasis _____

(f) **uretero**/reno/scopy _____
(Note the difference between -scope and -scopy.)

(g) **uretero**/stomy _____

Using your Exercise Guide, build words that mean:

(h) formation of an opening _____
between the intestine and ureter

(i) formation of an opening _____
between the colon and ureter

Root   Cyst
*(From Greek **kystis**, meaning bladder.)*

Combining forms   **Cyst/o**

Note.   We have already used cyst/o in Unit 2 with cholecyst/o, meaning the bile (gall) bladder. Here we are using **cyst/o** alone to mean the urinary bladder, which stores urine until it is expelled from the body.

WORD EXERCISE 5

Without using your Exercise Guide, write the meaning of:

(a) **cyst**/itis _____
(There are many causes of this condition which may be acute or chronic, including injury and infection. As the bladder is open to the external

genitalia via the urethra, it is easy for microorganisms to enter from outside. Sometimes infections are transmitted into the urinary tract from sexual contact, for example, gonorrhoea and Chlamydia. Cystitis is more common in women due to their shorter urethras.)

(b) **cysto**/lith/ectomy _____

(c) **cysto**/pyel/itis _____

(d) **cysto**/ptosis _____

Using your Exercise Guide, find the meaning of:

(e) **cysto**/scope _____

(f) **cysto**/procto/stomy _____

Meter and **metr/o** originate from Greek *metron*, meaning a measure, and **metry** from *metrein*, meaning process of measuring. Use these to build words meaning:

(g) instrument to measure bladder (capacity or pressure within) _____

(h) technique of measuring the bladder (capacity and pressure of) _____

(i) a trace, picture or recording of the measured volume and pressure of the bladder (use metr/o) _____

A technique that applies an electric current to tissues, causing them to heat up, is known as **diathermy** (*dia* – meaning through and *thermy* – meaning heat). These can be combined here to make:

Cystodiathermy
The process of applying heat through the bladder. The heat is produced by an electric current and is used to destroy tumours in the bladder wall.

Root | **Vesic**
*(From Latin **vesica**, also meaning bladder.)*

Combining forms **Vesic/o**

WORD EXERCISE 6

Without using your Exercise Guide, build words that mean:

(a) the formation of an opening into the bladder _____

(b) incision into the bladder _____

Using your Exercise Guide, find the meaning of:

(c) **vesico**/clysis _____

(d) **vesic**/al _____

(e) **vesico**/sigmoido/stomy _____

Without using your Exercise Guide, write the meaning of:

(f) **vesico**/ureter/al _____

Catheterization of the bladder is required following some surgical operations and when there is difficulty in emptying the bladder owing to a neuromuscular disorder or physical damage to the spinal cord. The procedure involves inserting a catheter through the urethra into the bladder (Fig. 35). A urinary **catheter** consists of a fine tube that allows urine to drain from the bladder into an external container. Some self-retaining catheters are held in position by means of an inflated balloon.

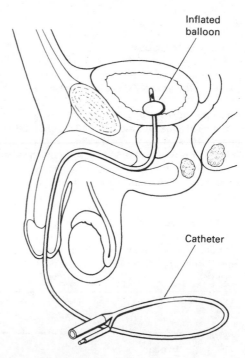

Inflated balloon

Catheter

Figure 35 Catheterization

Root | **Urethr**
*(From Greek **ourethro**, meaning urethra, the tube through which urine leaves the body from the bladder.)*

Combining forms **Urethr/o**

WORD EXERCISE 7

Without using your Exercise Guide, write the meaning of:

(a) **urethro**/metry _____

(b) **urethro**/trigon/itis _____
(Trigone refers to a triangular area at the base of the bladder, bounded by the openings of the ureters at the back and the urethral opening at the front.)

(c) **urethro**/pexy _____

Without using your Exercise Guide, build words that mean:

(d) condition of pain in the urethra _____

(e) condition of flow of blood from the urethra _____

(f) visual examination of the urethra _____

Using your Exercise Guide, find the meaning of:

(g) **urethro**/phyma _____

(h) **urethro**/tome _____

(i) **urethro**/stenosis _____

(j) **urethro**/dynia _____

> **Root**   **Urin**
> *(From a Latin word **urina**, meaning urine, the excretory product of the kidneys.)*
>
> *Combining forms*   **Urin/a/i/o**

WORD EXERCISE 8

Using your Exercise Guide, find the meaning of:

(a) **urini**/ferous _____

(b) **urina**/lysis _____

(This word refers to the technique of analysing urine. Detailed urinalysis is a valuable aid to the diagnosis of disease, e.g. the presence of high concentrations of glucose in the urine may indicate diabetes. Other components commonly analysed are colour, pH, specific gravity, ketone bodies, phenylketones, protein, bilirubin and solid casts of varying composition.)

Without using your Exercise Guide, write the meaning of:

(c) **urino**/meter _____
(This is used to estimate specific gravity of urine which can change in illness.)

> **Root**   **Ur**
> *(From a Greek word **ouron**, also meaning urine.)*
>
> *Combining forms*   **Ur/o**
> *(This form is also used to refer to the urinary tract and urination.)*

WORD EXERCISE 9

Without using your Exercise Guide, write the meaning of:

(a) **uro**/graphy _____
(Synonymous with intravenous pyelogram (IVP). The above procedure is also performed by injecting dye directly into the urinary tract rather than into a vein.)

Using your Exercise Guide, find the meaning of:

(b) **uro**/logist _____

(c) **uro**/genesis _____

(d) olig/**ur**/ia _____

(e) albumin/**ur**/ia _____

(f) azot/**ur**/ia _____

(g) poly/**ur**/ia _____

(h) dys/**ur**/ia _____

(i) haemat/**ur**/ia _____
(Am. hemat/ur/ia)

(j) py/**ur**/ia _____

(k) hyper/calci/**ur**/ia _____

Note.   The act of passing urine is known as micturition (from Latin *micturire*, meaning to pass water).

Root   Lith
*(From a Greek word **lithos**, meaning stone.)*

Combining forms   **Lith/o**

Here *lithos* refers to a kidney stone, which is a hard mass composed mainly of mineral matter present in the urinary system. Remember a stone is sometimes called a **renal calculus** (pl. **calculi**). Stones can prevent the passage of urine, causing pain and kidney damage. They need to be passsed or removed because they can seriously affect the functioning of the kidneys.

WORD EXERCISE 10

Without using your Exercise Guide, write the meaning of:

(a) **litho**/nephr/itis

(b) uro/**lith**/iasis

(c) **litho**/genesis

Using your Exercise Guide, find the meaning of:

(d) **litho**/trite

(e) **litho**/lapaxy

(f) **litho**/triptor
(This instrument focuses high energy shock waves generated by a high voltage spark on to a kidney stone. No surgery is required, as the stone disintegrates within the body and is passed in the urine. The procedure for using this instrument is called extra-corporeal shock wave lithotripsy (ECSL), *extra* meaning outside, *corporeal* meaning body.)

(g) **litho**/tripsy

(h) **lith**/uresis

Medical equipment and clinical procedures

WORD EXERCISE 11

Before completing Exercise 11, check the names of instruments and techniques of examination of the

urinary system mentioned in this unit. Revise -scope, -scopy, -tome, -metry, -meter and -thermy.

Match each term in Column A with a description from Column C by placing an appropriate number in Column B.

Column A	Column B	Column C
(a) diathermy		1. instrument for crushing stones
(b) cystoscope		2. device that separates wastes from the blood
(c) lithotriptor		3. instrument for cutting the urethra
(d) urinometer		4. visual examination of the ureter
(e) haemodialyser (Am. hemodialyzer)		5. instrument that measures the pressure and capacity of the bladder
(f) ureteroscopy		6. instrument to view the urethra
(g) urethrotome		7. device that destroys stones using shock waves
(h) cystometer		8. technique of heating a tissue by applying an electric current
(i) urethroscope		9. instrument for measuring specific gravity of urine
(j) lithotrite		10. instrument to view the bladder

ANATOMY EXERCISE

Now complete the Anatomy Exercise on page 76.

CASE HISTORY 7

The object of this exercise is to understand words associated with a patient's medical history.

To complete the exercise:

• read through the passage on urolithiasis; unfamiliar words are underlined and you can find their meaning using the Word Help

- write the meaning of the medical terms shown in bold print.

Urolithiasis

Mr G, an engineer recently returned from working in the Middle East, was admitted to Accident and Emergency in pain and clutching his right side. He had been awoken during the night by an excruciating pain in his right flank radiating to the iliac fossa and right testicle. In the past two days, he had developed severe **urethral** pain and **dysuria** associated with **haematuria**. Fluid intake made the pain worse and he had been vomiting. Mr G had recently been treated with antibiotics by his GP for bacteriuria and diagnosed as suffering from obstructive **uropathy**. His condition had become acute whilst waiting for his referral appointment. On admission he required immediate analgesia for severe pain and administered 10 mg morphine i.m. He was kept in overnight for observation and transferred to the Urology Unit the following morning.

The next day a dull pain was still present, and examination revealed loin tenderness and an enlarged palpable hydronephrotic right kidney. A plain abdominal radiograph identified a single calculus in the line of the right ureter. Excretion urography (intravenous **pyelography** IVP) confirmed the calculus to be obstructing the pelviureteric junction. The kidney outline appeared enlarged but smooth with no anatomical abnormalities of the calyces.

Mr G underwent extracorporeal shockwave **lithotripsy** (ESWL) and the calculus was successfully fragmented and excreted. His urinary catheter was left in place for one day, and he was discharged on 50 mg diclofenac t.i.d. His recovery was unremarkable and a follow-up KUB was arranged for two weeks through the Lithotripsy reception.

Mr G was advised that he should increase his fluid intake particularly when he returned to the Middle East. It was recommended that a urine output of 2–2.5 litres per day would be appropriate. Urine analysis indicated a slight **hypercalciuria,** and it was recommended that he restricted his intake of calcium and vitamin D. He was referred to the dietician for advice on food intake.

WORD HELP

analgesia condition of pain relief

calculus a stone/abnormal concretion

calyces cup-shaped divisions of the renal pelvis (sing. calyx)

catheter a tube for introducing or withdrawing fluid from the body

GP general practitioner (family doctor)

WORD HELP (Contd.)

hydronephrotic pertaining to hydronephrosis (a kidney swollen with water)

iliac fossa pertaining to the concave, upper and anterior part of the sacropelvic surface of the iliac bone. A fossa is a depression/recess below the general surface of a part

i.m. intramuscular (here meaning an injection into muscle)

KUB kidneys, ureters and bladder (X-ray/examination)

pelviureteric pertaining to a ureter and renal pelvis

radiograph an X-ray picture

t.i.d. three times daily (ter in die)

urography technique of recording/making an X-ray of the urinary tract

urology study of the urinary tract/system (here refers to a hospital department)

Now write the meaning of the following words from the case history without using your dictionary lists:

(a) urolithiasis _____

(b) urethral _____

(c) dysuria _____

(d) haematuria (Am. hematuria) _____

(e) uropathy _____

(f) pyelography _____

(g) lithotripsy _____

(h) hypercalciuria _____

(Answers to the case history exercise are given in the Answers to Word Exercises beginning on page 275.)

Quick Reference

Combining forms relating to the urinary system:

Albumin/o	albumin/albumen
Azot/o	urea/nitrogen
Cyst/o	bladder
Glomerul/o	glomerulus
Lith/o	stone
Nephr/o	kidney
Pyel/o	pelvis of kidney
Ren/o	kidney
Trigon/o	trigone

Quick Reference (Contd.)

Combining forms relating to the urinary system:

Ureter/o	ureter
Urethr/o	urethra
Urin/o	urine
Ur/o	urine/urinary tract
Vesic/o	bladder

Abbreviations

Some common abbreviations related to the urinary system are listed below. Note, some are not standard and their meaning may vary from one health care setting to another. There is a more extensive list for reference on page 307.

ARF	acute renal failure
BUN	blood urea nitrogen
CRF	chronic renal failure
CSU	catheter specimen of urine
Cysto	cystoscopy
HD	haemodialysis (Am. hemodialysis)
IVP	intravenous pyelogram
KUB	kidney, ureter, bladder
MSU	midstream urine
PCNL	percutaneous nephrolithotomy
U & E	urea and electrolytes
UTI	urinary tract infection

> **NOW TRY THE WORD CHECK** <

WORD CHECK

This self-check exercise lists all the word components used in this unit. First write down the meaning of as many word components as you can. Then check your answers using the Exercise Guide and Quick Reference box or the Glossary of Word Components (pp. 319–341).

Prefixes

ante-   *before*

dia-   *through*

dys-	*difficult/painful*
hyper-	*above*
intra-	*inside/into*
oligo-	*deficiency*
poly-	*much/many*
retro-	*backwards*

Combining forms of word roots

albumin/o	*albumin*
azot/o	*urea/nitrogen*
calc/i	*calcium*
col/o	*colon*
cyst/o	*bladder*
enter/o	*intestine*
gastr/o	*stomach*
glomerul/o	*glomerulus*
haem/o (Am. hem/o)	*blood*
hydr/o	*water*
lith/o	*stones*
nephr/o	*kidney*
proct/o	*anus/rectum*
pyel/o	*renal pelvis*
py/o	*pus*
ren/o	*kidney*
sigmoid/o	*sigmoid colon*
sten/o	*narrowing*
trigon/o	*trigone*
ureter/o	*ureter*
urethr/o	*urethra*

urin/o	urine
ur/o	urine/urinary tract
ven/o	vein
vesic/o	bladder

Suffixes

-al	pertaining to
-algia	condition of pain
-cele	hernia/swelling
-clysis	injection/infusion
-dynia	condition of pain
-ectasis	dilation/stretching
-ectomy	removal of
-ferous	pertaining to carrying
-genesis	formation
-gram	x-ray/recording
-graphy	technique of making x-ray
-iasis	abnormal condition of
-ic	pertaining to
-itis	inflammation of
-lapaxy	wash out/evacuate
-lithiasis	ab. cond. of stones
-logist	specialist who studies
-lysis	breakdown/disintegration
-meter	measuring instrument
-metry	technique of measuring
-osis	ab. cond. of
-ous	pertaining to
-pexy	surgical fixation
-phyma	tumour/boil

-plasty	surg. repair of
-ptosis	downward displacement of
-rrhage	excessive flow
-rrhaphy	suturing
-sclerosis	ab. cond. of hardening
-scope	viewing instrument
-scopy	technique of viewing
-stomy	formation of opening into
-thermy	heat
-tome	cutting instrument
-tomy	incision into
-tripsy	technique of crushing using shock waves
-triptor	instrument to crush
-trite	instrument to crush
-uresis	to urinate/excrete in urine

> ## NOW TRY THE SELF-ASSESSMENT <

SELF-ASSESSMENT

Test 7A

Below are some combining forms that refer to the anatomy of the urinary system. Indicate which part of the system they refer to by putting a number from the diagram (Fig. 36) next to each word.

(a)	ureter/o	4
(b)	nephr/o	2
(c)	glomerul/o	1
(d)	pyel/o	3
(e)	urethr/o	7

(f) lith/o   _6_

(g) cyst/o   _5_

(h) urin/o   _8_

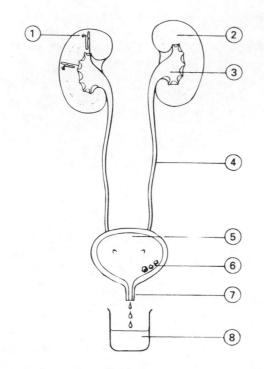

Figure 36   The urinary system

Score

8
8

Test 7B

Prefixes and suffixes

Match each prefix or suffix in Column A with a meaning in Column C by inserting the appropriate number in Column B.

Column A	Column B	Column C
(a) ante-	_9_	1. technique of breaking stones with shock waves
(b) -cele	_7_	2. measuring instrument

Column A	Column B	Column C
(c) -clysis	_15_	3. crushing instrument
(d) dia-	_16_	4. abnormal condition of urine
(e) dys-	_14_	5. technique of measuring
(f) -ferous	_11_	6. backward
(g) -iasis	_12_	7. protrusion/ swelling/ hernia
(h) intra-	_17_	8. tumour/boil
(i) -lapaxy	_18_	9. before
(j) -meter	_2_	10. to fall/ displace
(k) -metry	_5_	11. pertaining to carrying
(l) oligo-	_13_	12. abnormal condition of
(m) -phyma	_8_	13. too little/few
(n) poly-	_19_	14. difficult/ painful
(o) -ptosis	_10_	15. infusion/ injection into
(p) retro-	_6_	16. through
(q) -thermy	_20_	17. within/inside
(r) -tripsy	_1_	18. evacuation/ wash out
(s) -trite	_3_	19. many
(t) -uresis	_4_	20. heat

Score

20
20

Test 7C

Combining forms of word roots

Match each combining form in Column A with a meaning in Column C by inserting the appropriate number in Column B.

Column A	Column B	Column C
(a) col/o	17	1. blood
(b) cyst/o	8/9	2. kidney (i)
(c) gastr/o	11	3. kidney (ii)
(d) glomerul/o	15	4. sigmoid colon
(e) haemat/o (Am. hemat/o)	1	5. pus
(f) lith/o	19	6. trigone/base of bladder
(g) nephr/o	2/3	7. urethra
(h) proct/o	18	8. bladder (i)
(i) pyel/o	12	9. bladder (ii)
(j) py/o	5	10. vein
(k) ren/o	3/2	11. stomach
(l) sigmoid/o	4	12. pelvis/trough
(m) sten/o	20	13. urine
(n) trigon/o	6	14. urine/urinary tract
(o) ureter/o	16	15. glomeruli (of kidney)
(p) urethr/o	7	16. ureter
(q) urin/o	13	17. colon
(r) ur/o	14	18. anus/rectum
(s) ven/o	10	19. stone
(t) vesic/o	9/8	20. narrowing

Score

20
20

Test 7D

Write the meaning of:

(a) nephropyelolithotomy — incision to remove stones from renal pelvis + kidney

(b) ureterostenosis — abs. cond. of narrowing of the ureter.

(c) cystourethrography — tech. of x-ray the urethra + bladder.

(d) vesicocele — herniation of the bladder.

(e) pyelectasis — dilation of the renal pelvis.

Score

5
5

Test 7E

Build words that mean:

(a) dilatation of a ureter — ureterectasis

(b) formation of an opening between the ureter and sigmoid colon — sigmoidoureterostomy

(c) technique of making an X-ray of the bladder (use cyst/o) — cystography

(d) X-ray picture of the urinary tract — urogram

(e) abnormal condition of hardening of the kidney — nephrosclerosis

Score

5
5

Check answers to Self-Assessment Tests on page 299.

8 The nervous system

Objectives

Once you have completed Unit 8 you should be able to:

- understand the meaning of medical words relating to the nervous system

- build medical words relating to the nervous system

- associate medical terms with their anatomical position

- understand medical abbreviations relating to the nervous system.

Exercise Guide

Use this list of word components and their meanings to complete the word exercises in this unit.

Prefixes

a-	without/not
acro-	extremities/point
agora-	open place
an-	without/not
di-	two/double
dys-	difficult/disordered
epi-	above/upon/on
hemi-	half
hyper-	above
hypo-	below
intra-	within/inside
macro-	large
meso-	middle
micro-	small
para-	beside/near
polio-	grey matter (of CNS)
poly-	many
post-	after/behind
pre-	before/in front of
quadri-	four
sub-	under
tetra-	four

Roots/Combining forms

aqua-	water
cancer/o	cancer
ech/o	echo/reflected sound
electr/o-	electrical
fibr/o	fibre
haemat/o	blood
hemat/o (Am.)	blood
hydro-	water
necr/o	death (dead tissue)
py/o	pus
somat/o	body
syring/o	pipe/tube/cavity

Suffixes

-al	pertaining to
-algia	condition of pain
-cele	swelling/protrusion/hernia
-centesis	surgical puncture to remove fluid
-cyte	cell
-ectomy	removal of
-form	having the form of
-genic	pertaining to formation/originating in
-gram	X-ray picture/tracing/recording
-graph	usually an instrument that records
-graphy	technique of recording/making an X-ray
-gyric	pertaining to circular motion
-ia	condition of
-iatr(y)	doctor/medical treatment
-ic	pertaining to/in pharmacology a drug
-itis	inflammation of
-logist	specialist who studies ...
-logy	study of
-malacia	condition of softening
-meter	measuring instrument
-metry	process of measuring
-oma	tumour/swelling
-osis	abnormal condition/disease of
-ous	pertaining to
-pathy	disease of
-phthisis	wasting away
-plasia	condition of growth/formation (of cells)
-rrhagia	condition of bursting forth of blood/bleeding
-schisis	cleaving/splitting/parting
-sclerosis	abnormal condition of hardening
-scopy	visual examination
-stomy	to form a new opening or outlet
-therapy	treatment
-tic	pertaining to
-tomy	incision into
-trauma	injury/wound
-trophy	nourishment/development
-tropic	pertaining to affinity for/stimulating/changing in response to a stimulus
-us	thing/structure

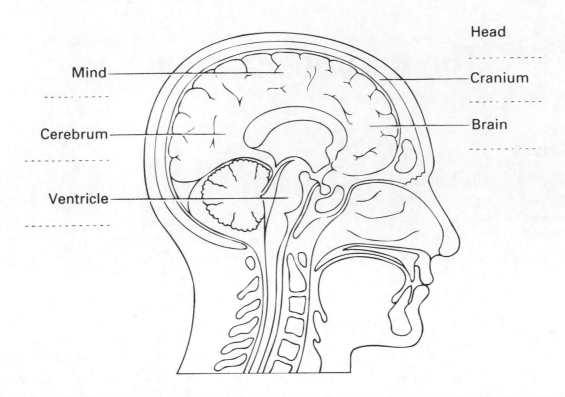

Mind

Cerebrum

Ventricle

Head

Cranium

Brain

| Figure 37 | Sagittal section through the head |

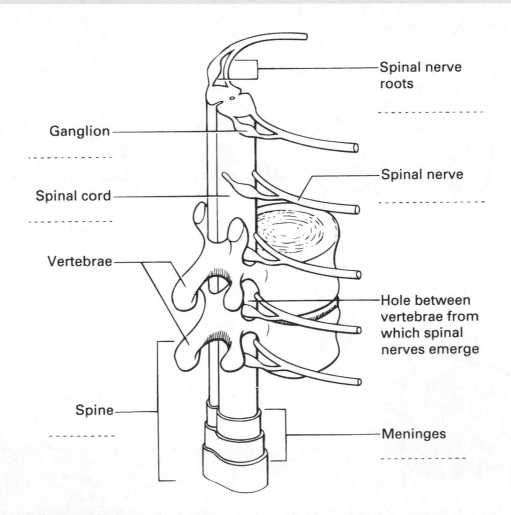

Spinal nerve roots

Ganglion

Spinal nerve

Spinal cord

Vertebrae

Hole between vertebrae from which spinal nerves emerge

Spine

Meninges

| Figure 38 | Section through the spine |

ANATOMY EXERCISE

When you have finished Word Exercises 1–21, look at the word components listed below. Complete Figures 37 and 38 by writing the appropriate combining form on each dotted line – more than one component may relate to the same position. (You can check their meanings in the Quick Reference box on p. 101.)

Cephal/o	Gangli/o	Psych/o
Cerebr/o	Mening/i/o	Rachi/o
Crani/o	Myel/o	Radicul/o
Encephal/o	Neur/o	Ventricul/o

The nervous system

Humans have a complex nervous system with a brain that is large in proportion to their body size. The brain and spinal cord are estimated to contain at least 10^{10} cells with vast numbers of connections between them. The nervous system performs three basic functions:

- It receives, stores and analyses information from sense organs such as the eyes and ears, making us aware of our environment. This awareness enables us to think and make responses that will aid our survival in changing conditions.

- It controls the physiological activities of the body systems and maintains constant conditions (homeostasis) within the body.

- It controls our muscles, enabling us to move and speak.

Because of its complexity, the nervous system has been difficult to study and progress in understanding its common disorders has been slow. However, recently developed imaging techniques are improving the diagnosis and treatment of nervous disorders.

The structure of the nervous system

For convenience of study medical physiologists have divided the system into the:

Central nervous system (CNS)
The CNS consists of the brain and spinal cord.

Peripheral nervous system (PNS)
The PNS is composed of 12 pairs of cranial nerves and 31 pairs of spinal nerves that connect the CNS with sense organs, muscles and glands.

Autonomic nervous system (ANS)
The ANS describes certain peripheral nerves that send impulses to internal organs and glands.

We begin our study of medical terms by examining the cells that form the system.

Root   **Neur**
*(From a Greek word **neuron**, meaning nerve.)*

Combining forms   **Neur/o**

Neurons are the basic structural units of the nervous system. They are specialized cells, elongated for the transmission of nerve impulses. Each neuron consists of a cell 'body' plus long extensions known as dendrons or dendrites and axons (Fig. 39).

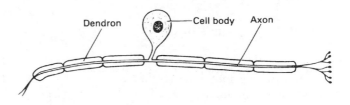

Dendron — Cell body — Axon

Figure 39   Neuron (sensory)

There are three basic types of neuron:

The sensory neuron
The sensory neuron transfers nerve impulses from sense organs to the central nervous system (CNS) (*sensory* – meaning pertaining to sensation).

The motor neuron
The motor neuron transmits nerve impulses away from the central nervous system to muscle cells or glands (*motor* – meaning pertaining to action).

The connector neurons (interneurons)
The connector neuron joins sensory neurons to motor neurons in the brain and spinal cord.

Note. As sensory neurons are transferring nerve impulses towards the CNS they are sometimes referred to as **afferent** neurons (from Latin *affere* – to bring). Motor neurons are sometimes referred to as **efferent** neurons because they carry nerve impules away from the CNS (from Latin *effere* – to carry away).

Use the Exercise Guide at the beginning of this unit to complete Word Exercises 1–21 unless you are asked to work without it.

WORD EXERCISE 1

Using your Exercise Guide, find the meaning of:

(a) **neuro**/logy   _____

(b) **neuro**/pathy   _____

(c) **neur**/algia   _____

(d) **neuro**/fibr/oma   _____

(e) poly/**neur**/itis   _____

(f) **neuro**/genic   _____

Using your Exercise Guide, build words that mean:

(g) hardening of a nerve   _____

(h) condition of softening of a nerve   _____

(i) person who specializes in the study of nerves and their disorders   _____

Using your Exercise Guide, find the meaning of:

(j) **neuro**/phthisis   _____

(k) **neuro**/tropic   _____

(l) **neuro**/trauma   _____

The neurons of the central nervous system are supported by another type of cell that sticks to them. These are known as **neuroglia** (glia is from a Greek word *glia*, meaning glue). **Neurogli/o** refers to a neurogliocyte/ neurogliacyte

Without using your Exercise Guide, write the meaning of:

(m) **neuroglio**/cyte   _____

Root   **Plex**
*(From a Latin word **plexus**, meaning a network of nerves, it is used to mean a nerve plexus.)*

Combining forms   **Plex/o**

WORD EXERCISE 2

Without using your Exercise Guide, write the meaning of:

(a) **plexo**/pathy   _____

(b) **plexo**/genic   _____

Root   **Cephal**
*(From a Greek word **kephale**, meaning head.)*

Combining forms   **Cephal/o**

WORD EXERCISE 3

Using your Exercise Guide, find the meaning of:

(a) **cephalo**/cele   _____

(b) a/**cephal**/ous   _____
(This refers to an abnormal, dead fetus.)

(c) **cephal**/haemat/oma   _____
(Am. cephal/hemat/oma)

(d) hydro/**cephal**/us   _____
(Fig. 40; this is characterized by an excess of cerebro-spinal fluid in the brain and results in enlarged head, compression of the brain and mental retardation if not corrected.)

Using your Exercise Guide, build words that mean:

(e) pertaining to a very small head   _____

(f) X-ray picture of the head   _____

(g) measurement of the head   _____

Using your Exercise Guide, find the meaning of:

(h) macro/**cephal**/us   _____

(i) **cephalo**/gyric   _____

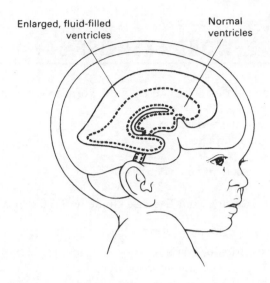

Enlarged, fluid-filled ventricles   Normal ventricles

Figure 40   Hydrocephalus

Root   **Encephal**
(From a Greek word **encephalos***, meaning brain.)*

Combining forms   **Encephal/o -encephalon** is also used to mean the brain

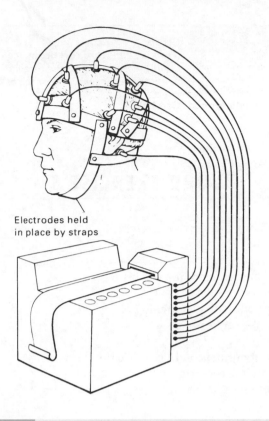

Electrodes held in place by straps

Figure 41   Electroencephalograph

WORD EXERCISE 4

Without using your Exercise Guide, write the meaning of:

(a) **encephal**/oma _____

Using your Exercise Guide, find the meaning of:

(b) **encephalo**/py/osis _____

(c) an/**encephal**/ic _____

(d) electro/**encephalo**/graph _____
    (Fig. 41)

This instrument records the electrical activity of the brain through electrodes placed on the surface of the scalp. The electroencephalogram is traced on to a recording paper and appears as a series of waves. Analysis of the waves can be used to diagnose epilepsy, localize intracranial lesions and confirm brain death.

Using your Exercise Guide, build a word that means:

(e) technique of X-raying/ _____
    recording the brain

Sometimes air or gas is injected into the spaces within the brain after removal of some cerebrospinal fluid. This assists in visualizing the fluid-filled spaces of the brain. A medical term that describes this process can be formed by using **pneumo-** as a prefix with the term you have just built. Remember *pneuma* means air/gas/wind.

Without using your Exercise Guide, build words that mean:

(f) technique of X-raying brain _____
    following injection of gas into
    spaces within brain

(g) technique of making a trace/ _____
    recording of the electrical
    activity of the brain

(h) disease of the brain _____

(i) protrusion or hernia of brain _____

Using your Exercise Guide, find the meaning of:

(j) echo/**encephalo**/gram _____
    (Ultrasonic soundwaves are used.)

(k) mes/**encephalon** _____

(l) polio/**encephal**/itis _____

Root   Cerebr
(From a Latin word **cerebrum,** *meaning brain. Here it refers to the cerebral hemispheres or cerebrum of the brain.)*

Combining forms   **Cerebr/o**

WORD EXERCISE 6

Using your Exercise Guide, build words that mean:

(a) visual examination of the ventricles _____

(b) incision into the ventricles _____

Without using your Exercise Guide, write the meaning of:

(c) **ventriculo**/graphy _____
    (Air, gas or radio-opaque dyes are injected into the ventricles during this procedure.)

Use the Latin root **cisterna**, meaning a closed space serving as a reservoir for fluid, and your Exercise Guide, to write the meaning of the word below. The closed space referred to here is the subarachnoid space outside the brain.

(d) **ventriculo**/cisterno/stomy _____
    (This is an operation for hydrocephalus.)

WORD EXERCISE 5

Without using your Exercise Guide, build words that mean:

(a) hardening of the cerebrum _____

(b) condition of softening of the cerebrum _____

(c) abnormal condition/disease of the cerebrum _____

Cerebrovascular accident

Cerebrovascular means pertaining to the blood vessels of the cerebrum (*vascul/o* meaning vessel, *-ar* meaning pertaining to) rupturing or blocking of these vessels results in a **stroke** or **apoplexy**. A reduction or holding back of blood flow (ischaemia) within the cerebrum causes nerve cells to die because of lack of oxygen and nutrients. As cells in the cerebrum control movements of many parts of the body, paralysis of limbs and loss of speech are common symptoms of strokes. The severity of symptoms depends on the area of brain tissue damaged. Sometimes there is a recovery, and the patient is left with slight paralysis or **paresis**.

Root   Crani
(From Greek **kranion** *and Latin* **cranium,** *meaning skull. The bones of the skull protect the soft brain beneath.)*

Combining forms   **Crani/o**

WORD EXERCISE 7

The cerebral cortex

The outer layer of the cerebrum is known as the cerebral cortex (*cortex* is from Latin, meaning rind/bark). It is extensively folded into fissures, giving it a large surface area. This part of the brain contains motor and sensory areas and is the site of consciousness and intelligence.

Using your Exercise Guide, build words that mean:

(a) incision into the skull _____

(b) the measurement of skulls _____

(c) pertaining to within the cranium _____
    (use *-al*)

Root   Ventricul
(From a Latin word **ventriculum,** *meaning ventricle or chamber. Here it refers to the cavities in the brain filled with cerebrospinal fluid, the cerebral ventricles.)*

Combining forms   **Ventricul/o**

Root   Gangli
(From a Greek word **ganglion,** *meaning swelling. Here it refers to knots of nerve cell bodies located outside the central nervous system known as ganglia.)*

Combining forms   **Gangli/o,** *note that root* **-ganglion-** *is also used*

WORD EXERCISE 8

Without using your Exercise Guide, build a word using **gangli/o** that means:

(a) tumour of a ganglion _____

Using your Exercise Guide, find the meaning of:

(b) pre/**ganglion**/ic _____

(c) post/**ganglion**/ic _____

(d) **ganglion**/ectomy _____

Root	**Mening**
	(From a Greek word **meningos***, meaning membrane. It refers to the meninges, the three membranes that surround the brain and spinal cord.)*

Combining forms   **Mening/i/o**

WORD EXERCISE 9

Without using your Exercise Guide, build words using **mening/o** that mean:

(a) inflammation of the meninges _____

(b) hernia or protrusion of the meninges _____

(c) condition of bursting forth (of blood) from meninges _____

Without using your Exercise Guide, write the meaning of:

(d) **meningo**/encephalo/cele _____

(e) **meningo**/encephal/itis _____

(f) **meningo**/encephalo/pathy _____

(g) **meningi**/oma _____

The outer of the three membranes of the meninges is known as the **dura mater**. The injection of local anaesthetic into the spine above the dura, i.e. into the epidural space, is known as an epidural block. It is often used for a forceps birth or caesarean section delivery (epi- means above or upon).

Using your Exercise Guide, find the meaning of:

(h) epi/**dur**/al _____

(i) sub/**dur**/al haemat/oma _____
    (Fig. 42) (Am. hemat/oma)

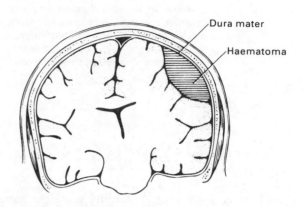

Dura mater

Haematoma

Figure 42   Subdural haematoma (Am. hematoma)

This is a common condition seen by neurologists following head injuries. It requires surgery via the cranium to seal leaking blood vessels and remove the blood clot. Surgery also relieves pressure on the brain tissue preventing further damage.

The two inner meninges, the **pia mater** and the **arachnoid membrane**, are thin. When these are inflamed the condition is known as **leptomeningitis** (from a Greek word *leptos*, meaning thin/slender). When the thick outer dura mater is inflamed it is known as **pachymeningitis** (pachy meaning thick). When meningitis is caused by a bacterium, the coccus *Neisseria meningitidis*, it is referred to as **meningo**coccal **mening**itis.

Root	**Radicul**
	(From a Latin word **radicula***, meaning root. Here we are using it to mean the spinal nerve roots that emerge from the spinal cord.)*

Combining forms   **Radicul/o**

WORD EXERCISE 10

Without using your Exercise Guide, write the meaning of:

(a) **radiculo**/ganglion/itis _____

(b) **radiculo**/neur/itis _____

Another combining form **radic/o** is also derived from this root, e.g.

(c) **radico**/tomy _____

Root **Myel**
(From a Greek word **myelos**, meaning marrow. It is used in reference to marrow within bones and also to spinal marrow, i.e. the soft spinal cord within the spine. Here we use it to mean the spinal cord.)

Combining forms   **Myel/o**

WORD EXERCISE 11

Without using your Exercise Guide, write the meaning of:

(a) **myelo**/mening/itis _____

(b) meningo/**myelo**/cele _____

(c) **myelo**/radicul/itis _____

(d) **myelo**/encephal/itis _____

(e) **myelo**/phthisis _____

(f) polio/**myel**/itis _____

Without using your Exercise Guide, build words that mean:

(g) hardening of the spinal marrow _____

(h) condition of softening of the spinal marrow _____

(i) technique of making an X-ray of the spinal cord _____

Using your Exercise Guide, find the meaning of:

(j) **myelo**/dys/plasia _____

(k) **myel**/a/trophy _____

(l) syringo/**myel**/ia _____

Root **Rachi**
(From a Greek word **rhachis**, meaning spine.)

Combining forms   **Rachi/o**

WORD EXERCISE 12

Using your Exercise Guide, find the meaning of:

(a) **rachio**/meter _____

(b) **rachio**/centesis _____

Rachiocentesis (Fig. 43) is performed to obtain a sample of cerebrospinal fluid (CSF) from the subarachnoid space in the lumbar region of the spinal cord. This procedure is commonly known as a **lumbar puncture** or **spinal tap**.

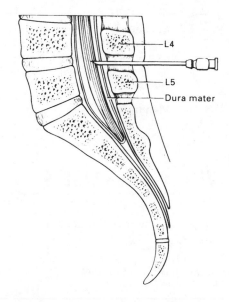

Figure 43 Lumbar puncture

Using your Exercise Guide, find the meaning of:

(c) **rachi**/schisis _____
(synonymous with spina bifida)

Root **Pleg**
(From Greek **plege**, meaning a blow, it is now used to mean a paralysis. Strokes, i.e. cerebrovascular accidents, are often the cause of this condition; these occur when a blockage or haemorrhage in the brain leads to destruction of cells that control motor activities.)

Combining forms   **pleg-** used as the suffix **-plegia**

WORD EXERCISE 13

Using your Exercise Guide, find the meaning of:

(a) quadri/**pleg**/ia _____
    (paralysis of limbs)

(b) hemi/**pleg**/ia _____
    (paralysis of right or
    left side of the body)

(c) para/**pleg**/ia _____
    (paralysis of lower limbs)

(d) di/**pleg**/ia _____
    (paralysis of like parts
    on either side of body)

(e) tetra/**pleg**/ia _____

Root	Aesthesi

*(From Greek **aisthesis**, meaning perception or sensation.)*

Combining forms   **Aesthe/s/i/o, Esthe/s/i/o** *(Am.)*

WORD EXERCISE 14

Without using your Exercise Guide, write the meaning of:

(a) an/**aesthes**/ia _____
    (Am. an/esthes/ia)

(b) an/**aesthe**/tic _____
    (Am. an/esthe/tic)

(c) an/**aesthesio**/logy _____
    (Am. an/esthesio/logy)

(d) an/**aesthesio**/logist _____
    (Am. an/esthesio/logist)

(e) hemi/an/**aesthes**/ia _____
    (Am. hemi/an/esthes/ia;
    refers to one side of the body)

Using your Exercise Guide, find the meaning of:

(f) hypo/**aesthes**/ia _____
    (Am. hypo/esthes/ia)

(g) hyper/**aesthes**/ia _____
    (Am. hyper/esthes/ia)

The term par**aesthes**ia (Am. paresthesia) is used to mean any abnormal sensations, such as 'pins and needles' (from Greek word *para*, meaning near).

Without using your Exercise Guide, build words that mean:

(h) pertaining to following/after _____
    anaesthesia (Am. anesthesia)

(i) pertaining to before anaesthesia _____
    (Am. anesthesia)

Root	Narc

*(From a Greek word **narke**, meaning stupor; it is used in medicine to refer to an abnormally deep sleep induced by a drug (narcotic). This is a different level of consciousness from anaesthesia (Am. anesthesia); patients are not oblivious to pain and can be woken up.)*

Combining forms   **Narc/o**

WORD EXERCISE 15

Without using your Exercise Guide, write the meaning of:

(a) **narc**/osis _____

Using your Exercise Guide, find the meaning of:

(b) **narco**/therapy _____

Root	Alges

*(From a Greek word **algesis**, meaning a sense of pain.)*

Combining forms   **Alges/i/o**

WORD EXERCISE 16

Without using your Exercise Guide, write the meaning of:

(a) **alges**/ia _____

(b) an/**alges**/ia _____

(c) hyper/**alges**/ia _____

(d) an/**alges**/ic _____
    (a drug)

Psychiatry

Disorders that interfere with the normal functioning of the brain may affect behaviour and personality, i.e. the mind. The study of the mind and treatment of its disorders is a specialist branch of medicine known as psychiatry. A psychiatrist is a person with medical qualifications who has specialized in the study and treatment of mental disease. The following terms are used by psychiatrists:

Root	Psych
	(From Greek **psyche**, *meaning soul or mind.)*
Combining forms	**Psych/o**

WORD EXERCISE 17

Without using your Exercise Guide, write the meaning of:

(a) **psycho**/logy _____

Note. A psychologist is not usually medically qualified and cannot treat disorders by means of drugs or surgery. Psychologists study human behaviour: for example, an educational psychologist may study intelligence and behaviour of school children.

(b) **psych**/ic _____

(c) **psycho**/pathy _____

Note. A psychopath is a person with a specific type of personality disorder in which he/she exhibits antisocial behaviour.

(d) **psych**/osis _____

Note. Psychoses originate in the mind itself, in contrast to neuroses which are mental conditions believed to arise because of stresses and anxieties in the patient's environment. Neurotic comes from *neur/o* meaning nerves and *tic*, meaning pertaining to; in psychiatry it means pertaining to a neurosis.

(e) **psycho**/tropic drug _____

Using your Exercise Guide, find the meaning of:

(f) **psycho**/somat/ic _____

(g) **psych**/iatry _____

Root	Phob
	(From a Greek word **phobos**, *meaning fear.)*
Combining forms	**phob-**, used in the suffix **-phobia**

WORD EXERCISE 18

Using your Exercise Guide, find the meaning of:

(a) acro/**phob**/ia _____

(b) agora/**phob**/ia _____

(c) aqua/**phob**/ia _____

(d) cancero/**phob**/ia _____

(e) necro/**phob**/ia _____

Root	Epilept
	(From Greek **epileptikos**, *meaning a seizure. It refers to epilepsy, the disordered electrical activity of the brain that produces a 'fit' and unconsciousness.)*
Combining forms	**Epilept/i/o**

WORD EXERCISE 19

Without using your Exercise Guide, write the meaning of:

(a) **epilepto**/genic

(b) post/**epilept**/ic

Using your Exercise Guide, find the meaning of:

(c) **epilepti**/form

Modern treatments of mental disease involve drug treatments and occasionally surgery. One of the most useful physical methods of treatment that brings about improvement in depressive states, mania and stupor is **electroconvulsive therapy** (ECT). This involves the application of a high voltage to the head via electrodes placed on its surface.

Medical equipment and clinical procedures

Patients with suspected neurological (*neurolog-* meaning neurology, *-ical* meaning pertaining to) disorders are examined by neurologists. Much information about the state of health of the nervous system can be gained from relatively simple testing of reflex actions using a tendon hammer (Fig. 44). One such test you are probably familiar with is the knee jerk reflex where the sensory nerve endings in the patella (knee cap) are tapped with a hammer. In a healthy patient the response will be that muscles in the thigh will contract, causing the leg to jerk upwards. A normal reflex action will indicate that the nerve pathway from the knee through the spinal cord is working normally.

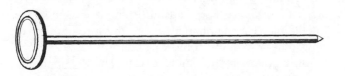

Figure 44	Tendon hammer

More detailed examinations of the nervous system require specialized equipment, described below.

Computerized tomography

This is a technique of making a recording using a **tomograph**, an X-ray machine that produces images of cross-sections through the body.

Positron Emission Tomography (PET)

This is a technique of imaging the distribution of positron emitting radioisotopes administered to the body. Particular isotopes can be taken up by active brain cells making this technique particularly useful for studying brain metabolism. More information about PET is included in Unit 18.

Electroencephalography

This is the technique of making a recording using an **electroencephalograph**, a machine that produces a tracing of the electrical activity of the brain. This procedure is used to aid diagnosis of epilepsy, brain tumours and other disorders of the brain (see Fig. 41).

Magnetic resonance imaging (MRI)

This recently developed technique using nuclear magnetic resonance is particularly useful for imaging the soft tissue of the brain and spinal cord. The patient is placed in an intense magnetic field, hydrogen atoms in the nerve tissue are excited with radio waves and signals from them are detected and computed into a picture. The procedure does not have the risks associated with X-rays.

The stereotaxic instrument

This is a device used in neurosurgery to locate precise positions within the brain by three-dimensional measurement. The stereotaxic instrument is fixed to the skull and is used to guide probes that destroy or stimulate brain tissue in patients with serious neurological or psychological problems.

Revise the names of all instruments and examinations mentioned in this unit, and then try Exercises 20 and 21.

WORD EXERCISE 20

Match each term in Column A with a description from Column C by placing an appropriate number in Column B.

Column A	Column B	Column C
(a) encephalography	5	1. instrument for testing reflexes
(b) pneumoencephalography	4	2. instrument that images serial sections of body using X-rays
(c) ventriculoscopy	6	3. measurement of the cranium
(d) tendon hammer	1	4. technique of making X-ray/recording of the brain after injection of air into ventricles
(e) tomograph	2	5. technique of making X-ray/recording of the brain
(f) craniometry	3	6. technique of viewing ventricles

WORD EXERCISE 21

Match each term in Column A with a description from Column C by placing an appropriate number in Column B.

Column A	Column B	Column C
(a) magnetic resonance imaging	3	1. technique of imaging serial sections of body using X-rays

Column A	Column B	Column C
(b) lumbar puncture	6	2. technique of making a recording of the electrical activity of the brain
(c) myelography	5	3. technique of imaging soft tissues of brain and spinal cord without using X-rays
(d) computed axial tomography	1	4. technique of making an X-ray/recording of brain ventricles
(e) electroence-phalography	2	5. technique of making an X-ray/recording of the spinal cord
(f) ventriculo-graphy	4	6. technique of removing cerebrospinal fluid from spinal cord

ANATOMY EXERCISE

Now complete the Anatomy Exercise on page 91.

CASE HISTORY 8

The object of this exercise is to understand words associated with a patient's medical history.

To complete the exercise:

- read through the passage on cerebrovascular accident; unfamiliar words are underlined and you can find their meaning using the Word Help

- write the meaning of the medical terms shown in bold print.

Cerebrovascular accident (Stroke)

Mr H, a single 56-year-old white male, became ill early in the day of admission whilst eating his breakfast. He had felt dizzy, developed a headache and complained of impaired vision in one eye. These symptoms were later followed by signs of a right-sided **hemiplegia**, **hemiparasthesia** and aphasia. Three weeks prior to his illness he had suffered a TIA in which he developed mild, right **hemisensory loss** in his arm and a sudden, transient hemianopia. His GP suspected a **cerebral** infarction or **intracranial** haemorrhage (Am. hemorrhage) and he was referred to the **neurology** unit for assessment.

On admission in the evening, Mr H's right arm and leg were flaccid and **hyper-reflexic**. A CT scan demonstrated a low density area (an infarct) without a mass effect. There was a loud localized bruit in his neck and digital subtraction angiography (DSA) detected a tight stenosis of the left internal carotid artery. Following diagnosis of a stroke caused by internal carotid artery occlusion; he was given anticoagulant therapy. Two weeks later he underwent a successful internal carotid endarterectomy.

The long term prognosis of Mr H's neurological deficit is uncertain. Three weeks following surgery he showed signs of recovery and had sufficient language to be intelligible. He maintained a rigorous programme of physiotherapy (Am. physical therapy) and speech therapy following initial recovery. The occupational therapist visited his home and advised on the installation of aids that will assist his rehabilitation. Unfortunately, Mr H is severely depressed following his resignation as a structural engineer with a building company.

WORD HELP

aphasia condition of being without speech

bruit abnormal sound upon auscultation (listening to body sounds)

CT computerized tomography, technique of imaging a 'slice' through the body using X-rays

DSA digital subtraction angiography. Technique of making two X-rays, one taken before an injection of dye into a blood vessel. The original computerized image is subtracted from the first, producing a clear image

endarterectomy removal of the inside of a blood vessel to remove a blockage and open its lumen

flaccid relaxed, flabby and soft

GP general practitioner (family doctor)

haemorrhage (Am. hemorrhage) bursting forth of blood from a vessel

hemianopia loss of half the vision in each eye (loosely used to mean half the vision in one eye)

infarction process of forming an infarct, a piece of dead tissue formed by the failure of its blood supply

neurological pertaining to neurology

occlusion state of being closed up

occupational therapist specialist in providing treatment/assistance aimed at helping people with physical and/or mental disability to become independent

physiotherapy (Am. physical therapy) employment of physical measures (massage/exercise etc.) to restore function following injury or disease

rehabilitation re-education that allows a sick or injured person to take his or her place in the world or gain some independence

stenosis abnormal condition of narrowing

TIA transient ischaemic (Am. ischemic) attack (i.e. insufficient blood supply to the brain)

Now write the meaning of the following words from the case history without using your dictionary lists:

(a) cerebrovascular   _____

(b) hemiplegia   _____

(c) hemiparaesthesia   _____
    (Am. hemiparesthesia)

(d) hemisensory loss   _____

(e) cerebral   _____

(f) intracranial   _____

(g) neurology   _____

(h) hyper-reflexic   _____

(Answers to the case history exercise are given in the Answers to Word Exercises beginning on page 275.)

Abbreviations

Some common abbreviations related to the nervous system and psychiatry are listed below. Note, however, some are not standard and their meaning may vary from one health care setting to another. There is a more extensive list for reference on page 307.

CAT	computerized axial tomography
CN	cranial nerve
CSF	cerebrospinal fluid
CVA	cerebrovascular accident
ECT	electroconvulsive therapy
EEG	electroencephalogram
ICP	intracranial pressure
KJ	knee jerk
MRI	magnetic resonance imaging
NCVs	nerve conduction velocities
PR	plantar reflex
SDH	subdural haematoma (Am. hematoma)

Quick Reference

Combining forms relating to the nervous system:

Aesthesi/o	sensation
Alges/i	sense of pain
Cephal/o	head
Cerebr/o	cerebrum/brain
Cistern/o	cistern/subarachnoid space
Crani/o	cranium
Dur/o	dura mater
Encephal/o	brain
Epilept/o	epilepsy
Esthesi/o (Am.)	sensation
Gangli/o	ganglion
Gli/a/o	gluelike/neuroglial cells
Mening/o	meninges
Motor	action/moving/set in motion
Myel/o	marrow/spinal cord
Narc/o	stupor/numbness
Neur/o	nerve
Plex/o	network, e.g. of nerves
Psych/o	mind
Rachi/o	spine
Radicul/o	nerve root
Somat/o	body
Syring/o	tube/cavity
Ventricul/o	ventricle

> **NOW TRY THE WORD CHECK** <

WORD CHECK

This self-check exercise lists all the word components used in this unit. First write down the meaning of as many word components as you can. Then check your answers using the Exercise Guide and Quick Reference box or the Glossary of Word Components (pp. 319–341).

Prefixes

a-   *without*

acro-   *extremities/point*

agora-   *open place*

an-   *without*

di-   *two/double*

dys-   *painful/difficult*

electro- *electrical*

epi-   *above/upon*

hemi-	half
hyper-	above normal
hypo-	below normal
lepto-	
macro-	large
meso-	middle
micro-	small
pachy-	thick
para-	beside
polio-	grey matter (CNS)
poly-	many
post-	after
pre-	before
quadri-	four
sub-	below/under
tetra-	four

Combining forms of word roots

aesthesi/o (Am. esthesi/o)	feeling/sensation
alges/i	sense of pain
aqua-	water
cancer/o	cancer
cephal/o	head
cerebr/o	cerebrum
cistern/o	cistern/subarachnoid space)
crani/o	skull
cyt/o	cell
dur/o	dura mater
ech/o	echo/reflected sound
encephal/o	brain
epilept/o	epilepsy

fibr/o	fibre
gangli/o	ganglion
gli/a/o	glue-like
haemat/o (Am. hemat/o)	blood
hist/o	tissue
hydro-	water
iatr/o	med. tx/ doctor
mening/o	meninges
motor	action/movement
myel/o	spinal cord
narc/o	stupor/numbness
necr/o	death
neur/o	nerve
plex/o	network eg. of nerves
pneum/o	air
psych/o	mind
py/o	pus
rachi/o	spine
radicul/o	nerve root
somat/o	body
syring/o	tube/cavity
ventricul/o	ventricles

Suffixes

-al	pert. to
-algia	cond. of pain
-cele	hernia/swelling
-centesis	surg. puncture to remove fluid
-cyte	cell
-ectomy	removal of
-form	resembles

-genic	pert to forming
-gram	x-ray/recording
-graph	inst to x-ray
-graphy	tech of making x-ray
-gyric	pert to circular motion
-ia	cond of
-ic	pert to
-ical	pert to
-itis	infl of
-logist	spec who studies
-logy	study of
-malacia	cond of softening
-meter	inst to measure
-metry	tech of measuring
-oma	tumour/swelling
-osis	abn cond of
-ous	pert to
-pathy	disease of
-phobia	cond of fear
-phthisis	wasting away
-plasia	cond of growth
-plegia	cond of paralysis
-rrhagia	cond of bursting forth
-schisis	cleaving/splitting
-sclerosis	abn cond of hardening
-scopy	tech of viewing
-stomy	formation of an opening
-therapy	tx
-tomy	incision into
-tic	pert to
-trauma	injury/wound

-trophy	nourishment/development
-tropic	pert to stimulating
-us	thing/structure

▷ NOW TRY THE SELF-ASSESSMENT ◁

SELF-ASSESSMENT

Test 8A

Below are some combining forms that refer to the anatomy of the nervous system. Indicate which part of the system they refer to by putting a number from the diagrams (Figs 45 and 46) next to each word.

(a) crani/o

(b) encephal/o

(c) meningi/o

(d) neur/o

(e) rachi/o

(f) gangli/o

(g) ventricul/o

(h) radicul/o

(i) cephal/o

(j) myel/o

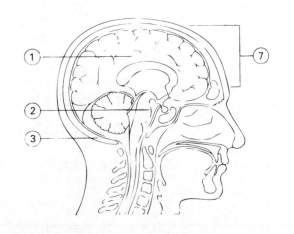

Figure 45   Sagittal section through the head

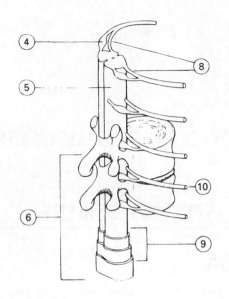

Column A	Column B	Column C
(l) meso-	_____	12. grey matter
(m) micro-	_____	13. half
(n) pachy-	_____	14. thin/slender
(o) para-	_____	15. open space
(p) polio-	_____	16. upon/above
(q) post-	_____	17. small
(r) pre-	_____	18. two/double
(s) quadri-	_____	19. point/extremity
(t) tetra-	_____	20. beside/near

Score

20

Figure 46 Section through the spine

Score

10

Test 8B

Prefixes

Match each prefix in Column A with a meaning in Column C by inserting the appropriate number in Column B.

Column A	Column B	Column C
(a) a-	_____	1. after/behind
(b) acro-	_____	2. middle
(c) agora-	_____	3. water (i)
(d) an-	_____	4. water (ii)
(e) aqua-	_____	5. thick
(f) di-	_____	6. large
(g) epi-	_____	7. without/not (i)
(h) hemi-	_____	8. without/not (ii)
(i) hydro-	_____	9. four (i)
(j) lepto-	_____	10. four (ii)
(k) macro-	_____	11. before/in front of

Test 8C

Combining forms of word roots

Match each combining form in Column A with a meaning in Column C by inserting the appropriate number in Column B.

Column A	Column B	Column C
(a) aesthesi/o (Am. esthesi/o)	_____	1. spine
(b) cephal/o	_____	2. mind
(c) cistern/o	_____	3. gas/wind/air
(d) crani/o	_____	4. stupor/deep sleep
(e) dur/o	_____	5. body
(f) encephal/o	_____	6. membranes of CNS
(g) epilept/o	_____	7. ganglion
(h) gangli/o	_____	8. cranium/skull
(i) gli/a/o	_____	9. ventricles of brain
(j) mening/o	_____	10. head

Column A	Column B	Column C
(k) motor	_____	11. dura mater
(l) myel/o	_____	12. fit/seizure/epilepsy
(m) narc/o	_____	13. cistern/reservoir/ subarachnoid space
(n) neur/o	_____	14. root (of spinal nerve)
(o) pneum/o	_____	15. nerve
(p) psych/o	_____	16. marrow (of spine)
(q) rachi/o	_____	17. pertaining to action
(r) radicul/o	_____	18. glue (cell)
(s) somat/o	_____	19. brain
(t) ventricul/o	_____	20. sensation

Score

20

Test 8D

Suffixes

Match each suffix in Column A with a meaning in Column C by inserting the appropriate number in Column B.

Column A	Column B	Column C
(a) -centesis	_____	1. condition of paralysis
(b) -form	_____	2. abnormal condition/ disease of
(c) -genic	_____	3. technique of recording/making an X-ray
(d) -gram	_____	4. pertaining to the body
(e) -graphy	_____	5. pertaining to affinity for/ stimulating

Column A	Column B	Column C
(f) -gyric	_____	6. formation of an opening into ...
(g) -malacia	_____	7. having form of
(h) -osis	_____	8. condition of increase in cell formation/number of cells
(i) -phobia	_____	9. nourishment
(j) -phthisis	_____	10. hardening
(k) -plasia	_____	11. wasting away/decay
(l) -plegia	_____	12. condition of softening
(m) -schisis	_____	13. recording/ tracing/X-ray
(n) -sclerosis	_____	14. puncture
(o) -somatic	_____	15. treatment
(p) -stomy	_____	16. splitting
(q) -therapy	_____	17. condition of fear
(r) -trauma	_____	18. pertaining to movement around a centre
(s) -trophy	_____	19. formation/ originating in
(t) -tropic	_____	20. injury/shock

Score

20

Test 8E

Write the meaning of:

(a) neuromyelitis _____

(b) rachiotomy _____

(c) meningomalacia _____

(d) encephalomyelopathy _____

(e) ventriculoscope _____

Score

5

Test 8F

Build words that mean:

(a) disease of the meninges _____

(b) instrument for measuring the head _____

(c) inflammation of the spinal cord and spinal nerve roots _____

(d) condition of bursting forth (of blood) from the brain _____

(e) study of cells of the nervous system _____

Score

5

Check answers to Self-Assessment Tests on page 299.

9 The eye

Objectives

Once you have completed Unit 9 you should be able to:

- understand the meaning of medical words relating to the eye

- build medical words relating to the eye

- associate medical terms with their anatomical position

- understand medical abbreviations relating to the eye.

Exercise Guide

Use this list of word components and their meanings to complete the word exercises in this unit.

Prefixes

a-	without
ambly-	dull/dim
an-	without
aniso-	unequal
bin-	two each/double
dia-	through
diplo-	double
dys-	difficult/painful
en-	in/within
ex-	out/out of/away from
hemi-	half
iso-	same/equal
mono-	one
pan-	all
presby-	old man/old age
uni-	one
xero-	dry

Roots/Combining forms

aden/o	gland
aesthesi/o	sensation
blast/o	immature germ cell/cell that forms ...
blenn/o	mucus
chromat/o	colour
cyst/o	bladder
electr/o	electrical
esthesi/o (Am.)	sensation
helc/o	ulcer
lith/o	stone
motor	action
my/o	muscle

myc/o	fungus
nas/o	nose
neur/o	nerve
py/o	pus
rhin/o	nose
ton/o	tone/tension

Suffixes

-agogic	pertaining to inducing/stimulating
-al	pertaining to
-algia	condition of pain
-ar	pertaining to
-cele	swelling/protrusion/hernia
-centesis	puncture
-chalasis	slackening/loosening
-conus	cone-like protrusion
-dialysis	separating
-ectasis	dilatation/stretching
-ectomy	removal of
-edema (Am.)	swelling due to fluid
-erysis	drag/draw/suck out
-gram	X-ray/tracing/recording
-graph	usually an instrument that records
-graphy	technique of recording/making an X-ray
-gyric	pertaining to circular motion
-ia	condition of
-itis	inflammation of
-kinesis	movement
-logist	specialist who studies ...
-malacia	condition of softening
-meter	measuring instrument
-metrist	specialist who measures
-metry	process of measuring
-mileusis	to carve
-nyxis	perforation/pricking/puncture
-oedema	swelling due to fluid
-oma	tumour/swelling
-osis	abnormal condition/disease/abnormal increase
-pathy	disease of
-pexy	fixation (by surgery)
-plasty	surgical repair/reconstruction
-plegia	condition of paralysis
-ptosis	falling/displacement/prolapse
-rrhaphy	suture/stitch/suturing
-rrhea (Am.)	excessive flow
-rrhoea	excessive flow
-schisis	cleavage/splitting/parting
-sclerosis	abnormal condition of hardening
-scope	viewing instrument
-scopy	visual examination
-spasm	involuntary muscle contraction
-stenosis	abnormal condition of narrowing
-stomy	formation of an opening into ...
-synechia	condition of adhering together
-thermy	heat
-tome	cutting instrument
-tomy	incision into

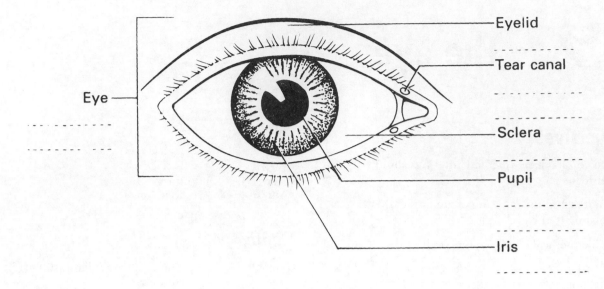

Figure 47 The eye

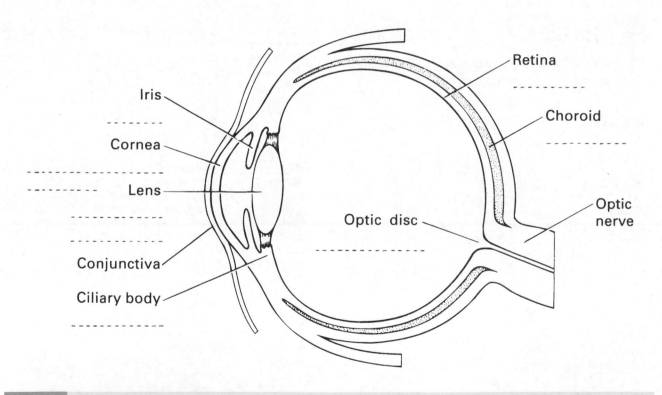

Figure 48 Section through the eye

ANATOMY EXERCISE

When you have finished Word Exercises 1–21, look at the word components listed below. Complete Figure 47 and 48 by writing the appropriate combining form on each dotted line – more than one component may relate to the same position. (You can check their meanings in the Quick Reference box on p. 117.)

Blephar/o	Ir/o	Papill/o
Choroid/o	Lacrim/o	Pupill/o
Corne/o	Irid/o	Phac/o
Cor/e/o	Kerat/o	Phak/o
Cycl/o	Ocul/o	Retin/o
Dacry/o	Ophthalm/o	Scler/o

The eye

The eyes are our main sense organs. Light enters the eye through the pupil and transparent cornea, it passes through the lens and is focused on to the light-sensitive retina. In the retina light stimulates receptors (rods and cones) to generate nerve impulses in sensory neurons; these impulses travel via neurons in the optic nerve to areas of the brain concerned with vision. In the visual cortex of the brain the impulses are interpreted as an image.

Use the Exercise Guide at the beginning of this unit to complete Word Exercises 1–21 unless you are asked to work without it.

Root — **Ophthalm**
*(From a Greek word **ophthalmos**, meaning eye.)*

Combining forms **Ophthalm/o**
(Be careful with spelling ophth.)

WORD EXERCISE 1

Using your Exercise Guide, build words that mean:

(a) an instrument to view the eye

(b) a medically qualified person who specializes in the study of the eye and its disorders

(c) condition of paralysis of the eye

(d) inflammation of the eye (synonymous with ophthalmia)

(e) abnormal condition of fungal infection of the eye

Using your Exercise Guide, find the meaning of:

(f) **ophthalm**/algia

(g) **ophthalmo**/gyric

(h) **ophthalmo**/neur/itis

(i) pan/**ophthalm**/itis

(j) **ophthalmo**/tono/meter
(This instrument is used to detect raised pressure within the eye and is used in the diagnosis of glaucoma. Sometimes **tonometer** is used alone and **tonography** is used to mean the technique of using a tonometer.)

(k) blenn/**ophthalm**/ia

(l) xer/**ophthalm**/ia

(m) en/**ophthalmos**

(n) ex/**ophthalmos**

Root — **Ocul**
*(From Latin **ocularis**, meaning of the eye.)*

Combining forms **Ocul/o**

WORD EXERCISE 2

Using your Exercise Guide, find the meaning of:

(a) mon/**ocul**/ar

(b) uni/**ocul**/ar _____

(c) bin/**ocul**/ar _____

(d) **oculo**/motor nerve _____

(e) **oculo**/nas/al _____

(f) electro/-**oculo**/gram _____
(This is produced from an electrodiagnostic test; it
also records eye position and movement.)

Without using your Exercise Guide, write the meaning
of:

(g) **oculo**/gyric _____

Root | **Opt**
*(From **optikos**, a Greek word meaning
sight. The words optical and optician are
derived from this root. Optical means
pertaining to sight; optician refers to a
person who prescribes spectacles to
correct defects in sight.)*

Combining forms **Opt/o**

WORD EXERCISE 3

Without using your Exercise Guide, write the meaning
of:

(a) **opto**/meter _____

Using your Exercise Guide, find the meaning of:

(b) **opto**/metry _____

(c) **opto**/metrist _____

(d) **opto**/myo/meter _____

(e) **opto**/aesthes/ia _____
(Am. opto/esthes/ia)

Orthoptics means pertaining to the study and treatment of muscle imbalances of the eye (squints). *Ortho*
means straight, therefore orthoptics refers to making
eyes and sight straight.

The combining form **optic/o** is also derived from
the same root as **opt/o**. It also means pertaining to sight
but it is sometimes used to mean optic nerve, e.g.
optico-pupillary – pertaining to the pupil and optic
nerve.

Root | **Op**
*(From Greek **ops**, also meaning eye. It
is usually used as the suffix -opsia to
mean a condition of defective vision.
Many focusing defects can be
corrected by prescribing appropriate
spectacles.)*

Combining forms **Op-**, *used in the suffixes* **-opia** *and* **-opsia**

WORD EXERCISE 4

Using your Exercise Guide, find the meaning of:

(a) dipl/**op**/ia _____

(b) presby/**op**/ia _____
(refers to a condition in which the lens loses
its elasticity; near point approximately 1 m)

(c) ambly/**op**/ia _____

(d) hemi/a/chromat/**ops**/ia _____

Three other common words that use -opia are difficult to understand from their word components. These
are:

Hypermetropia
Describes long-sightedness in which light rays are
focused beyond the retina (*hyper* – beyond/above).
The light rays when measured focus beyond the retina
(*metr* – measure).

Myopia
Short-sightedness. *My* comes from *myein*, meaning to
close. Presumably the eye tends to close when trying
to view a distant object.

Emmetropia
Light falls directly on to the retina in its correct
position, with no errors. This word refers to
normal/ideal vision (*em* meaning in, *metr* meaning
measure).

(e) dys/**op**/ia _____

(f) hemi/an/**op**/ia _____

Root | **Blephar**
*(From a Greek word **blepharon**, meaning
eyelid, sometimes used for eyelash.)*

Combining forms **Blephar/o**

WORD EXERCISE 5

Without using your Exercise Guide, build a word that means:

(a) condition of paralysis of the eyelid   _____

Using your Exercise Guide, build words that mean:

(b) spasm of the eyelid   _____

(c) falling/displacement of the eyelid   _____

(d) suturing of an eyelid   _____

Using your Exercise Guide, find the meaning of:

(e) **blepharo**/pyo/rrhoea (Am. blepharo/pyo/rrhea)   _____

(f) **blepharo**/aden/itis (refers to meibomian glands lying in grooves on inner surface of eyelids)   _____

(g) **blepharo**/synechia   _____

(h) **blepharo**/chalasis   _____

Root   Scler
(From Greek **skleros**, *meaning hard. Here it is used to mean the sclera, the tough, outer white part of the eye. The sclera is continuous with the transparent cornea at the front of the eye.)*

Combining forms   **Scler/o**

WORD EXERCISE 6

Using your Exercise Guide, find the meaning of:

(a) **sclero**/tomy   _____

(b) **scler**/ectasis   _____

(c) **sclero**/tome   _____

Root   Kerat
(From a Greek word **keras**, *meaning horn, here it is used to mean the cornea. The cornea, located at the front of the eye, provides strength, refractive power and transmits light into the eye.)*

Combining forms   **Kerat/o**

WORD EXERCISE 7

Without using your Exercise Guide, write the meaning of:

(a) sclero/**kerat**/itis   _____

(b) **kerato**/metry   _____

(c) **kerato**/tome   _____

Using your Exercise Guide, find the meaning of:

(d) **kerato**/plasty   _____

(e) **kerato**/centesis   _____

(f) **kerato**/helc/osis   _____

(g) **kerato**/nyxis   _____

(h) **kerato**/mileusis (actually an operation for correction of myopia or short-sightedness)   _____

(i) **kerato**/conus (See Fig. 49)   _____

The word cornea comes from the Latin word *corneus*, also meaning horny. Corneoplasty is synonymous with keratoplasty, an operation performed to replace a diseased or damaged cornea with a corneal graft.

Abnormal curvatures of the cornea cause light rays to focus on the retina unevenly. This is known as **astigmatism**.

The sclera and cornea are covered at the front of the eye with a delicate, transparent membrane that also lines the inner surface of the eyelids. This membrane is the **conjunctiva**; it is prone to irritation and infection, giving rise to **conjunctivitis**.

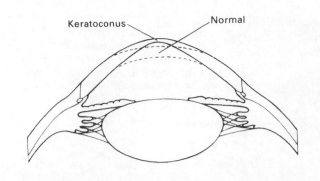

Figure 49   Keratoconus

 Root   **Ir**
*(From a Greek word **iris**, meaning rainbow. It refers to the iris, the circular, coloured membrane surrounding the pupil of the eye. Contraction of its muscle fibres regulates the size of the aperture (pupil) within the iris, thereby regulating the amount of light entering the eye.)*

Combining forms   **Ir/o, irid/o**

WORD EXERCISE 8

Without using your Exercise Guide, build words using irid/o that mean:

(a) falling/displacement of the iris   _____

(b) inflammation of the cornea and iris (use kerat/o)   _____

Using your Exercise Guide, find the meaning of:

(c) **irido**/kinesis   _____

(d) **irido**/dialysis   _____

(e) **irido**/cele   _____

Without using your Exercise Guide, write the meaning of:

(f) sclero/**irido**/dialysis   _____

(g) sclero/**irido**/tomy   _____

(h) kerato/**ir**/itis   _____

Root   **Cycl**
*(From a Greek word **kyklos**, meaning circle. Here it is used to mean the circular ciliary body of the eye.)*

Combining forms   **Cycl/o**

The ciliary body, a structure composed of muscles and processes, lies behind the iris (see Fig. 48). It connects the circumference of the iris to the choroid (the middle layer of the eyeball), changes the shape of the lens and secretes a watery fluid, aqueous humor, into the anterior chamber. Study Figure 50 which shows the anterior cavity in front of the lens and the posterior cavity behind the lens. The anterior cavity is sub-divided into the anterior chamber in front of both lens and iris and the posterior chamber between the lens and iris. The ciliary body continuously secretes aqueous humor into the anterior chamber. The fluid is drained into veins in the sclera at the same rate that it is produced. A raised intraocular pressure due to the accumulation of excess aqueous humor may result in **glaucoma,** a common eye disorder that causes pain and damage. The posterior cavity is filled with vitreous humor, a soft jelly-like material which maintains the spherical shape of the eyeball.

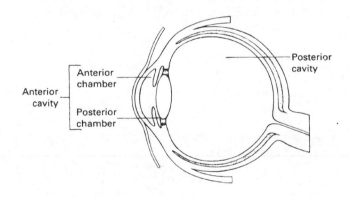

Figure 50   Section through the eye

WORD EXERCISE 9

Without using your Exercise Guide, write the meaning of:

(a) irido/**cycl**/itis   _____

(b) **cyclo**/plegia   _____

Using your Exercise Guide, find the meaning of:

(c) **cyclo**/dia/thermy

Root

Goni
*(From a Greek word **gonia**, meaning angle. Here it means the peripheral angle of the anterior chamber. This angle is observed when evaluating types of glaucoma.)*

Combining forms   **Goni/o**

WORD EXERCISE 10

Without using your Exercise Guide, build words that mean:

(a) instrument to measure the angle of the anterior chamber

(b) instrument to view the angle of the anterior chamber

(c) operation to make an incision into the angle of the anterior chamber (for glaucoma)

Root

Pupill
*(From a Latin word **pupilla**, meaning the pupil or aperture of the eye.)*

Combining forms   **Pupill/o**

WORD EXERCISE 11

Without using your Exercise Guide, write the meaning of:

(a) **pupillo**/plegia _____

(b) **pupillo**/metry _____

Root

Cor
*(From a Greek word **kore**, meaning pupil of the eye.)*

Combining forms   **Cor/e/o**

WORD EXERCISE 12

Using your Exercise Guide, find the meaning of:

(a) iso/**cor**/ia _____

(b) an/iso/**cor**/ia _____

(c) **coreo**/pexy _____

Without using your Exercise Guide, write the meaning of:

(d) **coreo**/plasty _____

Root

Choroid
*(From a Greek word **choroeides**, meaning like a fetal membrane. It is used to mean the choroid, the middle pigmented vascular coat of the posterior five-sixths of the eyeball. The choroid absorbs light and stops reflections within the eye.)*

Combining forms   **Choroid/o**

WORD EXERCISE 13

Without using your Exercise Guide, write the meaning of:

(a) **choroido**/cycl/itis _____

(b) sclero/**choroid**/itis _____

The word **uvea** from Latin *uva*, meaning grape, is used when referring to the pigmented parts of the eye. These parts include the iris, ciliary body and choroid. **Uveitis** refers to inflammation of all pigmented parts of the eye.

Root

Retin
*(From a Medieval/Latin word **retina**, probably derived from rete, meaning net. It refers to the retina, the light-sensitive area of the eye. Light is focused on to the retina by the lens.)*

Combining forms   **Retin/o**

WORD EXERCISE 14

Using your Exercise Guide, find the meaning of:

(a) **retino**/blast/oma _____

(b) **retino**/malacia _____

(c) **retino**/schisis _____

(d) **retino**/pathy _____

(e) **retino**/scopy _____

Without using your Exercise Guide, build words that mean:

(f) picture/recording of the
electrical activity of the retina _____

(g) inflammation of the
choroid and retina _____

(h) inflammation of the
retina and choroid _____

Note. The words in (g) and (h) above are synonymous. Remember, when building words, we add the components as we read the meaning, e.g. in (g) we begin with **-itis**, then add **choroid/o**, followed by **retin/o**; in (h) we begin with **-itis**, but then add **retin/o**, followed by **choroid/o**, thus making two different words that have the same meaning.

Root   **Papill**
*(From a Latin word **papilla**, meaning nipple-shaped.)*

Combining forms   **Papill/o**

Sensory neurons leaving the retina travel through the optic nerve at the back of the eye. Where the sensory neurons collect and form the optic nerve there is a disc-shaped area (visible through the pupil) in the retina. This area is known as the optic disc or optic papilla. **Papill/o** refers to the optic disc.

WORD EXERCISE 15

Using your Exercise Guide, find the meaning of:

(a) **papill**/oedema _____
(Am. papill/edema)

Without using your Exercise Guide, build a word that means:

(b) inflammation of the optic _____
disc and retina

A common disorder of the lens is the development of a cataract, an opacity of the lens or lens capsule. There are many types of cataract. Two common ones are hard

cataracts, that tend to form in the elderly, and soft cataracts, that occur at any age. The lens can be removed by **phako**-emulsification. In this process ultrasonic vibrations liquefy the lens and it is then sucked out. The lens is replaced with an intraocular implant, i.e. a plastic lens.

Root   **Phak**
*(From a Greek word **phakos**, meaning lentil. It refers to the lentil-shaped lens of the eye. The lens is a crystalline structure surrounded by the lens capsule. The shape of the lens and its focus are changed by ligaments connected to muscles in the ciliary body. The ability to change focus of the lens is known as accommodation.)*

Combining forms   **Phac/o or phak/o**

WORD EXERCISE 16

Without using your Exercise Guide, build words using phac/o that mean:

(a) condition of softening of a lens _____
(i.e. a soft cataract)

(b) instrument to view the lens _____
(actually to view changes in
its shape)

Using your Exercise Guide, build words that mean:

(c) hardening of a lens _____
(i.e. a hard cataract)

(d) condition of without _____
a lens (use a-)

Using your Exercise Guide, find the meaning of:

(e) **phaco**/cyst/ectomy _____

(f) **phaco**/erysis _____

Root   **Scot**
*(From a Greek word **skotos**, meaning darkness. It is used to refer to a scotoma, i.e. normal and abnormal blind spots in the visual field where vision is poor.)*

Combining forms   **Scot/o, also used as scotoma**

WORD EXERCISE 17

Without using your Exercise Guide, write the meaning of:

(a) **scoto**/meter _____

(b) **scoto**/metry _____

Using your Exercise Guide, find the meaning of:

(c) **scotoma**/graph _____

Root	Lacrim

Lacrim
(From a Latin word **lacrima**, meaning tear. Here it is used to mean lacrimal apparatus.)

Combining forms **Lacrim/o**

The eye is cleansed and lubricated by the lacrimal apparatus (Fig. 51) consisting of a gland, sac and ducts. The gland produces lacrimal fluid that washes over the eyeball and drains into the lacrimal sac through lacrimal ducts. The lacrimal sac in turn drains the fluid into the nose through the nasolacrimal duct.

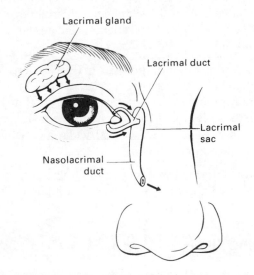

Lacrimal gland

Lacrimal duct

Lacrimal sac

Nasolacrimal duct

Figure 51 Lacrimal apparatus

WORD EXERCISE 18

Without using your Exercise Guide, build words that mean:

(a) incision into the lacrimal _____
apparatus

(b) pertaining to the lacrimal _____
apparatus and nose (use nas/o)

 Root **Dacry**
(From a Greek word **dakryon**, also meaning tear or lacrimal apparatus.)

Combining forms **Dacry/o**

WORD EXERCISE 19

Using your Exercise Guide, find the meaning of:

(a) **dacryo**/cyst _____
(refers to lacrimal sac)

(b) **dacryocysto**/graphy _____

(c) **dacryocysto**/rhino/stomy _____

(d) **dacryo**/lith _____

(e) **dacryo**/stenosis _____

(f) **dacry**/agogic _____

Without using your Exercise Guide, write the meaning of:

(g) **dacryocysto**/blenno/rrhoea _____
(Am. dacryo/cysto/blenno/rrhea)

(h) **dacryocysto**/py/osis _____

Medical equipment and clinical procedures

Before completing Exercises 20 and 21, revise the names of instruments and examinations used in this unit.

Match each term in column A with a description from column C by placing an appropriate number in Column B.

WORD EXERCISE 20

Column A	Column B	Column C
(a) ophthalmoscope	_____	1. X-ray picture of lacrimal apparatus
(b) dacryocystogram	_____	2. measurement of scotomas
(c) keratome	_____	3. instrument that measures tension within the eye

Column A	Column B	Column C
(d) pupillometry	_____	4. instrument for visual examination of the eye
(e) optometry	_____	5. instrument to cut the cornea
(f) scotometry	_____	6. instrument for measuring power of ocular muscles
(g) ophthalmotono-meter	_____	7. technique of measuring sight
(h) optomyometer	_____	8. technique of measuring pupils (width)

WORD EXERCISE 21

Match each term in column A with a description from Column C by placing an appropriate number in Column B.

Column A	Column B	Column C
(a) sclerotome	_____	1. visual examination of retina
(b) optometer	_____	2. technique of recording raised pressure/tension in the eye
(c) keratometry	_____	3. technique of making an X-ray of tear (lacrimal) sac
(d) pupillometer	_____	4. instrument to measure sight
(e) phacoscope	_____	5. instrument to cut the sclera
(f) retinoscopy	_____	6. measurement of cornea (curvature)
(g) tonography	_____	7. instrument to view the lens
(h) dacryocysto-graphy	_____	8. instrument that measures pupils (width)

ANATOMY EXERCISE

Now complete the Anatomy Exercise on page 109.

CASE HISTORY 9

The object of this exercise is to understand words associated with a patient's medical history.

To complete the exercise:

- read through the passage on optic neuritis; unfamiliar words are underlined and you can find their meaning using the Word Help

- write the meaning of the medical terms shown in bold print.

Optic neuritis

Mr I, a 22-year-old physics researcher, consulted his **optometrist** complaining of **diplopia** whilst driving and reading. He had also experienced dizziness and **ophthalmalgia** when moving his eyes. He thought his symptoms were caused by his inappropriate, old spectacles. The optometrist observed **optic neuritis** involving the head of the optic disc (**papillitis**) and perimetry detected a central **scotoma**. She contacted Mr I's GP and he was sent to the neurologist.

Examination revealed the pupils were equal, round and reactive to light but there was a mild paradoxic dilation of the left pupil to the swinging flashlight test. Vertical gaze was normal. There was an abnormal **ocular** movement on lateral gaze, when he attempted to look left, his right eye failed to adduct and although the left eye abducted, it showed a coarse horizontal nystagmus. When he looked to the right, there was no abnormality in the movement of the left eye but the right eye failed to abduct. His abdominal reflexes were absent and his gait was unsteady and wide.

Clinical examination indicated Mr I had lesions in the right medial longitudinal fasciculus (MLF) of the midbrain producing an internuclear **ophthalmoplegia** and sixth nerve palsy. This was confirmed with an MRI scan that revealed small periventricular foci within the pons in the region of the MLF.

Mr I was informed that he had multiple sclerosis (MS) and received appropriate counselling for his condition.

WORD HELP

abducted to move away from the median line (an imaginary line running down the centre of the body)

adduct to move towards the median line or midline of the body

foci centre of disease process (visible on the MRI scan)

gait manner of walking

GP general practitioner (family doctor)

internuclear between nuclei (here nucleus refers to a collection of nerve cells that control eye movement)

lateral gaze looking to the side

MLF medial longitudinal fasciculus, a region of the midbrain that controls eye movement

MRI magnetic resonance imaging

WORD HELP (Contd.)

multiple sclerosis nervous system disease characterized by loss of the myelin sheaths of nerve fibres and their replacement with scar (hard) tissue; the sclerotic (hard) patches being found at numerous sites in the brain, spinal cord and optic nerves (synonymous with disseminated sclerosis)

nystagmus involuntary rapid jerky eye movement

palsy paralysis

paradoxic dilation contradictory occurrence (here the left pupil dilates in response to light)

perimetry measuring acuity (clearness of vision) throughout the visual field

periventricular pertaining to around a ventricle (fluid-filled cavity in the brain)

pons part of the hind brain above the medulla

swinging flashlight test a test in which a flashlight is used to detect a pupillary defect

vertical gaze looking up and down

Now write the meaning of the following words from the case history without using your dictionary lists:

(a) optometrist _____

(b) diplopia _____

(c) ophthalmalgia _____

(d) optic neuritis _____

(e) papillitis _____

(f) scotoma _____

(g) ocular _____

(h) ophthalmoplegia _____

(Answers to the case history exercise are given in the Answers to Word Exercises beginning on page 275.)

Quick Reference

Combining forms relating to the eye:

Blephar/o	eyelid
Choroid/o	choroid
Chromat/o	colour
Conjunctiv/o	conjunctiva
Cor/e/o	pupil
Corne/o	cornea
Cycl/o	ciliary body
Dacry/o	tear/lacrimal apparatus/ducts etc.

Quick Reference (Contd.)

Combining forms relating to the eye:

Goni/o	angle (of anterior chamber)
Ir/o	iris
Irid/o	iris
Kerat/o	cornea
Lacrim/o	tear/lacrimal apparatus/ducts etc.
Ocul/o	eye
Ophthalm/o	eye
Optic/o	optic nerve
Opt/o	sight
Papill/o	optic disc
Phac/o	lens
Phak/o	lens
Pupill/o	pupil
Retin/o	retina
Scler/o	sclera
Scot/o	dark
Ton/o	tone/tension
Uve/o	uvea (pigmented part of eye)

Abbreviations

Some common abbreviations related to the eye are listed below. Note, some are not standard and their meaning may vary from one health care setting to another. There is a more extensive list for reference on page 307.

Accom	accommodation of eye
Astigm	astigmatism of eye
Em	emmetropia/good vision
IOFB	intraocular foreign body
My	myopia/short sight
OD	oculus dexter/right eye
OS	oculus sinister/left eye
OU	oculus unitas/both eyes together
POAG	primary open angle glaucoma
PERLAC	pupils equal, react to light, accommodation consensual
VA	visual acuity
VF	visual field

 NOW TRY THE WORD CHECK

WORD CHECK

This self-check exercise lists all the word components used in this unit. First write down the meaning of as many word components as you can. Then check your answers using the Exercise Guide and Quick Reference box or the Glossary of Word Components (pp. 319–341).

Prefixes

a-	without
ambly-	dull/dim
an-	without
bin-	two each/double
dia-	through
diplo-	double
dys-	painful/difficult
electro-	electrical
em-	in
en-	in/within
ex-	out
hemi-	half
hyper-	above normal
iso-	same/equal
mono-	one
ortho-	straight
pan-	all
presby-	old man's eyes
uni-	one
xero-	dry

Combining forms of word roots

aesthesi/o (Am. esthesi/o)	sensation
aden/o	gland

blast/o	immature germ cell
blenn/o	mucous
blephar/o	eyelid
choroid/o	choroid
chromat/o	colour
conjunctiv/o	conjunctiva
cor/e/o	pupil
cycl/o	ciliary body
cyst/o	bladder
dacry/o	tear/lacrimal apparatus
goni/o	angle
helc/o	ulcer
ir/o	iris
irid/o	iris
kerat/o	cornea
lacrim/o	tear/lacrimal apparatus
lith/o	stone
motor	action
myc/o	fungus
my/o	muscle
my (from myein)	muscle
nas/o	nose
neur/o	nerve
ocul/o	eye
ophthalm/o	eye
optic/o	optic nerve
opt/o	sight
papill/o	optic disc
phak/o, phac/o	lens
pupill/o	pupil

py/o	pus
retin/o	retina
rhin/o	nose
scler/o	sclera
scot/o	dark
sten/o	narrow
ton/o	tone / tension
uve/o	

Suffixes

-agogic	pertaining to stimulating
-al	pert. to
-algia	cond. of pain
-cele	hernia / swelling
-centesis	surg. puncture
-chalasis	slackening / loosening
-conus	cone-like protrusion
-desis	fixation
-dialysis	separating
-ectasis	dilation / stretching
-ectomy	removal of
-erysis	such out
-gram	x-ray / recording
-graph	instrument to record
-graphy	technique of recording
-gyric	pert. to circular motion
-ia	condition of
-itis	inflammation of
-kinesis	movement
-logist	specialist who studies
-malacia	cond. of softening

-meter	measuring instrument
-metrist	person who measures
-metry	process of measuring
-mileusis	to carve
-nyxis	perforation / puncture
-oedema (Am. -edema)	swelling due to fluid
-oma	tumour / swelling
-opia	cond. of vision
-osis	abnormal cond. of.
-pathy	disease of
-pexy	surg. fixation
-phobia	cond. of fear
-plasty	surg. repair / recon.
-plegia	cond. of paralysis
-ptosis	downward displacement
-rrhaphy	suturing
-rrhoea (Am. -rrhea)	excessive flow / discharge
-schisis	splitting / parting
-sclerosis	ab cond. of hardening
-scope	viewing instrument
-scopy	tech. of viewing
-spasm	involuntary muscle spasm
-synechia	cond. of adhering together, contraction
-thermy	heat
-tome	cutting instrument
-tomy	incision into

> **NOW TRY THE SELF-ASSESSMENT** <

SELF-ASSESSMENT

Test 9A

Below are some combining forms that refer to the anatomy of the eye. Indicate which parts of the eye they refer to by putting a number from the diagrams (Figs 52 and 53) next to each word:

(a) irid/o _3_

(b) scler/o _4_

(c) pupill/o _2_

(d) lacrim/o _5_

(e) blephar/o _1_

(f) phac/o _7_

(g) papill/o _8_

(h) retin/o _9_

(i) kerat/o _6_

(j) ophthalmoneur/o _10_

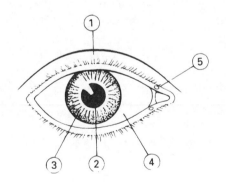

Figure 52 The eye

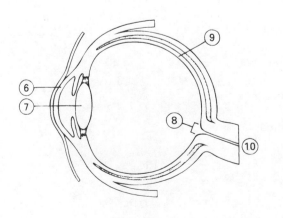

Figure 53 Section through the eye

Test 9B

Prefixes and suffixes

Match each prefix or suffix in Column A with a meaning in Column C by inserting the appropriate number in Column B.

Column A	Column B	Column C
(a) -agogic	12	1. dragging/drawing/sucking out
(b) ambly-	10	2. splitting
(c) -dialysis	18	3. swelling (due to fluid)
(d) electro-	19	4. one (i)
(e) -erysis	1	5. one (ii)
(f) -graph	14	6. person who measures
(g) -gyric	13	7. old man, old age
(h) hemi-	20	8. all
(i) -kinesis	15	9. condition of sticking together
(j) -metrist	6	10. dulled/made dim
(k) -mileusis	16	11. condition of vision (defective)
(l) mono-	4/5	12. pertaining to inducing/stimulating
(m) -oedema (Am. -edema)	3	13. pertaining to turning/circular movement
(n) -opia	11	14. instrument that records
(o) pan-	8	15. movement
(p) presby-	7	16. to carve
(q) -rrhaphy	17	17. suturing/stitching

Column A	Column B	Column C
(r) -schisis	2	18. separating
(s) -synechia	9	19. electrical
(t) uni-	5/4	20. half

Score

20

Column A	Column B	Column C
(q) pupill/o	5	17. eyelid
(r) retin/o	8	18. conjunctiva
(s) scotom/o	13	19. tear (i)
(t) uve/o	7	20. tear (ii)

Score

20

Test 9C

Combining forms of word roots

Match each combining form in Column A with a meaning in Column C by inserting the appropriate number in Column B.

Column A	Column B	Column C
(a) blephar/o	17	1. cone (shaped)
(b) choroid/o	14	2. cornea
(c) chromat/o	9	3. optic disc
(d) conjunctiv/o	18	4. iris (rainbow)
(e) conus	1	5. pupil
(f) cycl/o	12	6. sight/vision
(g) dacry/o	19/20	7. pigmented area of eye (uvea)
(h) helc/o	10	8. retina
(i) irid/o	4	9. colour
(j) kerat/o	2	10. ulcer
(k) lacrim/o	20/19	11. lens
(l) ocul/o	15/16	12. ciliary body
(m) ophthalm/o	16/15	13. darkness/blind spot
(n) optic/o	6	14. choroid
(o) papill/o	3	15. eye (i)
(p) phak/o	11	16. eye (ii)

Test 9D

Write the meaning of:

(a) ophthalmoplasty — surg. recast. of eye.

(b) retinopexy — surg. fixation. of retina

(c) dacryopyorrhoea (Am. dacryopyorrhea) — excessive pus for lacrimal apparatus

(d) sclero-iritis — infl of iris + sclera.

(e) oculomotor nerve — nerve that stimulates movement of eye.

Score

5

Test 9E

Build words that mean:

(a) visual examination of the eye — ophthalmoscopy

(b) inflammation of eyelid — blepharitis

(c) any disease of cornea — keratopathy

(d) instrument to view the retina — retinoscope

(e) condition of paralysis of iris — iridoplegia

Score

5

Check answers to Self-Assessment Tests on page 299.

10 The ear

Objectives

Once you have completed Unit 10 you should be able to:

- understand the meaning of medical words relating to the ear

- build medical words relating to the ear

- associate medical terms with their anatomical position

- understand medical abbreviations relating to the ear.

Exercise Guide

Use this list of word components and their meanings to complete the word exercises in this unit.

Prefixes

bin-	two each/double
endo-	within/inside
macro-	large
micro-	small

Roots/Combining forms

electr/o	electrical
laryng/o	larynx
myc/o	fungus
pharyng/o	pharynx

py/o	pus
rhin/o	nose
ten/o	tendon

Suffixes

-al	pertaining to
-algia	condition of pain
-ar	pertaining to
-centesis	puncture to remove fluid
-eal	pertaining to
-ectomy	removal of
-emphraxis	blocking/stopping up
-genic	pertaining to formation/ originating in
-gram	X-ray tracing/picture/recording
-graphy	technique of recording/making an X-ray
-ia	condition of
-itis	inflammation of
-logy	study of
-meter	measuring instrument
-metry	process of measuring
-osis	abnormal condition/disease/ abnormal increase
-plasty	surgical repair/reconstruction
-rrhea (Am.)	excessive discharge/flow
-rrhoea	excessive discharge/flow
-sclerosis	abnormal condition of hardening
-scope	instrument to view
-scopy	technique of viewing/ examining
-stomy	formation of an opening/an opening
-tome	cutting instrument
-tomy	incision into

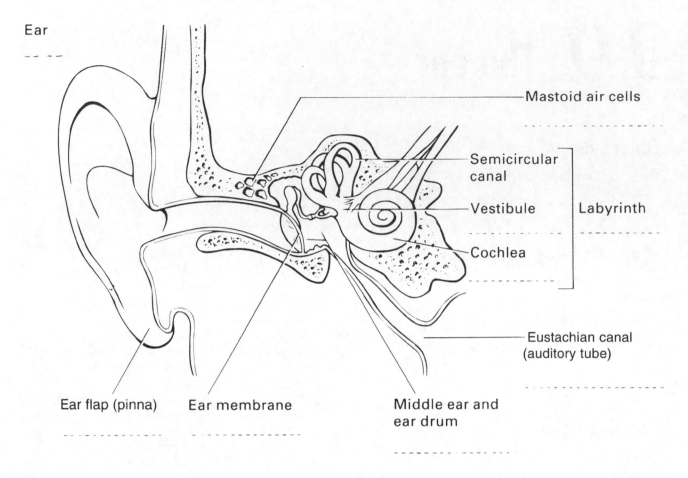

Ear

Mastoid air cells

Semicircular canal

Vestibule

Labyrinth

Cochlea

Eustachian canal (auditory tube)

Ear flap (pinna)   Ear membrane   Middle ear and ear drum

Figure 54   Section through the ear

ANATOMY EXERCISE

When you have finished Word Exercises 1–14, look at the word components listed below. Complete Figure 54 by writing the appropriate combining form on each dotted line – more than one component may relate to the same position. (You can check their meanings in the Quick Reference box on p. 131.)

Auricul/o	Mastoid/o	Salping/o
Cochle/o	Myring/o	Tympan/o
Labyrinth/o	Ot/o	Vestibul/o

The ear

The ear is a major sense organ concerned with two important functions:

1. hearing
2. balance.

The ear provides an auditory input into the brain. Sound waves in the air cause vibrations in the ear drum and these are transmitted to the fluid-filled cochlea in the inner ear. The cochlea is the organ of hearing and contains special receptor cells that generate nerve impulses in response to sound. Nerve impulses from the cochlea are relayed via sensory neurons to auditory areas in the brain where they are interpreted as sounds. The possession of two ears enables us to sense the direction of sound.

The vestibular apparatus of the inner ear contains receptors that detect changes in velocity and position of the body. Sensory impulses from the vestibular apparatus are relayed via sensory neurons to centres in the cerebellum and other regions of the brain where they are used in the neural processes that allow us to maintain our balance and upright posture.

Use the Exercise Guide at the beginning of this unit to complete Word Exercises 1–14 unless you are asked to work without it.

Root   Ot
*(From Greek word **ous**, meaning ear.)*

Combining forms   **Ot/o**

WORD EXERCISE 1

Using your Exercise Guide, build words that mean:

(a) the study of the ear

(b) instrument to view the ear

(c) abnormal condition of hardening of the ear (actually due to new bone formation in the middle ear)

(d) abnormal condition of pus in the ear

Using your Exercise Guide, find the meaning of:

(e) **oto**/scopy

(f) **oto**/rhino/laryngo/logy

(g) **oto**/myc/osis

(h) **oto**/pyo/rrhoea
(Am. oto/pyo/rrhea)

(i) micr/**ot**/ia

(j) macr/**ot**/ia

The ear can be divided into three areas, the external, middle and inner ear. Infection and inflammation (**ot**itis) can occur in any of these areas. The following terms are used to describe the position of the inflammation:

Otitis externa
   inflammation of the external ear.
Otitis media
   inflammation of the middle ear.
Otitis interna
   inflammation of the inner ear.

Infection commonly begins in the middle ear because it is connected to the **nasopharynx** by a short tube known as the **Eustachian tube** (**auditory tube** or **pharyngo-tympanic tube**). This tube functions to equalize the pressure on either side of the ear drum but it also provides an entrance for microorganisms such as those present in upper respiratory tract infections.

Root   Aur
*(From a Latin word **auris**, meaning ear.)*

Combining forms   **Aur/i**

WORD EXERCISE 2

Without using your Exercise Guide, build a word that means:

(a) instrument to view the ear (otoscope) (Fig. 55)

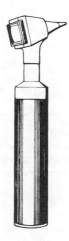

Figure 55   Otoscope/auriscope

Viewing of the ear canal and tympanic membrane is improved by using an **aural speculum** (Fig. 56), a device that is inserted into the external ear before examining with an **auriscope**.

The auriscope is used to examine the external ear canal and the ear membrane. Occasionally, the ear canal can become blocked by excessive wax production by the cerumenous (wax) glands in its lining. Wax can be removed by washing the ear with warm water using an aural syringe (Fig. 57) or using wax solvents to bring about cerumenolysis.

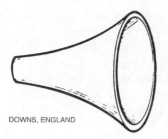

Figure 56 Aural speculum

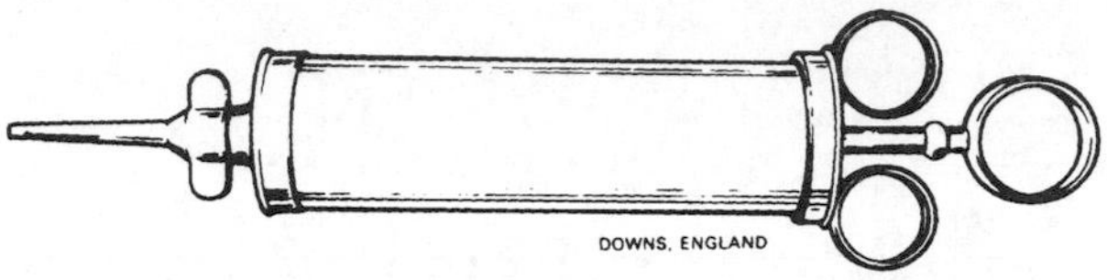

Figure 57 Aural syringe

Using your Exercise Guide, find the meaning of:

(b) bin/**aur**/al _____

(c) end/**aur**/al _____

The Latin word *auricula* refers to the ear flaps (pinnae) of the external ear.

(d) bin/**auricul**/ar _____

Root

Myring
*(A New Latin word **myringa**, meaning membrane. It refers to the tympanic membrane or ear drum.)*

Combining forms **Myring/o**

 WORD EXERCISE 3

Using your Exercise Guide, build words that mean:

(a) incision into the ear membrane _____
(allows air to enter to aid drainage)

(b) instrument used to cut the ear _____
membrane

Without using your Exercise Guide, build a word that means:

(c) abnormal condition of fungal _____
infection of the ear membrane

Sometimes the tympanic membrane is surgically punctured to assist the drainage of fluid from the middle ear (as in glue ear). Once an opening is made in the membrane, fluid drains through the Eustachian tube (auditory tube) into the nasopharynx. A small plastic grommet (Fig. 58) can be fixed into the membrane to equalize the air pressure on either side of the membrane and allow drainage through the Eustachian tube for an extended period. The grommet eventually falls out and the membrane heals.

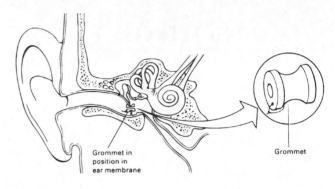

Figure 58 Grommet

Root

Tympan
*(From a Greek word **tympanon**, meaning drum. Here it refers to the tympanum, i.e. the cavity of the middle ear. It is also used to mean tympanic membrane.)*

Combining forms **Tympan/o**

 WORD EXERCISE 4

Using your Exercise Guide, build words that mean:

(a) reconstructive surgery of _____
the tympanum

(b) puncture of the tympanic _____
membrane

(c) opening into the tympanum/ _____
tympanic membrane

Without using your Exercise Guide, write the meaning of:

(d) **tympan**/itis _____

(e) **tympano**/tomy _____

Root   **Salping**
*(From Greek **salpigx**, meaning trumpet tube. Here it refers to the trumpet-shaped Eustachian tube that connects the middle ear to the nasopharynx. The Eustachian tube is also called the auditory tube or pharyngotympanic tube.)*

Combining forms   **Salping/o**

WORD EXERCISE 5

Using your Exercise Guide, find the meaning of:

(a) **salping**/emphraxis _____

(b) **salpingo**/pharyng/eal _____

Within the middle ear we find the smallest bones in the body, the ear ossicles (Fig. 59). These have been named **malleus, incus** and **stapes**. Their function is to transmit vibrations from the tympanic membrane to the oval window of the inner ear. Behind the oval window is a fluid-filled structure known as the **cochlea**, the organ of hearing. Within the cochlea are sensory hair cells (receptors) that respond to vibrations in the fluid by producing nerve impulses. The auditory area of the brain interprets nerve impulses from the cochlea as sound, enabling us to hear.

Root   **Stapedi**
*(From a Latin word **stapes**, meaning stirrup, it refers to the stapes, the stirrup-shaped ear ossicle.)*

Combining forms   **Staped/i/o**

WORD EXERCISE 6

Using your Exercise Guide, build a word that means:

(a) removal of the stapes _____

Using your Exercise Guide, find the meaning of:

(b) **stapedio**/teno/tomy _____

Root   **Malle**
*(From a Latin word **malleus**, meaning hammer. It refers to the malleus, the hammer-shaped ear ossicle.)*

Combining forms   **Malle/o**

WORD EXERCISE 7

Without using your Exercise Guide, write the meaning of:

(a) **malleo**/tomy _____

Root   **Incud**
*(From a Latin word **incus**, meaning anvil. It refers to the incus, the anvil-shaped ear ossicle.)*

Combining forms   **Incud/o**

WORD EXERCISE 8

Without using your Exercise Guide, write the meaning of:

(a) **incudo**/mall/eal _____

(b) **incudo**/stapedi/al _____

(c) malleo/**incud**/al _____

ANATOMY EXERCISE

Write the appropriate combining form for each ossicle on the dotted lines of Figure 59.

Sometimes the ear bones are referred to in a more general way, using **ossicle**, to mean small ear bones, e.g. **ossicul**ectomy for removal of one or more ossicles, **ossiculo**tomy for incision into the ear ossicles. The ossicles can be replaced by a plastic prosthesis that will transmit vibrations to the inner ear and restore hearing.

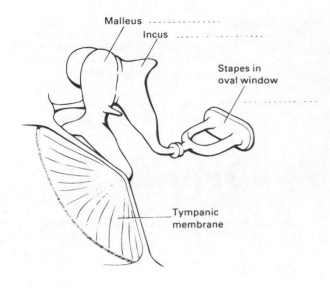

Malleus

Incus

Stapes in
oval window

Tympanic
membrane

Figure 59 Ear ossicles

The membranous labyrinth lies within the bony labyrinth and is also filled with fluid. Distension of the membranous labyrinth with excess fluid gives rise to **Ménière's** disease, symptoms of which include vertigo (dizziness) and deafness.

The portions of the inner ear concerned with balance are collectively known as the vestibular apparatus.

WORD EXERCISE 10

Without using your Exercise Guide, build words that mean:

(a) inflammation of a labyrinth _____

(b) removal of a labyrinth _____

Root Cochle
(From a Latin word **cochlea***, meaning snail. It refers to the cochlea, the snail shell-shaped anterior bony labyrinth of the inner ear.)*

Combining forms **Cochle/o**

WORD EXERCISE 9

Using your Exercise Guide, build words that mean:

(a) an opening into the cochlea _____

(b) technique of recording the cochlea's electrical activity _____

Root Labyrinth
(From a Greek word **labyrinthos***, meaning maze or anything twisted or spiral-shaped. Here it refers to the labyrinth of the inner ear.)*

Combining forms **Labyrinth/o**

The inner ear consists of bony and membranous labyrinths. The bony labyrinth is a series of canals in the temporal bone filled with fluid. It consists of the cochlea (organ of hearing), vestibule and semicircular canals (organs of equilibrium).

Root Vestibul
(From the Latin word **vestibulum***, meaning entrance. It refers to the vestibule, the oval cavity in the middle of the bony labyrinth.)*

Combining forms **Vestibul/o**

WORD EXERCISE 11

Without using your Exercise Guide, write the meaning of:

(a) **vestibulo**/tomy _____

Using your Exercise Guide, find the meaning of:

(b) **vestibulo**/genic _____

Root Mast
(From a Greek word **mastos***, meaning breast. It refers to the nipple-shaped air cells or the air space within the mastoid process. The mastoid process is a bone located behind the external ear.)*

Combining forms **Mastoid/o**

WORD EXERCISE 12

Using your Exercise Guide, build a word that means:

(a) condition of pain in the mastoid region _____

Without using your Exercise Guide, build words that mean:

(b) incision into the mastoid bone _____

(c) removal of tissue from the mastoid process _____

(d) inflammation of the mastoid process and tympanum _____

Root Audi
(From a Latin word **audire**, *meaning to hear.)*

Combining forms **Audi/o**

WORD EXERCISE 13

Without using your Exercise Guide, build a word that means:

(a) the science dealing with the study of hearing _____

Note. An **audiometrist** is a technician who has specialized in the study of hearing. He or she tests and measures a patient's hearing ability (*-ist* meaning a specialist who …).

Using your Exercise Guide, find the meaning of:

(b) **audio**/meter _____

(c) **audio**/gram _____

(d) **audio**/metry _____

Medical equipment and clinical procedures

Revise the names of all instruments and examinations used in this unit before completing Exercise 14.

WORD EXERCISE 14

Match each term in Column A with a description in Column C by placing an appropriate number in Column B.

Column A	Column B	Column C
(a) audiometer	_____	1. technique of measuring hearing
(b) audiometry	_____	2. instrument for viewing ear
(c) aural speculum	_____	3. technique of viewing ear
(d) auriscope	_____	4. device for removing wax from ear
(e) otoscopy	_____	5. device to aid drainage of fluid from ear
(f) aural syringe	_____	6. instrument that measures hearing
(g) grommet	_____	7. device that holds ear canal open

ANATOMY EXERCISE

Now complete the Anatomy Exercise on page 124.

CASE HISTORY 10

The object of this exercise is to understand words associated with a patient's medical history.

To complete the exercise:

• read through the passage on otitis media with effusion; unfamiliar words are underlined and you can find their meaning using the Word Help

• write the meaning of the medical terms shown in bold print.

Otitis media with Effusion (OME, 'Glue Ear')

Miss J, a 5-year old infant, presented to her GP with persistent **otalgia**. She had a previous history of acute otitis media with perforation in the left ear and had been treated with broad-spectrum antibiotics. Her parents were concerned that her hearing and speech were impaired. Miss J's nursery teacher reported that she was inattentive in class and seemed 'in a world of her own'. Her mother had also noticed her snoring and had been worried about her breathing during a recent cold. Her tonsils were very large, she had a poor nasal airway and was breathing through her mouth, signs consistent with adenoid hypertrophy.

Pneumatic **otoscopy** by her GP revealed bilateral otitis media with effusion (non-suppurative OM) and she was referred to the **audiometrist** for a hearing assessment. She cooperated well and a pure-tone **audiogram** was obtained indicating a mild loss of 20–30 decibels in hearing threshold. Over the next 6 months she received several courses of antibiotic therapy. Initially, there were signs of improvement but her condition did not resolve and she was referred to the paediatric **otology** clinic.

The consultant otologist confirmed the diagnosis. Her tympanic membranes were dull, retracted and lacked mobility. Fluid containing air bubbles was visible in the right ear, and she had a negative Rinne test.

Tympanometry revealed a flat tympanogram characteristic of glue ear with reduced compliance and a negative middle ear pressure. Her audiogram indicated conductive deafness across the entire frequency range of 35–40 decibels.

Miss J underwent adenoidectomy and anterior, bilateral **myringotomy** under general anaesthesia. A thick mucoid secretion was aspirated from both ears and grommets (**tympanostomy** tubes) inserted into her tympanic membranes. Six months later the grommets were still in position and her hearing and speech were much improved.

WORD HELP

acute symptoms/signs of short duration

adenoid resembling a gland (here refers to an enlarged pharyngeal tonsil seen in the nasopharynx of children)

adenoidectomy removal of an adenoid

anterior pertaining to towards the front

aspirated withdrawal by suction of fluid

bilateral pertaining to two sides

broad-spectrum affecting a wide range (of infective organisms)

WORD HELP (Contd.)

compliance quality of yielding to pressure (here referring to the movement of the ear drum in relation to pressure)

conductive deafness deafness caused by impairment of conduction of sound waves through the normal route

decibel unit used for measurement of intensity of sound

effusion a fluid discharge into a part/escape of fluid into an enclosed space

GP general practitioner (family doctor)

grommet plastic tube inserted into the ear drum to ventilate the middle ear

hypertrophy increase in size of cells in a tissue (above normal growth/nourishment)

mucoid resembling mucus

otitis media condition of inflammation of the middle ear

otologist specialist who studies the ear and its disorders

paediatric pertaining to medical care and treatment of children

perforation a hole made through a membrane or similar tissue

pneumatic pertaining to air (pneumatic otoscopy refers to viewing the ear membrane whilst stimulating it with a puff of air to observe its movement)

Rinne test test using a tuning fork for diagnosis of conductive deafness

suppurative having a tendency to produce pus

tympanogram recording of the compliance and impedance of the tympanic membrane

Now write the meaning of the following words from the case history without using your dictionary lists:

(a) otalgia

(b) otoscopy

(c) audiometrist

(d) audiogram

(e) otology

(f) tympanometry

(g) myringotomy

(h) tympanostomy

(Answers to the case history exercise are given in the Answers to Word Exercises beginning on page 275.)

answers using the Exercise Guide and Quick Reference box or the Glossary of Word Components (pp. 319–341).

Quick Reference

Combining forms relating to the ear:

Audi/o	hearing
Aur/i	ear
Auricul/o	ear flap
Cochle/o	cochlea
Incud/o	incus (an ear ossicle)
Labyrinth/o	labyrinth (of inner ear)
Malle/o	malleus (an ear ossicle)
Mastoid/o	mastoid process/mastoid air cells
Myring/o	ear membrane (drum)
Ossicul/o	ossicle
Ot/o	ear
Salping/o	Eustachian/auditory tube
Stapedi/o	stapes (an ear ossicle)
Tympan/o	ear drum/middle ear
Vestibul/o	vestibular apparatus (of inner ear)

Prefixes

bin-

electro-

endo-

macro-

micro-

Combining forms of word roots

audi/o

aur/i

auricul/o

cochle/o

incud/o

labyrinth/o

laryng/o

malle/o

mastoid/o

myc/o

myring/o

ossicul/o

ot/o

pharyng/o

py/o

rhin/o

salping/o

stapedi/o

ten/o

tympan/o

vestibul/o

Abbreviations

Some common abbreviations related to the ear are listed below. Note, however, some are not standard and their meaning may vary from one health care setting to another. There is a more extensive list for reference on page 307.

AC	air conduction
AD	auris dextra (right ear)
AS	auris sinistra (left ear)
ASOM	acute suppurative otitis media
aud	audiology
BC	bone conduction
CSOM	chronic suppurative otitis media
ENT	ear, nose and throat
ETF	Eustachian tube function
OE	otitis externa
OM	otitis media
oto	otology

> **NOW TRY THE WORD CHECK** <

WORD CHECK

This self-check exercise lists all the word components used in this unit. First write down the meaning of as many word components as you can. Then check your

Suffixes

-al

-algia

-ar

-aural

-centesis

-eal

-ectomy

-emphraxis

-externa

-genic

-gram

-ia

-interna

-ist

-itis

-media

-logy

-meter

-metry

-osis

-plasty

-rrhoea
(Am. -rrhea)

-sclerosis

-scope

-stomy

-tome

-tomy

> **NOW TRY THE SELF-ASSESSMENT** <

SELF-ASSESSMENT

Test 10A

Below are some combining forms that refer to the anatomy of the ear. Indicate which part of the system they refer to by putting a number from the diagram (Fig. 60) next to each word.

(a) ot/o

(b) myring/o

(c) tympan/o

(d) nasopharyng/o

(e) ossicul/o

(f) labyrinth/o

(g) cochle/o

(h) mastoid/o

(i) salping/o

(j) vestibul/o

| **Figure 60** | Section through the ear |

Score

10

Test 10B

Prefixes and suffixes

Match each prefix or suffix in Column A with a meaning in Column C by inserting the appropriate number in Column B.

Column A	Column B	Column C
(a) -al	_____	1. incision into
(b) -ar	_____	2. flow/discharge
(c) -aural	_____	3. external
(d) -eal	_____	4. instrument that cuts
(e) electro-	_____	5. hardening
(f) -emphraxis	_____	6. inner/internal
(g) endo-	_____	7. middle
(h) -externa	_____	8. pertaining to (i)
(i) -gram	_____	9. pertaining to (ii)
(j) -ia	_____	10. pertaining to (iii)
(k) -interna	_____	11. small
(l) macro-	_____	12. in/within
(m) -media	_____	13. abnormal condition/ disease of
(n) -metry	_____	14. pertaining to the ear
(o) micro-	_____	15. picture/ X-ray/tracing
(p) -osis	_____	16. electrical
(q) -rrhoea (Am. -rrhea)	_____	17. condition of
(r) -sclerosis	_____	18. large
(s) -tome	_____	19. to block/stop up
(t) -tomy	_____	20. measurement

Score

20

Test 10C

Combining forms of word roots

Match each combining form in Column A with a meaning in Column C by inserting the appropriate number in Column B.

Column A	Column B	Column C
(a) audi/o	_____	1. stapes
(b) aur/i	_____	2. larynx
(c) auricul/o	_____	3. nose
(d) incud/o	_____	4. Eustachian tube
(e) labyrinth/o	_____	5. ear (i)
(f) laryng/o	_____	6. ear (ii)
(g) malle/o	_____	7. ear flap (pinna)
(h) mastoid/o	_____	8. ear drum/ middle ear
(i) myc/o	_____	9. vestibular apparatus
(j) myring/o	_____	10. malleus
(k) ossicul/o	_____	11. fungus
(l) ot/o	_____	12. hearing
(m) pharyng/o	_____	13. ear membrane
(n) py/o	_____	14. tendon
(o) rhin/o	_____	15. incus
(p) salping/o	_____	16. pharynx
(q) stapedi/o	_____	17. mastoid
(r) ten/o	_____	18. ear bones/ossicles
(s) tympan/o	_____	19. pus
(t) vestibul/o	_____	20. labyrinth of inner ear

Score

20

Test 10D

Write the meaning of:

(a) otolaryngology _____

(b) tympanosclerosis _____

(c) stapediovestibular _____

(d) tympanomalleal _____

(e) vestibulocochlear _____

Score

5

Test 10E

Build words that mean:

(a) puncture of mastoid process _____

(b) removal of the ear membrane _____

(c) surgical repair of the ear _____

(d) condition of pain in ear _____

(e) originating in the middle ear _____

Score

5

Check answers to Self-Assessment Tests on page 299.

11 The skin

Objectives

Once you have completed Unit 11 you should be able to:

- understand the meaning of medical words relating to the skin

- build medical words relating to the skin

- associate medical terms with their anatomical position

- understand medical abbreviations relating to the skin.

Exercise Guide

Use this list of word components and their meanings to complete the word exercises in this unit.

Prefixes

a-	without
an-	without/not
auto-	self
crypto-	hidden
dys-	difficult/painful
epi-	above/upon/on
hyper-	above/excessive
hypo-	below/deficient
intra-	within/inside
pachy-	thick
para-	beside/near
sub-	under/below
xantho-	yellow
xero-	dry

Roots/Combining forms

aden/o	gland
aesthe/s/i/o	sensation/sensitivity
esthe/s/i/o (Am.)	sensation/sensitivity
lith/o	stone
motor	action
myc/o	fungus
phyt(e)	plant (fungus)
schiz/o	split/cleft

Suffixes

-al	pertaining to
-auxis	increase
-cyte	cell
-ia	condition of
-ic	pertaining to
-itis	inflammation of
-logist	specialist who studies
-lysis	breakdown/disintegration
-oma	tumour/swelling
-osis	abnormal condition/disease/ abnormal increase
-phagia	condition of eating
-plasty	surgical repair/reconstruction
-poiesis	formation
-rrhexis	break/rupture
-rrhea (Am.)	excessive discharge/flow
-rrhoea	excessive discharge/flow
-schisis	splitting/parting/cleaving
-tic	pertaining to
-tome	cutting instrument
-trophy	nourishment/development
-tropic	pertaining to stimulating/affinity for

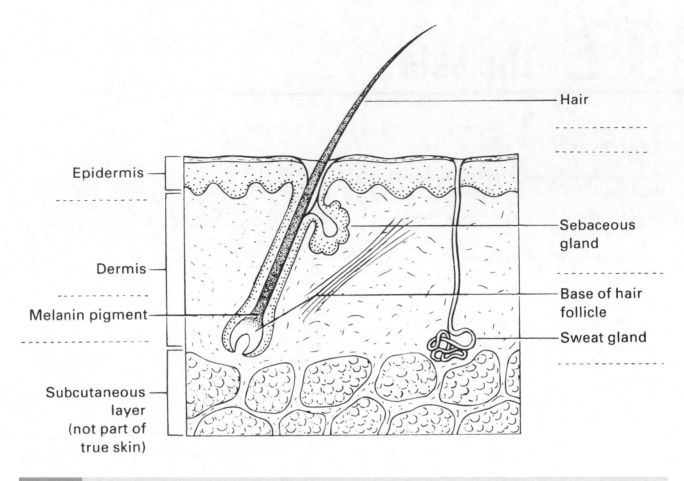

Hair

Epidermis

Sebaceous
gland

Dermis

Base of hair
follicle

Melanin pigment

Sweat gland

Subcutaneous
layer
(not part of
true skin)

Figure 61   Section through the skin

ANATOMY EXERCISE

When you have finished Word Exercises 1–9, look at the word components listed below. Complete Figure 61 by writing the appropriate combining form on each dotted line – more than one component may relate to the same position. (You can check their meanings in the Quick Reference box on p. 142.)

Derm/o	Melan/o	Seb/o
Hidraden/o	Pil/o	Trich/o
Kerat/o		

The skin

The skin can be regarded as the largest organ in the body; it consists of two layers, the outer **epidermis** and the inner **dermis**. The skin protects us from the environment and plays a major role in thermoregulation. In its protective role, it prevents the body dehydrating, resists the invasion of microorganisms and provides protection from the harmful effects of ultraviolet light. Cells in the epidermis enable the surface of the skin to continuously regenerate, and the presence of elastic fibres and collagen fibres in the dermis make the skin tough and elastic.

Use the Exercise Guide at the beginning of this unit to complete Word Exercises 1–9 unless you are asked to work without it.

Root	**Derm** *(From a Greek word* **derma**, *meaning skin.)*
Combining forms	**Derm/a/t/o**, also used as the suffix **-derma**

The medical specialty concerned with the diagnosis and treatment of skin disease is known as **dermatology** (*-logy* meaning study of).

WORD EXERCISE 1

Using your Exercise Guide, find the meaning of:

(a) **dermat**/osis _____

Actinic dermatoses are conditions in which the skin is abnormally sensitive to light (from a Greek word *aktis*, meaning ray).

(b) epi/**dermis** _____

The **epidermis** forms the outer layer of the body and it functions to protect the underlying layer called the **dermis**. Note the dermis and epidermis form the skin; the underlying (subcutaneous) fatty tissue often studied with them is not regarded as part of the true skin.

The epidermis can be subdivided into five distinct layers, the outermost forming a layer of tough dead cells (scales), known as the stratum corneum. At the surface, the cells of the epidermis fit together like the scales of a fish; for this reason it is known as a stratified **squamous** epithelium (squamous from Latin *squama*, meaning scale of a fish or reptile). The word epithelium (combining form epitheli/o) refers to a type of tissue formed from one or more layers of cells that cover and line internal and external surfaces of the body. As the epidermis consists of many layers of cells it is described as a stratified epithelium.

(c) **dermato**/phyte _____

(d) pachy/**derma** _____

(e) xantho/**derma** _____

(f) **dermato**/auto/plasty _____

(g) xero/**derm**/ia _____

(h) **dermato**/logist _____

Using your Exercise Guide, build words that mean:

(i) abnormal condition of fungi _____
in the skin (use dermat/o
and myc/o)

(j) an instrument to cut skin _____
for grafts (use derm/a)

(k) pertaining to below _____
the skin (use derm/a)

(l) pertaining to within the skin _____
(use derm/a)

Note. There are a few words in use derived from *cutis*, the Latin for skin, e.g. **cutaneous** – pertaining to the skin (from cutane/o meaning skin and -ous meaning pertaining to); **cuticle** – the epidermis (from cuti- meaning skin and -cle meaning small).

Root	Kerat
	*(From a Greek word **keras**, meaning horn. We have already used this word to mean the cornea of the eye. Here it is used to mean the outer, horny layer of the skin, i.e. the epidermis.)*

Combining forms   **Kerat/o**

WORD EXERCISE 2

Without using your Exercise Guide, write the meaning of:

(a) actinic **kerat**/osis _____
(pertaining to the sun's rays)

Using your Exercise Guide, find the meaning of:

(b) hyper/**kerato**/tic _____

(c) **kerat**/oma _____

(d) **kerato**/lysis _____

Note. There is no way of telling whether a medical term containing the root **kerat** refers to the cornea or epidermis except by noting the context in which it is written.

The cells of the outer layer of the epidermis are said to be **keratinized** because they contain the waterproof protein **keratin** that gives the epidermis its ability to protect the underlying dermis. (The combining form **keratin/o** refers to the protein keratin.)

Other disorders of the epidermis include:

Ichthyosis
A disorder in which there is abnormal keratinization, giving rise to a dry scaly skin (**ichthy/o** from Greek, meaning fish, i.e. fish-like skin).

Acanthosis
A thickening of the prickle cell layer of the epidermis (**acanth/o** from Greek, meaning spike).

The skin appendages

The multiplication of cells in the basal layer of the epidermis gives rise to the appendages of the skin: hairs, sebaceous glands, sweat glands and nails. Here we use terms associated with each appendage:

> **Root** **Pil**
> *(From a Latin word **pilus**, meaning hair or composed of hair. Hairs grow from depressions in the epidermis known as follicles.)*
>
> Combining forms **Pil/o**

WORD EXERCISE 3

Using your Exercise Guide, find the meaning of:

(a) **pilo**/motor nerve _____
(This nerve stimulates the arrector pili muscles to contract, causing erection of the hair in cold conditions.)

A technique known as electrolysis is used to destroy hairs permanently by heating the base of a hair to destroy its dividing cells. The heating is achieved by passing an electric current through the hair follicle. This technique is also used by beauty therapists for the removal of excess hair and is known as e**pil**ation (e- meaning out from, i.e. the hair out of its follicle).

Hairs can also be removed by using a de**pil**atory paste that dissolves hair (de- meaning away). The hairs regrow following depilation as the base of the hair is not destroyed.

> **Root** **Trich**
> *(From a Greek word **trichos**, meaning hair.)*
>
> Combining forms **Trich/o**

WORD EXERCISE 4

Without using your Exercise Guide, write the meaning of:

(a) **tricho**/phyt/osis _____

(b) **trich**/osis _____

Using your Exercise Guide, find the meaning of:

(c) **tricho**/aesthes/ia _____
(Am. tricho/esthes/ia)

(d) schizo/**trich**/ia _____

(e) **tricho**/rrhexis _____

> **Root** **Seb**
> *(From a Latin word **sebum**, meaning fat or grease. It is used to mean sebum, the secretion of the sebaceous glands or sebaceous gland.)*
>
> Combining forms **Seb/o**

The sebaceous glands open directly on to the skin or more usually into the side of a hair follicle (a pilo**seb**aceous follicle). They produce an oily secretion, known as sebum, that lubricates and waterproofs the hair and skin. Sebum is mildly bacteriostatic and fungistatic enabling the skin to resist infection.

Excessive production of sebum at puberty gives rise to **acne vulgaris**, a condition in which the skin becomes inflamed and develops pus-filled pimples.

WORD EXERCISE 5

Using your Exercise Guide, find the meaning of:

(a) **sebo**/rrhoea _____
(Am. sebo/rrhea)

(b) **sebo**/lith _____

(c) **sebo**/tropic _____

> **Root** **Hidr**
> *(From a Greek word **hidros**, meaning sweat.)*
>
> Combining forms **Hidr/o**

WORD EXERCISE 6

Without using your Exercise Guide, write the meaning of:

(a) **hidr**/osis _____

(b) hyper/**hidr**/osis _____

Using your Exercise Guide, find the meaning of:

(c) **hidro**/poiesis _____

(d) an/**hidr**/osis _____

(e) **hidr**/aden/itis _____

Sweat glands are also known by their Latin name of sudoriferous glands (*sudor* meaning sweat, *ferous* meaning carrying).

> ## Root   Onych
> *(From a Greek word **onychos**, meaning nail.)*
>
> Combining forms   **Onych/o**

WORD EXERCISE 7

Using your Exercise Guide, find the meaning of:

(a) **onycho**/crypt/osis _____

(b) **onych**/auxis _____

(c) **onycho**/dys/trophy _____

(d) **onych**/a/trophy _____

(e) par/**onych**/ia _____

(f) **onycho**/schisis _____

(g) **onycho**/phagia _____

Without using your Exercise Guide, build words that mean:

(h) breaking down/disintegration _____
of nails
(Here the nail comes away from the nail bed.)

(i) fungal condition of nails _____

(j) inflammation of nails _____
(synonymous with **onych**ia)

Without using your Exercise Guide, write the meaning of:

(k) **onycho**/rrhexis _____

(l) an/**onych**/ia _____

(m) pachy/**onych**/ia _____

> ## Root   Melan
> *(From a Greek word **melanos**, meaning black. Here we are using it to mean melanin, a black pigment found in skin, hair and the choroid of the eye.)*
>
> Combining forms   **Melan/o**

WORD EXERCISE 8

Without using your Exercise Guide, build words that mean:

(a) a pigment cell _____

(b) abnormal condition of excessive _____
black/pigment

Without using your Exercise Guide, write the meaning of:

(c) **melan**/oma _____

Malignant melanoma is on the increase, and this is believed to be the effect of solar damage caused by excessive sunbathing. Sometimes melanomas develop from pigmented naevi (moles). They are highly malignant, and once the tumour cells have spread, they become difficult to eradicate. Malignant melanoma can be fatal unless treated early in its development. 5-year survival rate can be related to the depth of the tumour in the skin at first presentation.

Note.   Naevus (pl. naevi; Am. nevus, pl. nevi) is the medical name for a mole or birthmark on the body. Naevi arise from melanocytes or developmental abnormalities of blood vessels.

Medical equipment and clinical procedures

Suspicious lesions of skin need to be examined microscopically for signs of malignancy. Small samples of skin are removed during an excision **biopsy** (*bio* meaning life, *opsis* meaning vision, biopsy = observation of living tissue). These are then sectioned and stained in the histology laboratory. The biopsy tissue is examined by a histologist/pathologist to determine whether the cells are **benign** or **malignant** (benign means innocent/harmless; malignant means virulent and dangerous to life).

Benign lesions can be removed if they are causing a problem or are unsightly. Malignant lesions threaten life and are treated by surgical excision, radiotherapy and chemotherapy.

Treatment of skin disorders using lasers

Developments in physics have led to the development of medical **lasers** which are playing a prominent role in the treatment of skin disorders. Here we examine a selection of their applications to dermatology. First we need to understand the meaning of the acronym laser.

LASER is built from the first letter of each of the following words: **L**ight **A**mplification by **S**timulated **E**mission of **R**adiation.

A laser is a device that produces an intense, coherent beam of monochromatic light in the visible region. All the light waves in the beam are in phase and do not diverge so it can be targeted precisely (see Fig. 62). The beam is capable of focusing intense heat and power when focused at close range.

The medical laser transfers energy in the form of light to the tissues. When the laser beam strikes living tissue it is heated and destroyed (**thermolysis**) in a fraction of a second. Some lasers can heat tissues to over 100°C, resulting in their complete vaporization.

The extent of destruction of a tissue depends on the presence of chemicals in cells that absorb the light. These are known as **chromatophores**. There are three main chromatophores found in tissues: water, melanin and haemoglobin. A skin lesion containing a large amount of melanin, such as a mole, can be specifically targeted and destroyed by a laser with little destruction of the surrounding tissue.

There are many types of medical laser, each one emitting a beam of specific wavelength. The wavelength of the radiation emitted depends on the medium used by the laser, which may be a gas, liquid or solid. In the laser, the atoms of the medium are excited electrically and are stimulated to emit energy in the form of light. Besides laser light, other forms of radiation are used to treat chronic skin disorders. Here are three examples of lasers used by dermatologists:

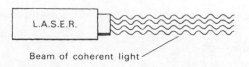

L.A.S.E.R.

Beam of coherent light

Figure 62   Laser

Treatment of psoriasis

Psoriasis is a common chronic skin condition in which there is an increased rate of production of skin cells. The excess skin cells form plaques of silvery scales that continuously flake off, exposing erythematous (reddened) skin that shows pinpoint bleeding. A large proportion of a dermatologist's time may be concerned with this disorder as it affects approximately 2% of the population. There is no cure and therapies are aimed at reducing the scaling and inflammation. A recent innovation is the technique known as:

PUVA (**P**soralen **U**ltra **V**iolet **A** light)

This is a form of **photochemotherapy** that uses a **psoralen** to sensitize the skin to light before it is irradiated with ultraviolet light (long wave A). After administration of the psoralen (taken orally) the patient is placed in a chamber illuminated with ultraviolet light. The treatment is convenient for patients; their skin shows dramatic improvement and the effect lasts for several months. Unfortunately, there is a risk of developing skin cancer because of excessive exposure to UVA; this risk is being evaluated.

WORD EXERCISE 9

Match each term in Column A with a description in Column C by placing an appropriate number in Column B.

Type of Laser	Medium	Wavelength	Chromatophore	Use
CO_2	Carbon dioxide gas	Infrared 10–600 nm	Water	Vaporizes/cuts tissue. Coagulates blood vessels. Bloodless surgery as it seals up cut vessels. Used to incise tissue and excise a variety of lesions
Argon	Ionized argon gas	Blue–green 488–514 nm	Melanin Haemoglobin	Penetrates epidermis and coagulates underlying pigments. Used to remove vascular and pigmented naevi (Am. nevi)
Dye	Various synthetic dyes	Can be tuned to any required wavelength	Melanin Haemoglobin	Removing tattoos. Removing pigmented tattoo inks, vascular lesions, moles, port wine stains, etc.

Column A	Column B	Column C
(a) excision biopsy	_____	1. removal of hair
(b) dermatome	_____	2. instrument that destroys tissue using a beam of coherent light
(c) medical laser	_____	3. destruction of tissue by heating with an electric current
(d) PUVA	_____	4. removal of living tissue from the body
(e) epilation	_____	5. instrument for cutting a thin layer of skin
(f) electrolysis	_____	6. technique of exposing photo-sensitized skin to light

ANATOMY EXERCISE

Now complete the Anatomy Exercise on page 136.

CASE HISTORY 11

The object of this exercise is to understand words associated with a patient's medical history.

To complete the exercise:

- read through the passage on psoriasis; unfamiliar words are underlined and you can find their meaning using the Word Help

- write the meaning of the medical terms shown in bold print.

Psoriasis

Mrs K, a 48-year-old woman, presented at the **dermatology** clinic with chronic plaque psoriasis and accompanying arthropathy. She had developed guttate psoriasis at the age of 12 following severe tonsillitis. This was self-limiting but shortly after psoriatic patches appeared on her legs and arms and then on the trunk. Since then the condition has persisted with exacerbations on her scalp, knees and arms, and over the last 5 years she has developed arthritis in her distal interphalangeal finger joints.

Mrs K's condition was reviewed by the **dermatologist**. She had developed large **hyperkeratotic** plaques on her trunk and extremities. Her scalp was also affected with some degree of erythema extending beyond the hair margin. Mrs K indicated that the severity of her arthritis

seemed to parallel the worsening of her **cutaneous lesions**.

Her nails were pitted with opaque yellow areas within the nail plates. Several nails were showing signs of **onycholysis** with **keratinous** debris under their free edges. Following assessment, Mrs K underwent a course of PUVA using 8-methoxypsoralen twice weekly for 6 weeks. She experienced drying of the skin and pruritus but showed considerable improvement. At the present she is receiving a single maintenance treatment every 3 weeks and her fair skin is being examined for presence of malignant **epitheliomas** (non-**melanoma** skin cancer being the major, slight, long-term risk factor).

WORD HELP

arthritis inflammation of the joints

arthropathy diseased joints

chronic pertaining to long term, continued

distal further away from point of attachment

erythema relating to erythema (reddening of the skin)

exacerbations increased severity of symptoms

guttate marked or covered with drop-like spots

interphalangeal pertaining to between the bones of the fingers or toes

lesion pathological change in a tissue

malignant dangerous, life threatening

8-methoxypsoralen a psoralen (drug) that sensitizes the skin to light

plaque flat area, a patch

pruritus itching

psoriasis chronic inflammatory disease of the skin exhibiting red patches in the epidermis covered with silvery scales

psoriatic pertaining to psoriasis

PUVA administration of a **p**soralen (a drug that sensitizes the skin to light) followed by exposure to **u**ltra**v**iolet light **A**

Now write the meaning of the following words from the case history without using your dictionary lists:

(a) dermatology _____

(b) dermatologist _____

(c) hyperkeratotic _____

(d) cutaneous _____

(e) onycholysis _____

(f) keratinous _____

(g) epithelioma _____

(h) melanoma _____

(Answers to the case history exercise are given in the Answers to Word Exercises beginning on page 275).

Quick Reference

Combining forms relating to the skin:

Acanth/o	spiny
Cutane/o	skin
Derm/at/o	skin/dermis
Epitheli/o	epithelium
Hidr/o	sweat
Hidraden/o	sweat gland
Ichthy/o	fish-like
Kerat/o	epidermis
Keratin/o	keratin
Melan/o	melanin
Onych/o	nail
Pil/o	hair
Seb/o	sebum/sebaceous gland
Squam/o	scaly
Trich/o	hair

Abbreviations

Some common abbreviations related to the skin are listed below. Note, however, some are not standard and their meaning may vary from one health care setting to another. There is a more extensive list for reference on page 307.

bx	biopsy
Derm	dermatology
Ez	eczema
KS	Karposi's sarcoma
SCC	squamous cell carcinoma
SED	skin erythema dose
SPF	sun protection factor
ST	skin test
STD	skin test dose
STU	skin test unit
Subcu	subcutaneous
ung	ointment (unguentum)

> ### NOW TRY THE WORD CHECK <

WORD CHECK

This self-check exercise lists all the word components used in this unit. First write down the meaning of as many word components as you can. Then check your answers using the Exercise Guide and Quick Reference box or the Glossary of Word Components (pp. 319–341).

Prefixes

a-	without
an-	without
auto-	self
crypto-	hidden
dys-	difficult/painful
epi-	above/upon
hyper-	above normal
hypo-	below normal
intra-	inside/within
pachy-	thick
para-	beside
sub-	below
xantho-	yellow
xero-	dry

Combining forms of word roots

acanth/o	spiny / spiky
aden/o	gland
aesthesi/o (Am. esthesi/o)	sensation
cutane/o	skin
cyt/o	cell
dermat/o	skin
epitheli/o	epithelium
hidr/o	sweat
ichthy/o	fish-like
kerat/o	epidermis
keratin/o	protein

lith/o	_stone_
melan/o	_melanin_
motor	_action_
myc/o	_fungus_
onych/o	_nail_
phyt(e)	
pil/o	_hair_
schizo-	
seb/o	_sebum_
squam/o	
trich/o	_hair_

Suffixes

-auxis	
-ia	_cond. of_
-ic	_pert. to_
-itis	_inflammation of_
-logist	_spec. who studies_
-logy	_study of_
-lysis	_breakdown/disintegration_
-oma	_tumour/swelling_
-osis	_ab. cond. of_
-ous	_pert. to_
-phagia	_cond. of eating_
-plasty	_surg. repair/reconstruction_
-poiesis	_formation_
-rrhexis	_break/rupture_
-rrhoea (Am. -rrhea)	_exc. flow/discharge_
-schisis	_splitting/parting_
-tic	_pert. to_

-tome	_cutting instrument_
-trophy	_nourishment_
-tropic	_pert. to stimulating_

> **NOW TRY THE SELF-ASSESSMENT** <

SELF-ASSESSMENT

Test 11A

Below are some combining forms that refer to the anatomy of the skin. Indicate which part of the system they refer to by putting a number from the diagram (Fig. 63) next to each word:

(a) hidraden/o _____

(b) seb/o _____

(c) trich/o _____

(d) melan/o _____

(e) kerat/o _____

(f) dermat/o _____

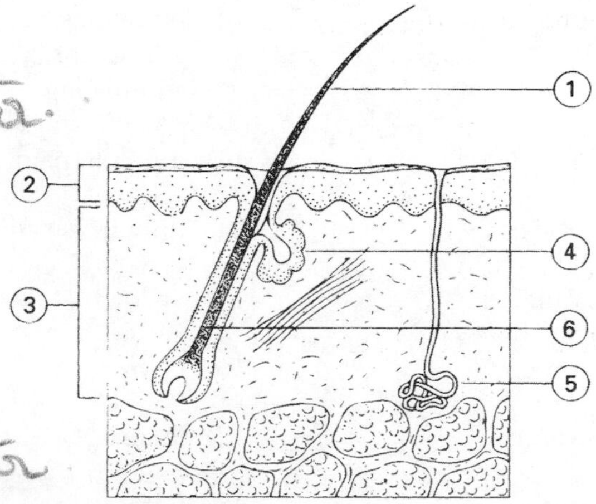

Figure 63 Section through the skin

Score

6

Test 11B

Prefixes and suffixes

Match each prefix or suffix in Column A with a meaning in Column C by inserting the appropriate number in Column B.

Column A	Column B	Column C
(a) a-		1. cutting instrument
(b) auto-		2. above
(c) -auxis		3. breakdown/ disintegration
(d) crypto-		4. within
(e) dys-		5. condition of eating/swallowing
(f) hyper-		6. thick
(g) hypo-		7. nourishment
(h) intra-		8. hidden/concealed
(i) -lysis		9. dry
(j) -oma		10. formation/ making
(k) pachy-		11. break/rupture
(l) -phagia		12. pertaining to affinity for/ stimulating
(m) -poiesis		13. difficult/painful
(n) -rrhexis		14. tumour/swelling
(o) -schizo		15. yellow
(p) -tome		16. below
(q) -trophy		17. increase
(r) -tropic		18. without/not
(s) xanth/o		19. self
(t) xer/o		20. split

Score

20

Test 11C

Combining forms of word roots

Match each combining form in Column A with a meaning in Column C by inserting the appropriate number in Column B.

Column A	Column B	Column C
(a) aden/o		1. horny/epidermis
(b) dermat/o		2. pertaining to action
(c) hidr/o		3. fungus
(d) kerat/o		4. hair (i)
(e) lith/o		5. hair (ii)
(f) motor		6. nail
(g) myc/o		7. skin
(h) onych/o		8. plant
(i) phyt/o		9. sweat
(j) pil/o		10. sebum
(k) seb/o		11. gland
(l) trich/o		12. stone

Score

12

Test 11D

Write the meaning of:

(a) dermatophytosis

(b) keratinocyte

(c) trichoanaesthesia (Am. trichoanesthesia)

(d) hidradenoma

(e) epidermomycosis

Score

5

Test 11E

Build words that mean:

(a) inflammation of the skin   _____

(b) abnormal condition of nails   _____

(c) condition of nails
     blackened with melanin   _____

(d) study of skin   _____

(e) condition of thick nails   _____

Score

5

Check answers to Self-Assessment Tests on page 299.

12 The nose and mouth

Objectives

Once you have completed Unit 12 you should be able to:

- understand the meaning of medical words relating to the nose and mouth

- build medical words relating to the nose and mouth

- associate medical terms with their anatomical position

- understand medical abbreviations relating to the nose and mouth.

Exercise guide

Use this list of word components and their meanings to complete the word exercises in this unit.

Prefixes

a-	without
dys-	difficult/painful
endo-	within/inside
intra-	inside
macro-	large
ortho-	straight/correct/normal
peri-	around
poly-	many
post-	after
prosth-	adding (replacement part)

Roots/Combining forms

aden/o	gland
aer/o	air/gas
angi/o	vessel
bronch/o	bronchi/bronchial tree
bucc/o	cheek
dynam/o	force
laryng/o	larynx
lith/o	stone
man/o	pressure
myc/o	fungus
nas/o	nose
ot/o	ear
pharyng/o	pharynx
trich/o	hair
tympan/o	middle ear/ear drum

Suffixes

-agogue	agent that induces/promotes
-al	pertaining to
-algia	condition of pain
-cele	swelling/protrusion/hernia
-dynia	condition of pain
-eal	pertaining to
-ectomy	removal of
-genic	pertaining to formation/originating in
-gram	X-ray tracing/picture/recording
-graphy	technique of recording/making an X-ray
-ia	condition of
-ic	pertaining to
-ist	specialist
-itis	inflammation of
-logy	study of
-meter	measuring instrument
-metry	process of measuring
-osis	abnormal condition/disease of
-pathy	disease of
-phagia	condition of eating
-phonia	condition of having voice
-phyma	tumour/boil
-plasty	surgical repair/reconstruction
-plegia	condition of paralysis
-rrhagia	condition of bursting forth (of blood)
-rrhaphy	suture/stitch/suturing
-rrhea (Am.)	excessive flow
-rrhoea	excessive flow
-schisis	cleaving/splitting/parting
-scope	viewing instrument
-scopy	technique of viewing/examining
-stomy	formation of an opening into ...
-tomy	incision into
-us	thing/structure/anatomical part

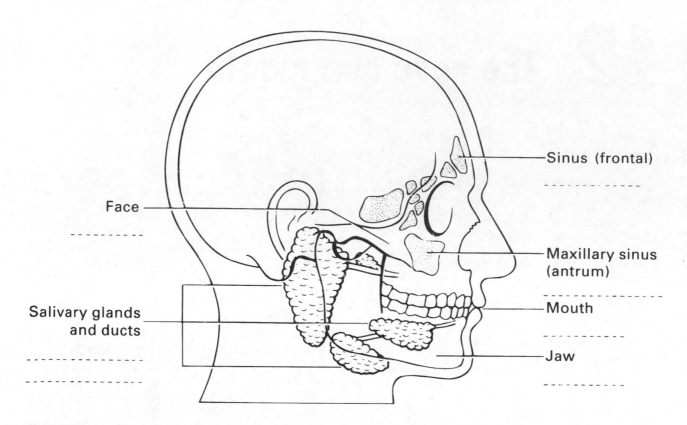

Face

Salivary glands
and ducts

Sinus (frontal)

Maxillary sinus
(antrum)

Mouth

Jaw

Figure 64   Sagittal section of the head showing sinuses and salivary glands

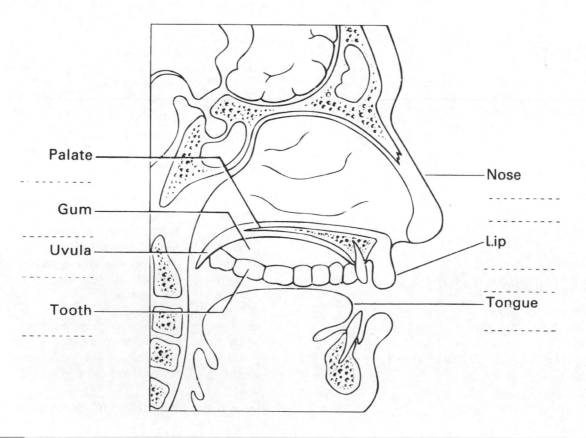

Palate

Gum

Uvula

Tooth

Nose

Lip

Tongue

Figure 65   Sagittal section of the nasal cavity

ANATOMY EXERCISE

When you have finished Word Exercises 1–18, look at the word components listed below. Complete Figures 64 and 65 by writing the appropriate combining form on each dotted line – more than one component may relate to the same position. (You can check their meanings in the Quick Reference box on p. 155.)

Antr/o	Labi/o	Sial/o
Cheil/o	Nas/o	Sin/o
Faci/o	Odont/o	Stomat/o
Gingiv/o	Palat/o	Uvul/o
Gloss/o	Ptyal/o	
Gnath/o	Rhin/o	

The nose and mouth

Receptors for the sense of smell are located in the olfactory epithelium which is in the roof of the nasal cavity. In order for us to smell a substance it must be volatile so it can be carried into the nose and then it must dissolve in the mucus covering the receptors. Humans can distinguish between 2000 and 4000 different odours.

Receptors for taste are located on the taste buds of the tongue. When a substance is eaten, four types of receptor can be stimulated, producing sensations for sweet, bitter, salty and sour. The sense of taste is known as gustation.

In this unit we will look at terms associated with the mouth and nose.

Use the Exercise Guide at the beginning of this unit to complete Word Exercises 1–18 unless you are asked to work without it.

Root | **Stomat**
*(From a Greek word **stomatos**, meaning mouth.)*

Combining forms **Stomat/o**

WORD EXERCISE 1

Using your Exercise Guide, find the meaning of:

(a) **stomato**/logy _____

(b) **stomato**/rrhagia _____

(c) **stomato**/pathy _____

Using your Exercise Guide, build words that mean:

(d) condition of pain in the mouth _____

(e) abnormal condition of fungi in the mouth _____

Root | **Or**
*(From a Latin word **oris**, meaning mouth.)*

Combining forms **Or/o**

WORD EXERCISE 2

Using your Exercise Guide, find the meaning of:

(a) **or**/al _____

(b) intra/**or**/al _____

(c) **oro**/pharyng/eal _____

(d) **oro**/nas/al _____

Root | **Gloss**
*(From a Greek word **glossa**, meaning tongue.)*

Combining forms **Gloss/o**

WORD EXERCISE 3

Without using your Exercise Guide, build words that mean:

(a) the study of the tongue _____

(b) condition of pain in the _____
tongue (use -dynia or -algia)

(c) pertaining to the pharynx _____
and tongue (use -eal)

Using your Exercise Guide, find the meaning of:

(d) **glosso**/plegia _____

(e) **glosso**/trich/ia _____

(f) **glosso**/cele _____

(g) macro/**gloss**/ia _____

(h) **glosso**/plasty _____

A Latin combining form **lingu/o** is also used to mean tongue, language or relationship to the tongue, e.g. **lingu**al – pertaining to the tongue, sub**lingu**al – under the tongue.

Disorders of the mouth, tongue, pharynx and palate give rise to problems with eating, swallowing and talking, e.g.

> **Dysphagia**
> A condition of difficulty in eating (from Greek *phagein* to eat).
>
> **Dyslalia**
> A condition of difficulty in talking (from Greek *lalein* to talk).

Root **Sial**
*(From a Greek word **sialon**, meaning saliva. It is also used to refer to salivary glands and ducts. Three pairs of salivary glands secrete saliva into the mouth. Saliva begins the digestion of starch in food.)*

Combining forms   **Sial/o**

 WORD EXERCISE 4

Using your Exercise Guide, find the meaning of:

(a) **sial**/aden/ectomy _____

(b) **sial**/angio/graphy _____

(c) poly/**sial**/ia _____

(d) **sialo**/gram _____

Using your Exercise Guide, build a word that means:

(e) stone in the saliva (duct or gland) _____

Using your Exercise Guide, find the meaning of:

(f) **sial**/agogue _____
(a drug)

(g) **sial**/aero/phagia _____

Root **Ptyal**
*(From a Greek word **ptyalon**, meaning saliva.)*

Combining forms   **Ptyal/o**

 WORD EXERCISE 5

Using your Exercise Guide, find the meaning of:

(a) **ptyalo**/genic _____

(b) **ptyalo**/rrhoea _____
(Am. ptyalo/rrhea)

Without using your Exercise Guide, write the meaning of:

(c) **ptyalo**/lith _____

Root **Gnath**
*(From a Greek word **gnathos**, meaning jaw.)*

Combining forms   **Gnath/o**

 WORD EXERCISE 6

Without using your Exercise Guide, build words that mean:

(a) condition of pain in the jaw _____

(b) plastic surgery of the jaw _____

(c) science dealing with the jaw/ _____
chewing apparatus

(d) pertaining to the jaw and mouth _____

Using your Exercise Guide, find the meaning of:

(e) **gnatho**/dynamo/meter _____

(f) **gnatho**/schisis _____
(refers to upper jaw and palate – a cleft palate)

(g) **gnath**/itis _____

Root | **Cheil**
*(From a Greek word **cheilos**, meaning lip.)*

Combining forms **Cheil/o**

WORD EXERCISE 7

Without using your Exercise Guide, write the meaning of:

(a) **cheilo**/stomato/plasty _____

(b) **cheilo**/schisis _____

Using your Exercise Guide, find the meaning of:

(c) **cheilo**/rrhaphy _____

Without using your Exercise Guide, build a word that means:

(d) inflammation of the lip _____

Root | **Labi**
*(From a Latin word **labium**, meaning lip.)*

Combining forms **Labi/o**

WORD EXERCISE 8

Using your Exercise Guide, find the meaning of:

(a) **labio**/glosso/laryng/eal _____

Without using your Exercise Guide, build a word that means:

(b) pertaining to pharynx, tongue and lips _____

Root | **Gingiv**
*(From a Latin word **gingiva**, meaning gum.)*

Combining forms **Gingiv/o**

WORD EXERCISE 9

Without using your Exercise Guide, build words that mean:

(a) inflammation of the gums _____

(b) removal of gum _____
(usually performed for pyorrhoea; Am. pyorrhea)

Without using your Exercise Guide, write the meaning of:

(c) labio/**gingiv**/al _____

Root | **Palat**
*(From Latin **palatum**. Here it refers to the palate.)*

Combining forms **Palat/o**

WORD EXERCISE 10

Without using your Exercise Guide, build words that mean:

(a) condition of paralysis of the soft palate _____

(b) pertaining to the jaw and palate _____

(c) split palate _____
(cleft palate)

Using your Exercise Guide, find the meaning of:

(d) post/**palat**/al _____

Root | **Uvul**
*(From a Latin word **uvula**, meaning grape. It refers to the uvula, the central tag-like structure extending downwards from the soft palate.)*

Combining forms **Uvul/o**

WORD EXERCISE 11

Without using your Exercise Guide, build a word that means:

(a) removal of the uvula _____

Without using your Exercise Guide, build a word that means:

(b) incision into the uvula _____

Root	Phas
	*(From a Greek word **phasis**, meaning speech.)*
Combining forms	**Phas/i/o**

WORD EXERCISE 12

Using your Exercise Guide, find the meaning of:

(a) a/**phas**/ia _____

(b) dys/**phas**/ia _____

There are many varieties and causes of aphasia. Common types are:

Motor aphasia
A condition due to an inability to move muscles involved in speech. (The word **aphonia** is also used to refer to a loss of voice.)

Sensory aphasia
A condition in which there is an inability to recognize spoken (or written) words.

Root	Odont
	*(From a Greek word **odontos**, meaning tooth.)*
Combining forms	**Odont/o**

WORD EXERCISE 13

(a) the scientific study of teeth (dentistry) _____

(b) any disease of teeth _____

(c) condition of toothache (pain) _____

Using your Exercise Guide, find the meaning of:

(d) peri/**odont**/ics _____
(includes all tissues supporting teeth)

(e) end/**odonto**/logy _____
(includes pulp and roots)

(f) orth/**odont**/ic(s) _____

(g) orth/**odont**/ist _____

(h) prosth/**odont**/ics _____

A prosthesis is any artificial replacement for a body part, in this case the replacement of lost teeth and associated structures.

Root	Rhin
	*(From a Greek word **rhinos**, meaning nose.)*
Combining forms	**Rhin/o**

We have already used **rhin/o** when studying the breathing system. Here we use the same combining form with new suffixes.

WORD EXERCISE 14

Using your Exercise Guide, find the meaning of:

(a) **rhino**/phonia _____

(b) **rhino**/mano/metry _____

(c) **rhino**/phyma _____

(d) **rhino**/scopy _____

(e) oto/**rhino**/laryngo/logy _____

Without using your Exercise Guide, write the meaning of:

(f) **rhino**/rrhagia _____
(also known as epistaxis)

Note. There is also a Latin word *nasus* meaning nose; its combining form **nas/o** is used in several exercises in this unit.

Root Sinus
(A Latin word meaning hollow/cavity. Here it is used to mean a sinus, a hollow cavity in a bone of the skull.)

Combining forms **Sin/o, sinus-**

WORD EXERCISE 15

Using your Exercise Guide, find the meaning of:

(a) **sin**/us _____

(b) **sino**/bronch/itis _____

Without using your Exercise Guide, write the meaning of:

(c) **sinus**/itis _____
(of the paranasal sinuses)

(d) **sino**/gram _____

Root Antr
*(From a Greek word **antron**, meaning cave. Here it refers to the superior maxillary sinus, the antrum of Highmore.)*

Combining forms **Antr/o**

WORD EXERCISE 16

Using your Exercise Guide, build words that mean:

(a) instrument to view the antrum _____

(b) inflammation of the tympanum and antrum _____

Without using your Exercise Guide, write the meaning of:

(c) **antro**/tomy _____
(usually performed to drain out infected fluid)

(d) **antro**/nas/al _____

(e) **antro**/cele _____

Using your Exercise Guide, find the meaning of:

(f) **antro**/bucc/al _____

(g) **antro**/stomy _____

Root Faci
*(From a Latin word **facies**, meaning face.)*

Combining forms **Faci/o**

WORD EXERCISE 17

Without using your Exercise Guide, write the meaning of:

(a) **faci**/al _____

(b) **facio**/plegia _____

(c) **facio**/plasty _____

Medical equipment and clinical procedures

Revise the names of all instruments and examinations used in this unit before completing Exercise 18.

WORD EXERCISE 18

Match each term in Column A with a description from Column C by placing an appropriate number in Column B.

Column A	Column B	Column C
(a) antroscope	_____	1. instrument that measures force of jaws
(b) sialangiography	_____	2. technique of recording the tongue (movement in speech)
(c) gnatho-dynamometer	_____	3. instrument for viewing maxillary antrum
(d) rhinomanometer	_____	4. an artificial part of the body, e.g. false tooth
(e) prosthesis	_____	5. technique of making an X-ray/recording of salivary ducts
(f) glossography	_____	6. instrument that measures air pressure in nose

ANATOMY EXERCISE

Now complete the Anatomy Exercise on page 149.

CASE HISTORY 12

The object of this exercise is to understand words associated with a patient's medical history.

To complete the exercise:

- read through the passage on acute sinusitis; unfamiliar words are underlined and you can find their meaning using the Word Help

- write the meaning of the medical terms shown in bold print.

Acute sinusitis

Mrs L, a 28-year-old mother, was brought into Accident and Emergency late at night by her husband concerned that she was seriously ill. She was recovering from a viral **rhinitis** when, on the morning of admission she was stricken with an excruciating frontal headache with pain in her cheek and upper teeth. She felt dizzy, and her right cheek was hot and tender to touch. There was no immediate history of any dental problems.

She was examined by the casualty registrar and found to have an elevated temperature and pulse. **Rhinoscopy** demonstrated reddened, oedematous mucous (Am. edematous) membranes and signs of a mucopurulent discharge from the middle meatus. Questioning of the patient revealed she had hyposmia and in the previous three days had become embarrassed by a cacosmia emanating from her nose.

A CT scan demonstrated fluid in her right maxillary sinus and excluded any orbital or intracranial involvement. A diagnosis of acute maxillary **sinusitis** was made by the registrar and she was prescribed decongestants and started on a course of antibiotic therapy. A sample of the discharge from her nose was sent to the microbiology laboratory for culture and sensitivity testing. Before leaving A and E she was given appropriate analgesia for her headache and referred to the department of **Otorhinolaryngology**.

Mrs L's follow up medical treatment with antibiotics and decongestants had limited success and her condition became chronic with a purulent nasal and **post-nasal** discharge. Pus from the maxillary sinus was removed by **antral** washout (antral lavage) following proof puncture through the nasal wall of the maxillary antrum. This was repeated on four occasions before the consultant advised surgery and the formation of an **intranasal antrostomy**. Functional endoscopic sinus surgery (FESS) was used to improve drainage of the maxillary sinus through its natural ostium.

Following her operation Mrs L showed great improvement; mucosal activity and the self-cleaning mechanism of her sinuses were restored.

WORD HELP

acute symptoms/signs of short duration

analgesia condition of without pain/prescribing of drugs that reduce pain

cacosmia condition of stench or unpleasant odour

chronic lasting/lingering for a long time

CT computed tomography

culture and sensitivity testing growing microorganisms in the laboratory and testing them for sensitivity to antibiotics

decongestant drug used for the relief of congestion

endoscopic pertaining to (using) an endoscope i.e. an instrument used to visually examine the body cavities

intracranial pertaining to within the cranium

hyposmia condition of reduced sense of smell (below normal)

maxillary sinus the sinus/antrum (air space) in the facial bone known as the maxilla

meatus a passage or opening

mucopurulent containing pus and mucus

mucosal pertaining to the mucosa (here the mucous membrane lining the maxillary sinus)

mucous pertaining to mucus (a viscous secretion)

oedematous pertaining to accumulation of fluid in a tissue (Am. edematous)

orbital pertaining to the orbit of the eye (bony eye-socket)

ostium a natural mouth or opening

proof evidence (here proving the antrum is infected)

purulent containing pus

Now write the meaning of the following words from the case history without using your dictionary lists:

(a) rhinitis _____

(b) rhinoscopy _____

(c) sinusitis _____

(d) otorhinolarygology _____

(e) post-nasal _____

(f) antral _____

(g) intranasal _____

(h) antrostomy _____

(Answers to the case history exercise are given in the Answers to Word Exercises beginning on page 275.)

Quick Reference

Combining forms relating to the nose and mouth:

Aden/o	gland
Antr/o	antrum/maxillary sinus
Bucc/o	cheek
Cheil/o	lip
Faci/o	face
Gingiv/o	gum
Gloss/o	tongue
Gnath/o	jaw
Labi/o	lip
Laryng/o	larynx
Lingu/o	tongue
Nas/o	nose
Odont/o	tooth
Or/o	mouth
Palat/o	palate
Phag/o	eating/consuming
Pharyng/o	pharynx
Ptyal/o	saliva/salivary gland/duct
Rhin/o	nose
Sial/o	saliva/salivary gland/duct
Sin/o	sinus
Sinus-	sinus
Stomat/o	mouth
Uvul/o	uvula

Abbreviations

Some common abbreviations related to the nose and mouth are listed below. Note, however, some are not standard and their meaning may vary from one health care setting to another. There is a more extensive list for reference on page 307.

dmft	decayed missing filled teeth (deciduous)
DMFT	decayed missing filled teeth (permanent)
ging	gingiva (gums)
La	labial (lips)
LaG	labia and gingiva (lips and gums)
NAS	nasal
NP	nasopharynx
NPO	non per os/nothing by mouth
odont	odontology
Os	mouth
po/PO	per os/by mouth
Subling	sublingual/under the tongue

▷ NOW TRY THE WORD CHECK ◁

WORD CHECK

This self-check exercise lists all the word components used in this unit. First write down the meaning of as many word components as you can. Then check your answers using the Exercise Guide and Quick Reference box or the Glossary of Word Components (pp. 319–341).

Prefixes

a- _____

dys- _____

endo- _____

intra- _____

macro- _____

ortho- _____

peri- _____

poly- _____

post- _____

prostho- _____

sub- _____

Combining forms of word roots

aden/o _____

aer/o _____

angi/o _____

antr/o _____

bronch/o _____

bucc/o _____

cheil/o _____

dynam/o _____

faci/o _____

gingiv/o _____

gloss/o _____

gnath/o _____

labi/o _____

laryng/o _____

lingu/o _____

lith/o _____

man/o _____

myc/o _____

nas/o _____

odont/o _____

or/o _____

ot/o _____

palat/o _____

phag/o _____

pharyng/o _____

ptyal/o _____

rhin/o _____

sial/o _____

sin/o, sinus- _____

stomat/o _____

trich/o _____

tympan/o _____

uvul/o _____

Suffixes

-agogue _____

-al _____

-algia _____

-cele _____

-dynia _____

-eal _____

-ectomy _____

-genic _____

-gram _____

-graphy _____

-ia _____

-ic _____

-ist _____

-itis _____

-lalia _____

-logy _____

-meter _____

-metry _____

-osis _____

-pathy _____

-phagia _____

-phasia _____

-phonia _____

-phyma _____

-plasty _____

-plegia _____

-rrhagia _____

-rrhaphy _____

-rrhoea (Am. -rrhea _____

-schisis _____

-scope _____

-scopy _____

-stomy _____

-tomy _____

-us _____

> **NOW TRY THE SELF-ASSESSMENT** <

 SELF-ASSESSMENT

Test 12A

Below are some combining forms that refer to the anatomy of the nose and mouth. Indicate which part of the system they refer to by putting a number from the diagrams (Figs 66 and 67) next to each word.

(a) gloss/o _____

(b) stomat/o _____

(c) cheil/o _____

(d) gingiv/o _____

(e) palat/o _____

(f) rhin/o _____

(g) odont/o _____

(h) faci/o _____

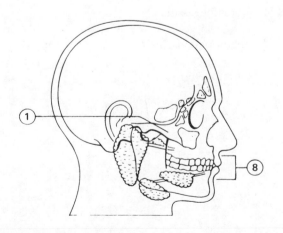

Figure 66 Sagittal section of the head showing sinuses and salivary glands

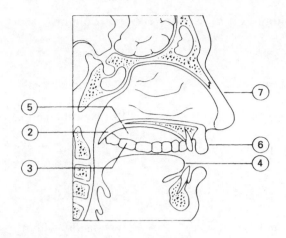

Figure 67 Sagittal section of the nasal cavity

Score

8

Test 12B

Prefixes and suffixes

Match the prefixes and suffixes in Column A with a meaning in Column C by inserting an appropriate number in Column B.

Column A	Column B	Column C
(a) -agogue	_____	1. condition of voice
(b) -cele	_____	2. split
(c) -dynia	_____	3. suturing/stitching
(d) -ectomy	_____	4. inflammation
(e) endo-	_____	5. condition of speech
(f) -itis	_____	6. condition of paralysis
(g) -logy	_____	7. straight
(h) -metry	_____	8. measurement
(i) ortho-	_____	9. disease
(j) -pathy	_____	10. condition of excessive flow (of blood)

Column A	Column B	Column C
(k) peri-	_____	11. many
(l) -phasia	_____	12. surgical repair
(m) -phonia	_____	13. condition of pain
(n) -plasty	_____	14. hernia/ protrusion/swelling
(o) -plegia	_____	15. removal of
(p) poly-	_____	16. inside/within
(q) prostho-	_____	17. study of
(r) -rrhagia	_____	18. around
(s) -rrhaphy	_____	19. inducing/ stimulating
(t) -schisis	_____	20. addition of artificial part

Score

20

Column A	Column B	Column C
(i) labi/o	_____	9. maxillary sinus/ antrum of Highmore
(j) laryng/o	_____	10. hair
(k) man/o	_____	11. mouth
(l) odont/o	_____	12. jaw
(m) palat/o	_____	13. cheek/inside mouth
(n) ptyal/o	_____	14. palate
(o) rhin/o	_____	15. lip (i)
(p) sial/o	_____	16. lip (ii)
(q) sin/o	_____	17. force
(r) stomat/o	_____	18. face
(s) trich/o	_____	19. saliva (i)
(t) uvul/o	_____	20. saliva (ii)

Score

20

Test 12C

Combining forms of word roots

Match each combining form in Column A with a meaning in Column C by inserting the appropriate number in Column B.

Column A	Column B	Column C
(a) antr/o	_____	1. gum
(b) bucc/o	_____	2. tooth
(c) cheil/o	_____	3. sinus
(d) dynam/o	_____	4. pressure (rare)
(e) faci/o	_____	5. larynx
(f) gingiv/o	_____	6. uvula
(g) gloss/o	_____	7. tongue
(h) gnath/o	_____	8. nose

Test 12D

Write the meaning of:

(a) glossodynamometer _____

(b) sialometry _____

(c) stomatoglossitis _____

(d) gnathopalatoschisis _____

(e) odontogenic _____

Score

5

Test 12E

Build words that mean:

(a) incision into a salivary gland (use sial/o) _____

(b) suturing of the palate _____

(c) condition of fungi in nose _____

(d) pertaining to the lips _____

(e) surgical repair of the palate _____

Score

5

Check answers to Self-Assessment Tests on page 299.

13 The muscular system

Objectives

Once you have completed Unit 13 you should be able to:

- understand the meaning of medical words relating to the muscular system

- build medical words relating to the muscular system

- associate medical terms with their anatomical position

- understand medical abbreviations relating to the muscular system.

Exercise Guide

Use this list of word components and their meanings to complete the word exercises in this unit.

Prefixes

dys-	difficult/disordered/painful
electro-	electrical
hyper-	above normal/excessive

Roots/Combining forms

aesthesi/o	sensation
cardi/o	heart
esthesi/o (Am.)	sensation
fibr/o	fibre
neur/o	nerve
paed/o	child
ped/o (Am.)	child
phren/o	diaphragm

Suffixes

-al	pertaining to
-algia	condition of pain
-ar	pertaining to
-genic	pertaining to formation/ originating in
-globin	protein
-gram	X-ray/tracing/recording
-graph	usually an instrument that records
-graphy	technique of recording/making an X-ray
-ia	condition of
-ic	pertaining to
-itis	inflammation of
-kymia	condition of involuntary twitching of muscle
-logy	study of
-lysis	breakdown/disintegration
-malacia	condition of softening
-meter	measuring instrument
-oma	tumour/swelling
-osis	abnormal condition/disease/ abnormal increase
-paresis	slight paralysis
-pathy	disease of
-plasty	surgical repair/reconstruction
-rrhaphy	suture/stitch/suturing
-rrhexis	break/rupture
-sclerosis	abnormal condition of hardening
-spasm	involuntary muscle contraction
-tome	cutting instrument
-tomy	incision into
-tonia	condition of tension/tone
-trophy	nourishment/development
-tropic	pertaining to affinity for/stimulating

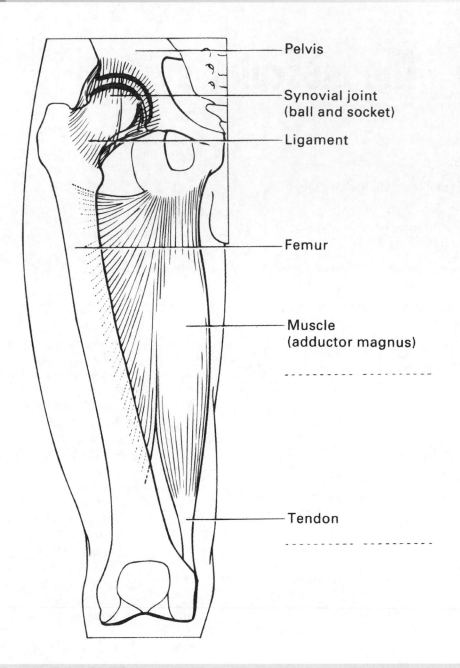

Pelvis

Synovial joint
(ball and socket)

Ligament

Femur

Muscle
(adductor magnus)

- - - - - - - - - - - - - - - - - -

Tendon

- - - - - - - - - - - - - - - - - -

Figure 68 Muscle arrangement in the thigh

ANATOMY EXERCISE

When you have finished Word Exercises 1–7, look at the word components listed below. Complete Figure 68 by writing the appropriate combining form on each dotted line – more than one component may relate to the same position. (You can check their meanings in the Quick Reference box on p. 166.)

Muscul/o   Tendin/o
My/o   Ten/o

The muscular system

Muscles compose 40–50% of the body's weight. The function of muscle is to effect the movement of the body as a whole and to move internal organs involved in the vital processes required to keep the body alive. There are three types of muscle tissue:

- Skeletal muscle – moves the vocal chords, diaphragm and limbs.
- Cardiac muscle – moves the heart.
- Smooth muscle – moves the internal organs, bringing about movement of food through the intestines and urine through the urinary tract. It is also found in the walls of blood vessels where it acts to maintain blood pressure.

Use the Exercise Guide at the beginning of this unit to complete Word Exercises 1–7 unless you are asked to work without it.

Root	**My**
	(From a Greek word **myos**, *meaning muscle.)*
Combining forms	**My/o, myos**

WORD EXERCISE 1

Using your Exercise Guide, find the meaning of:

(a) **myo**/neural ....

(b) **myo**/cardio/pathy ....

(c) **myo**/dys/trophy ....

(d) **myos**/itis ....

(e) **myo**/fibr/osis ....

Using your Exercise Guide, build words using my/o that mean:

(f) abnormal condition of hardening of a muscle ....

(g) tumour of a muscle ....

(h) muscle protein ....

(i) spasm of a muscle ....

The combining form **lei/o** (from Latin, meaning smooth) is added to myo to give **leiomy/o**, which refers to smooth muscle. A **leiomy**oma is a tumour/swelling of smooth muscle.

Using your Exercise Guide, find the meaning of:

(j) **myo**/kymia ....

(k) **myo**/tonia ....

(l) **myo**/paresis ....

(m) **myo**/rrhexis ....

(n) **myo**/malacia ....

The contraction of a muscle can be measured, using an instrument known as a **myo**graph.

Using your Exercise Guide, build words that mean:

(o) the technique of recording muscular contraction ....

(p) the technique of recording the electrical currents generated in muscular contraction ....

(q) trace/recording made by a myograph ....

Root	**Rhabd**
	(From a Greek word **rhabdos**, *meaning stripe. It is used with my/o when referring to striped/striated muscle.)*
Combining forms	**Rhabd/o**

WORD EXERCISE 2

Without using your Exercise Guide, write the meaning of:

(a) **rhabdo**/my/oma ....

Using your Exercise Guide, find the meaning of:

(b) **rhabdo**/myo/lysis ....

Root	**Muscul**
	(From a Latin word **musculus**, *meaning muscle.)*
Combining forms	**Muscul/o**

WORD EXERCISE 3

Using your Exercise Guide, find the meaning of:

(a) **musculo**/tropic ....

(b) **musculo**/phren/ic ....

Without using your Exercise Guide, write the meaning of:

(c) **muscul**/ar dys/trophy ....

Note. Loss or impairment of muscular movement due to a lesion in neural or neuromuscular mechanisms is known as a paralysis or palsy. A paresis is a partial paralysis and a pseudoparesis, a condition simulating paralysis (*pseudo-* meaning false). The latter is of hysterical (neurotic) origin and not due to organic disease within a muscle or nerve.

Root	**Kine** (From a Greek word **kinein**, meaning movement/motion.)
Combining forms	**Kine/s/i/o, kinet/o**

WORD EXERCISE 4

Using your Exercise Guide, find the meaning of:

(a) **kine**/aesthes/ia ....
    (Am. kin/esthes/ia)

(b) myo/**kinesi**/meter ....

(c) **kineto**/genic ....

(d) hyper/**kines**/ia ....

Without using your Exercise Guide, build a word using kines/o that means:

(e) condition of difficult/ ....
    painful movement

A Greek word *taxis* is sometimes used when describing an ordered movement in response to a stimulus. **Ataxia** refers to a disordered movement that is irregular and jerky (*a-* meaning without, i.e. condition of without normal movement). There are many types of ataxia, e.g. motor ataxia – an inability to control muscles; Friedreich's ataxia – an inherited movement disorder.

Root	**Ten** (From a Greek word **tenontos**, to stretch. It is used to mean tendon.)
Combining forms	**Ten/o, tenont/o** (Greek) **Tend/o, tendon/o, tendin/o** (Latin). Note that the combining forms **tend/o** and **tendin/o** are derived from Latin (**tendonis/tendines**, meaning tendon).

WORD EXERCISE 5

Using your Exercise Guide, find the meaning of:

(a) **ten**/algia ....

(b) **tendo**/tome ....

Without using your Exercise Guide, write the meaning of:

(c) **tendin**/itis ....

(d) **tenonto**/logy ....

Using your Exercise Guide, build words that mean:

(e) repair of a muscle and ....
    tendon (use ten/o)

(f) incision of a muscle and ....
    tendon (use ten/o)

A tendon is a fibrous non-elastic cord of connective tissue that is continuous with the fibres of a skeletal muscle; its function is to attach muscle to bone. Tendons must be strong in tension because they are used to pull bones and thereby move the body. If a tendon is wide and thin, it is known as an **aponeurosis**. This word is derived from *apo-* meaning detached/away from, *neuro-* tendon (also used to mean nerve) and *-osis* condition of.

Several words are used with **aponeur/o** meaning an aponeurosis.

Using your Exercise Guide, find the meaning of:

(g) **aponeuro**/rrhaphy ....

Without using your Exercise Guide, write the meaning of:

(h) **aponeur**/itis ....

Root	Orth
	(From a Greek word **orthos**, meaning straight)
Combining forms	**Orth/o**

WORD EXERCISE 6

Using your Exercise Guide, find the meaning of:

(a) **ortho**/paed/ic _____
(Am. ortho/ped/ic)
(Formerly this word just applied to the correction of deformities in children. It is now a branch of surgery dealing with all conditions affecting the locomotor system.)

Other common words related to this include:

> **Orthosis**
>   a structure/appliance used to correct a deformity.
>
> **Orthotics**
>   the knowledge of use of orthoses.

Medical equipment and clinical procedures

Revise the names of all instruments and examinations in this unit before completing Exercise 7.

WORD EXERCISE 7

Match each term in Column A with a description in Column C by placing an appropriate number in Column B.

Column A	Column B	Column C
(a) myography	_____	1. appliance used to straighten deformities of the locomotor system
(b) electromyography	_____	2. recording/trace of muscular movement
(c) myogram	_____	3. a recording of the electrical activity of muscle
(d) myokinesio-meter	_____	4. technique of recording electrical activity of muscle
(e) orthosis	_____	5. technique of making a recording of muscle (contraction)
(f) electromyo-gram	_____	6. instrument for measuring movement of muscle

ANATOMY EXERCISE

Now complete the Anatomy Exercise on page 162.

CASE HISTORY 13

The object of this exercise is to understand words associated with a patient's medical history.

To complete the exercise:

- read through the passage on Duchenne muscular dystrophy; unfamiliar words are underlined and you can find their meaning using the Word Help

- write the meaning of the medical terms shown in bold print.

Duchenne muscular dystrophy (DMD)

Miss M, a single parent, consulted her GP about her 4-year-old son R who appeared to have difficulty in climbing the stairs and running. Her son had been slow to sit up and walk and seemed less able than his peers. Her GP observed the child to have a 'waddling' gait and stand up by 'climbing up his legs' using his hands against his ankles, knees and thighs (Gower's sign). His calf muscles appeared to be bulky and lacking strength. He was referred to the Paediatric Hospital with suspected muscular **dystrophy**.

Detailed examination revealed R to have proximal weakness in his limbs and **pseudohypertrophy** of his calf muscles. A muscle biopsy showed **dystrophic** changes with muscle fibre necrosis and their replacement with fat. Immunochemical staining detected an absence of dystrophin. His serum creatine phosphokinase levels were grossly elevated. **Electromyography** indicated a **myopathic** pattern with short polyphasic action potentials.

R's mother was also investigated and also found to have raised serum creatine phosphokinase levels and an abnormal **electromyogram**. R was diagnosed as having Duchenne muscular dystrophy, a fatal sex-linked condition inherited from his mother. DMD is due to a mutant gene located on the X-chromosome and as there appeared to be no previous incidence of this condition in the family, it was likely this was a spontaneous mutation. Miss M was advised by the genetics counsellor that she was a carrier of DMD and if she produced another boy there was a 50% chance that he would also have DMD.

By the age of 10 R was severely disabled and receiving daily passive physiotherapy to help prevent contractures of his muscles. At 14 he was unable to move his arms and legs and his limb bones were long and thin (disuse **atrophy**). He died at the age of 16 from **myocardial** involvement and pulmonary infection.

WORD HELP

action potential electrochemical impulse generated by a muscle or nerve

biopsy removal and examination of living tissue

contractures abnormal shortening/contraction of muscle

dystrophin an essential structural protein found in muscle fibres

gait manner of walking

GP general practitioner (family doctor)

immunochemical pertaining to chemical basis of immunity

mutant gene that has changed from normal form resulting in a change to the organism inheriting it

mutation sudden change in the genetic material of cells (in this case in the mother's sex cells)

necrosis condition of localized death of tissue

passive not produced by the active effort of (the patient)

physiotherapy treatment using physical means to maintain or build physique or correct deformities due to injury or disease (AM. physical therapy)

polyphasic pertaining to many phases (here electrical potentials out of phase)

proximal near to origin/point of attachment

pulmonary pertaining to the lungs

serum clear fluid separated from blood when it is allowed to clot

sex-linked gene linked to a sex-chromosome (may result in increased frequency of certain disorders in one particular sex e.g. DMD affects boys only)

X-chromosome one of a pair of sex chromosomes that determine the sex of an individual

Now write the meaning of the following words from the case history without using your dictionary lists:

(a) dystrophy

(b) pseudohypertrophy

(c) dystrophic

(d) electromyography

(e) myopathic

(f) electromyogram

(g) atrophy

(h) myocardial

(Answers to the case history exercise are given in the Answers to Word Exercises beginning on page 275.)

Quick Reference

Combining forms relating to the muscular system:

Aponeur/o	aponeurosis
Fibr/o	fibre
Kinesi/o	movement
Lei/o	smooth (muscle)
Muscul/o	muscle
My/o	muscle
Paed/o	child
Ped/o (Am.)	child
Rhabd/o	striated (muscle)
Tax/o	ordered movement
Tendin/o	tendon
Tend/o	tendon
Ten/o	tendon
Tenont/o	tendon

Abbreviations

Some common abbreviations related to the muscular system are listed below. Note, however, some are not standard and their meaning may vary from one health care setting to another. There is a more extensive list for reference on page 307.

DTR	deep tendon reflex
EMG	electromyogram/electromyography
im	intramuscular
IMHP	intramuscular high potency
MAMC	mid-arm muscle circumference
MAP	muscle action potential
MD	muscular dystrophy
MFT	muscle function test
MNJ	myoneural junction
MS	muscle shortening/strength/musculoskeletal
Ortho	orthopaedics (Am. orthopedics)
TJ	triceps jerk

NOW TRY THE WORD CHECK

WORD CHECK

This self-check exercise lists all the word components used in this unit. First write down the meaning of as many word components as you can. Then check your answers using the Exercise Guide and Quick Reference box or the Glossary of Word Components (pp. 319–341).

Prefixes

a- — without

dys- — difficult/painful

electro- — electrical

hyper- — above normal

ortho- — straight

pseudo- — false

Combining forms of word roots

aesthesi/o (Am. esthesi/o) — feeling

aponeur/o — cond. of detached tendon

cardi/o — heart

fibr/o — fibre

kinesi/o — movement

lei/o — smooth muscle

muscul/o — muscle

my/o — muscle

neur/o — tendon / nerve

paed/o (Am. ped/o) — child

phren/o — diaphragm

rhabd/o — striated muscle

tax/o — ordered movement

tendin/o — tendon

tend/o — tendon

ten/o — tendon

tenont/o — tendon

Suffixes

-al — pert. to

-algia — cond. of pain

-genic — pert. to formation

-globin — protein

-gram — x-ray/recording

-graph — instrument to record

-graphy — tech. of recording

-ic — pert. to

-itis — inflammation of

-kymia — cond. of involuntary twitching of muscle

-logy — study of

-lysis — breakdown/disintegration

-meter — inst. to measure

-oma — tumour/swelling

-osis — ab. cond. of

-paresis — partial paralysis

-pathy — disease of

-rrhaphy — suture/stitching

-rrhexis — break/rupture

-sclerosis — ab. cond. of hardening

-spasm — involuntary muscle contraction

-taxia — cond. of ordered movement

-tome — cutting instrument

-tonia — cond. of tension/tone

-trophy — nourishment

-tropic — pert. to stimulating

> **NOW TRY THE SELF-ASSESSMENT** <

SELF-ASSESSMENT

Test 13A

Prefixes, suffixes and combining forms of word roots

Match each word component from Column A with a meaning in Column C by inserting the appropriate number in Column B.

Column A	Column B	Column C
(a) aesthesi/o (Am. esthesi/o)	18	1. child
(b) cardi/o	15	2. movement
(c) electro-	8	3. tumour/ swelling
(d) fibr/o	13	4. diaphragm
(e) -globin	9	5. slight paralysis/ weakness
(f) kinesi/o	2	6. rupture/ break
(g) muscul/o	16/17	7. condition of hardening
(h) my/o	17/16	8. electrical
(i) -oma	3	9. protein
(j) ortho-	19	10. involuntary contraction of muscle
(k) paed/o (Am. ped/o)	1	11. condition of continuous slight contraction of muscle
(l) paresis	5	12. nourishment
(m) phren/o	4	13. fibre
(n) -rrhexis	6	14. pertaining to affinity for/ acting on

Column A	Column B	Column C
(o) -sclerosis	7	15. heart
(p) -spasm	10	16. muscle (i)
(q) ten/o	20	17. muscle (ii)
(r) -tonia	11	18. sensation
(s) -trophy	12	19. straight
(t) -tropic	14	20. tendon

Score

20

Test 13B

Write the meaning of:.

(a) electromyograph *instr to record electrical activity of muscle*

(b) kinesiology *study of movement*

(c) myotenotomy *incision into tendon + muscle*

(d) myoatrophy *without nourishment of muscle*

(e) musculoaponeurotic *pert t. an aponeurosis + muscle*

Score

5

Test 13C

Build words that mean:

(a) condition of softening of muscle *myomalacia*

(b) pertaining to originating in muscle *myotropic*

(c) disease of muscle *myopathy*

(d) suturing of a tendon (use ten/o) *tenorrhaphy*

(e) cutting of a tendon (use ten/o) *tenotomy*

Score

5

Check answers to Self-Assessment Tests on page 299.

14 The skeletal system

Objectives

Once you have completed Unit 14 you should be able to:

- understand the meaning of medical words relating to the skeletal system

- build medical words relating to the skeletal system

- associate medical terms with their anatomical position

- understand medical abbreviations relating to the skeletal system.

Exercise Guide

Use this list of word components and their meanings to complete the word exercises in this unit.

Prefixes

dys-	bad/difficult/painful
endo-	within/inside
poly-	many

Roots/Combining forms

calcin/o	calcium
cost/o	rib
fibr/o	fibre
lith/o	stone
my/o	muscle
petr/o	stone/rock (brittle)
por/o	pore
py/o	pus

Suffixes

-al	pertaining to
-algia	condition of pain
-blast	cell that forms … /immature germ cell
-centesis	puncture to remove fluid
-clasis	breaking
-clast	a cell that breaks
-desis	fixation/bind together by surgery
-eal	pertaining to
-ectomy	removal of
-genesis	capable of causing/forming
-genic	pertaining to formation/originating in
-gram	X-ray/tracing/recording
-graphy	technique of recording/making an X-ray
-ic	pertaining to
-itis	inflammation of
-logist	specialist who studies …
-lysis	breakdown/disintegration
-lytic	pertaining to breakdown/disintegration
-malacia	condition of softening
-oid	resembling
-olisthesis	slipping
-oma	tumour/swelling
-osis	abnormal condition/disease/abnormal increase
-ous	pertaining to/of the nature of
-pathy	disease of
-phyte	plant/plant-like growth
-plasty	surgical repair/reconstruction
-scope	viewing instrument
-scopy	visual examination
-tome	cutting instrument
-trophy	nourishment/development

Details of synovial
joint

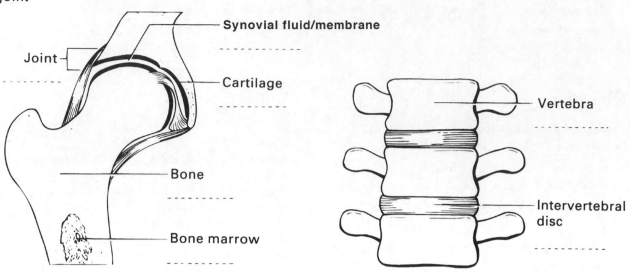

Figure 69   Joints

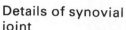

ANATOMY EXERCISE

When you have finished Word Exercises 1–10, look at the word components listed below. Complete Figure 69 by writing the appropriate combining form on each dotted line. (You can check their meanings in the Quick Reference box on p. 176.)

Arthr/o   Myel/o   Spondyl/o
Chondr/o   Oste/o   Synovi/o
Disc/o

The skeletal system

The supporting structure of the body consisting of 206 bones is known as the skeletal system. This system has five main functions:

- it supports all tissues
- it protects vital organs and soft tissues
- it manufactures blood cells
- it stores minerals that can be released into the blood
- it assists in movement.

Cartilage is found at the ends of bones and functions to form a smooth surface for the movement of one bone over another at a joint. In joints, bones are held together by tough fibrous connective tissues called ligaments. (The function of ligaments is to connect bone to bone.)

Use the Exercise Guide at the beginning of this unit to complete Word Exercises 1–10 unless you are asked to work without it.

Root   Oste
(From a Greek word **osteon**, *meaning bone.)*

Combining forms   **Oste/o**

WORD EXERCISE 1

Using your Exercise Guide, find the meaning of:

(a) **osteo**/phyte _____
(refers to a bony outgrowth at joint surface)

(b) **osteo**/por/osis _____
(refers to loss of calcium/phosphorus/bone density)

(c) **osteo**/petr/osis _____
(refers to spotty calcification of bone, which becomes brittle)

(d) **osteo**/clasis _____

(e) **osteo**/clast _____
(a type of cell, compare with osteoblast)

(f) **osteo**/dys/trophy _____

Using your Exercise Guide, build words that mean:

(g) a cell that forms bone _____

(h) pertaining to breaking down of bone _____

(i) instrument to cut bone _____

(j) specialist who studies bones _____

(*Osseus* is a Latin word meaning of bone. It is used in **osse**ous, meaning pertaining to bone/of the nature of bone, and **oss**ification, meaning to form bone.)

Root	Arthr
	(From a Greek word **arthron**, meaning joint or articulation, i.e. the point where two or more bones meet.)

Combining forms   **Arthr/o**

WORD EXERCISE 2

Using your Exercise Guide, find the meaning of:

(a) **arthro**/endo/scope _____

(b) **arthro**/py/osis _____

(c) **arthro**/graphy _____

(d) poly/**arthr**/itis _____

Rheumatoid arthritis refers to a polyarthritis accompanied by general ill health and varying degrees of crippling joint deformities, pain and stiffness (*rheumat/o* refers to rheumatism, a condition marked by inflammation, degeneration and metabolic disturbance of connective tissues especially those associated with joints).

(e) **arthro**/desis _____
(Also known as an artificial **ankylosis** (from Greek *agkylos* meaning bent/fusion). An arthrodesis is achieved by surgery; see Fig. 70.)

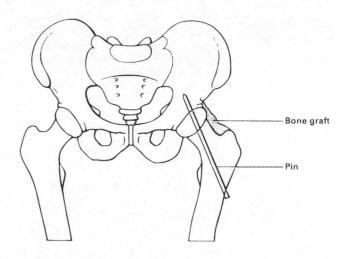

Bone graft

Pin

Figure 70	Arthrodesis of hip

Without using your Exercise Guide, write the meaning of:

(f) **arthro**/clasis _____

Using your Exercise Guide, build words that mean:

(g) technique of viewing a joint _____

(h) puncture of a joint _____

(i) X-ray picture of a joint _____

(j) disease of a joint _____

(k) stony material in a joint _____

(l) surgical repair of a joint _____
(This operation includes the formation of artificial joints, e.g. in a hip replacement where the natural joint is replaced with a metallic prosthesis; Fig. 71.)

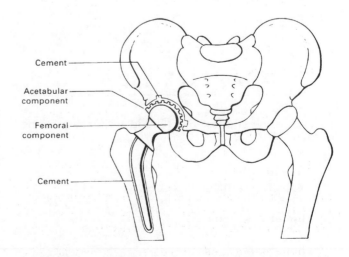

Cement

Acetabular component

Femoral component

Cement

Figure 71	Arthroplasty

Root

Synovi
*(From a New Latin word **synovia**, meaning the fluid secreted by the synovial membrane that lines the cavity of a joint. Here the combining form is used to mean synovial membrane.)*

Combining forms   **Synovi/o**

WORD EXERCISE 3

Without using your Exercise Guide, write the meaning of:

(a) arthro/**synov**/itis _____

Using your Exercise Guide, find the meaning of:

(b) **synov**/ectomy _____

(c) **synovi**/oma _____

Bursae are sacs of synovial fluid surrounded by a synovial membrane. They are found between tendons, ligaments and bones. Inflammation due to pressure, injury or infection results in **burs**itis (from Latin *bursa*, meaning purse).

 Root

Chondr
*(From a Greek word **chondros**, meaning cartilage, the plastic-like connective tissue found at the ends of bones, e.g. in joints where it forms a smooth surface for movement of a joint.)*

Combining forms   **Chondr/o**

WORD EXERCISE 4

Without using your Exercise Guide, write the meaning of:

(a) **chondro**/phyte _____
     (actually a cartilaginous growth)

(b) **chondr**/osse/ous _____

(c) **chondro**/por/osis _____

(d) **chondro**/dys/trophy _____

Using your Exercise Guide, find the meaning of:

(e) **chondro**/cost/al _____

(f) endo/**chondr**/al _____

Using your Exercise Guide, build words that mean:

(g) condition of pain in a
     cartilage _____

(h) condition of softening
     of cartilage _____

(i) formation of cartilage _____

(j) breakdown of cartilage _____

Using your Exercise Guide, find the meaning of:

(k) **chondro**/calcin/osis _____

A cartilage which is often damaged and removed is the crescent-shaped cartilage in the knee joint. The operation to remove this cartilage is known as **menisc**ectomy (from Latin *meniscus*, meaning crescent; combining forms **menisc/o**).

 Root

Spondyl
*(From Greek word **spondylos**, meaning vertebra or vertebral column.)*

Combining forms   **Spondyl/o**

WORD EXERCISE 5

Without using your Exercise Guide, write the meaning of:

(a) **spondyl**/algia _____

(b) **spondylo**/py/osis _____

Without using your Exercise Guide, build words that mean:

(c) breakdown/disintegration
     of vertebrae _____

(d) any disease of vertebrae _____

Using your Exercise Guide, find the meaning of:

(e) **spondyl**/olisthesis _____
     (this applies to lumbar vertebrae)

Here we need to mention three other conditions of the vertebrae:

Kyphosis
An abnormally curved spine (as viewed from the side), commonly called hunch/humpback or dowager's hump. (**Kyph/o** is from Greek *kyphos*, meaning crooked/hump.) See Figure 72(a).

Scoliosis
A lateral curvature of the vertebral column. (**Scoli/o** is from a Greek word *scoli*, meaning crooked/twisted.) See Figure 72(b).

Lordosis
A forward curvature of the spine in the lumbar region (from a Greek word meaning to bend the body forward).

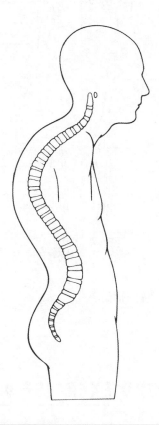

Figure 72   (a) Kyphosis

Two of these words can be combined as in:

Scoliokyphosis } both meaning lateral and
Kyphoscoliosis } posterior curvature of the spine.

Root   **Disc**
*(From a Latin word **diskus**, meaning disc. It refers to pads of connective tissue that act as shock absorbers between vertebrae, i.e. intervertebral discs.)*

Combining forms   **Disc/o, Disk/o (Am.)**

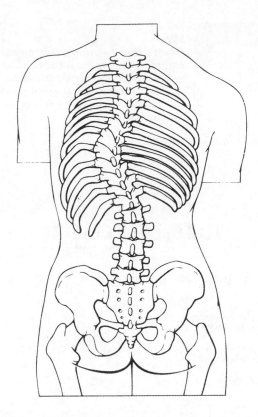

Figure 72   (b) Scoliosis

 WORD EXERCISE 6

Using your Exercise Guide, find the meaning of:

(a) **disc**/oid   _____

(b) **disco**/genic   _____

Without using your Exercise Guide, build words that mean:

(c) technique of making   _____
an X-ray of an
intervertebral disc

(d) removal of an   _____
intervertebral disc

The excision of degenerated intervertebral discs requires the removal of a thin layer of bone from the vertebral arch. This operation is termed a **lamin**ectomy (from Latin *lamina*, meaning thin plate; combining forms **lamin/o**).

Root | **Myel**
*(From a Greek word **myelos**, meaning marrow. Here we use it to mean the marrow of bones. Remember we have already used this root in reference to the spinal marrow and blood cells of the marrow cavities.)*

Combining forms **Myel/o**

WORD EXERCISE 7

Without using your Exercise Guide, write the meaning of:

(a) osteo/**myel**/itis _____

(b) **myelo**/fibr/osis _____

Medical equipment and clinical procedures

Revise the names of all instruments and clinical procedures used in this unit and then try Exercise 8.

WORD EXERCISE 8

Match each term in Column A with a description from Column C by placing an appropriate number in Column B.

Column A	Column B	Column C
(a) osteotome	4	1. puncture of a joint to withdraw synovial fluid
(b) arthrodesis	3	2. technique of making an X-ray of a joint
(c) replacement arthroplasty	5	3. fixation of a joint by surgery
(d) arthrocentesis	1	4. chisel-like instrument used to cut bone
(e) arthrography	2	5. insertion of a metallic prothesis to replace a joint

The skeleton

There are many terms that refer to specific bones within the skeleton. Look at the diagram (Fig. 73) and then complete Exercises 9 and 10.

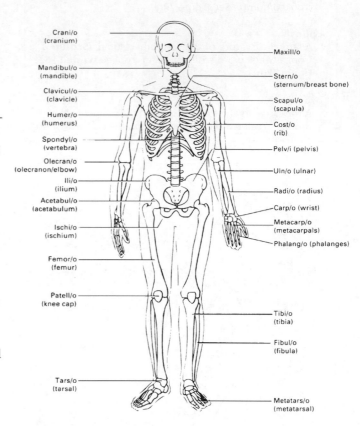

Figure 73 The skeleton

WORD EXERCISE 9

Without using your Exercise Guide, build words that mean:

(a) surgical repair/reconstruction of the collar bone   *claviculoplasty*

(b) condition of softening of the cranium   *craniomalacia.*

(c) pertaining to between the ribs   *intercostal*

(d) removal of a finger   *phalangectomy.*

(e) pertaining to the pelvis   *pelvic*

(f) inflammation of an elbow joint   *olecranarthritis.*

(g) pertaining to the femur and tibia   *tibiofemoral*

(h) surgical fixation of the scapula   *scapulodesis*

(i) condition of pain in the
metatarsal region   *metatarsalgia*

(j) surgical operation to reconstruct
the hip socket   *acetabuloplasty*

WORD EXERCISE 10

Using your Exercise Guide and Fig. 73, find the meaning of:

(a) inter/**phalang**/eal   _____

(b) **metatars**/algia   _____

(c) tarso/**metatars**/al   _____

(d) **metacarp**/al   _____

ANATOMY EXERCISE

Now complete the Anatomy Exercise on page 170.

CASE HISTORY 14

The object of this exercise is to understand words associated with a patient's medical history.

To complete the exercise:

- read through the passage on rheumatoid arthritis; unfamiliar words are underlined and you can find their meaning using the Word Help

- write the meaning of the medical terms shown in bold print.

Rheumatoid arthritis

Mrs N, a 58-year-old female, was referred to the **rheumatologist** by her GP with a generalized **arthralgia** and aggravating symptoms in her left shoulder. Her GP prescribed NSAIDs for 7 weeks bringing some relief. Five years previously she had a **bursitis** in the same shoulder that had been successfully treated. There was no history of rheumatoid arthritis in her family.

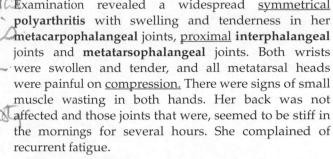

Examination revealed a widespread symmetrical **polyarthritis** with swelling and tenderness in her **metacarpophalangeal** joints, proximal **interphalangeal** joints and **metatarsophalangeal** joints. Both wrists were swollen and tender, and all metatarsal heads were painful on compression. There were signs of small muscle wasting in both hands. Her back was not affected and those joints that were, seemed to be stiff in the mornings for several hours. She complained of recurrent fatigue.

Mrs N had diminished movement of the chest with dullness on percussion; breath sounds were absent at the right base.

Joint radiography indicated an erosion in the 3rd metatarsophalangeal joint and a CXR confirmed a right sided pleural effusion. Haematology reported a high rheumatoid factor. A diagnosis of erosive rheumatoid arthritis with pleural effusion was made. Initial treatment of her inflammatory **arthropathy** was enteric coated aspirin 4 g/day; she was advised of possible side effects.

WORD HELP

aggravating making worse

base here it refers to the base/lower part of the right lung

compression pressing

CXR chest X-ray

effusion a fluid discharge into a part/escape of fluid into an enclosed space

enteric pertaining to the intestine, here refers to a coating on a pill or tablet that allows it to pass to the intestine without being affected in the stomach

erosion destruction (here of a piece of bone)

GP general practitioner (family doctor)

haematology the study of blood, here refers to the department that analyses blood

NSAID non-steroid anti-inflammatory drug

percussion striking the body to produce a sound (here striking the thoracic wall)

pleural pertaining to the pleura (membranes that surround the lungs)

proximal near to origin/point of attachment

radiography technique of making an X-ray/recording

rheumatoid resembling rheumatism (a painful condition marked by inflammation and degeneration of connective tissues especially around joints)

rheumatoid factor type of antibody found in the sera of patients with rheumatoid arthritis

symmetrical correspondence on opposite sides of the body/ equality of parts on either side of the midline of the body

Now write the meaning of the following words from the case history without using your dictionary lists:

(a) rheumatologist   _____

(b) arthralgia   _____

(c) bursitis

(d) polyarthritis

(e) metacarpophalangeal

(f) interphalangeal

(g) metatarsophalangeal

(h) arthropathy

(Answers to the case history exercise are given in the Answers to Word Exercises beginning on page 275.)

Quick Reference

Combining forms relating to the skeletal system:

Ankyl/o	fusion/adhesion/bent
Arthro	joint
Burs/o	bursa
Calcin/o	calcium
Chondr/o	cartilage
Cost/o	rib
Disc/o	intervertebral disc
Fibr/o	fibre
Kyph/o	crooked/humped
Lamin/o	lamina/part of vertebral arch
Lord/o	bend forward
Menisc/o	meniscus
Myel/o	bone marrow
Osse/o	bone
Oste/o	bone
Petr/o	stone/rock
Por/o	passage/pore
Scoli/o	crooked/twisted
Spondyl/o	vertebra
Synovi/o	synovial fluid/membrane

Abbreviations

Some common abbreviations related to the skeletal system are listed below. Note, however, some are not standard and their meaning may vary from one health care setting to another. There is a more extensive list for reference on page 307.

BM(T)	bone marrow trephine
C 1–7	cervical vertebrae 1–7

Abbreviations (Contd.)

CDH	congenital dislocation of the hip
Fx	fracture
L 1–5	lumbar vertebrae 1–5
OA	osteoarthritis
Osteo	osteomyelitis
PID	prolapsed intervertebral disc
RA	rheumatoid arthritis
RF (RhF)	rheumatoid factor
T 1–12	thoracic vertebrae 1–12
THR	total hip replacement

⟩ NOW TRY THE WORD CHECK ⟨

WORD CHECK

This self-check exercise lists all the word components used in this unit. First write down the meaning of as many word components as you can. Then check your answers using the Exercise Guide and Quick Reference box or the Glossary of Word Components (pp. 319–341).

Prefixes

dys-   *difficult/painful*

endo-   *inside/within*

inter-   *between*

poly-   *many*

Combining forms of word roots

ankyl/o   *fusion/bent*

arthro   *joint*

burs/o   *bursa*

calcin/o   *calcium*

chondr/o   *cartilage*

cost/o   *ribs*

disc/o   *disc*

fibr/o   *fibre*

kyph/o — crooked/humped.

lamin/o — lamina.

lith/o — stone

lord/o — bend forward

menisc/o — meniscus

myel/o — bone marrow

osse/o — bone

oste/o — bone

petr/o — stone/rock

phyt/o — plant/plant-like growth

por/o — pore/passage.

py/o — pus

rheumat/o — rheumatism

scoli/o — crooked/twisted

spondyl/o — vertebra

synovi/o — synovial fluid/membrane

-graphy — tech. of recording

-ic — pert. to

-itis — infl. of.

-logist — spec. who studies

-lysis — breakdown/disintegration

-lytic — pert. to breakdown.

-malacia — cond. of softening

-oid — resembling

-olisthesis — slipping

-oma — tumour/swelling

-osis — abs cond. of.

-pathy — disease of

-plasty — surg. rec.

-scope

-scopy

-tome

-trophy

Suffixes

-al — pert. to

-algia — cond. of pain.

-blast — immature germ cell.

-centesis — surg. puncture to remove fluid

-clasis — breaking.

-clast — a cell that breaks.

-desis — fixation (by surgery)

-eal — pert. to.

-ectomy — removal of.

-genesis — formation

-genic — pert. to formation

-gram — x-ray/recording

Combining forms referring to specific parts of the skeleton

acetabul/o

carp/o

clavicul/o

cost/o

crani/o

femor/o

fibul/o

humer/o

ili/o

ischi/o

mandibul/o

maxill/o

metacarp/o

metatars/o

olecran/o

patell/o

pelv/i

phalang/o

radi/o

scapul/o

spondyl/o

stern/o

tars/o

tarsometatars/o

tibi/o

uln/o

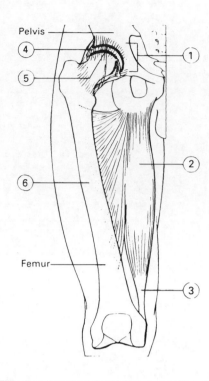

Figure 74   Muscle and skeletal arrangement in the thigh

Score

6

> **NOW TRY THE SELF-ASSESSMENT** <

SELF-ASSESSMENT

Test 14A

Below are some combining forms that refer to the anatomy of the skeletal system and its movement. Indicate which part of the system they refer to by putting a number from the diagram (Fig. 74) next to each word.

(a) synovi/o

(b) tendin/o

(c) my/o

(d) arthr/o

(e) oste/o

(f) chondr/o

Test 14B

Prefixes and suffixes

Match each prefix or suffix in Column A with a meaning in Column C by inserting the appropriate number in Column B.

Column A	Column B	Column C
(a) -al		1. resembling
(b) -algia		2. tumour/swelling
(c) -blast		3. slipping/ dislocation
(d) -centesis		4. condition of pain
(e) -clast		5. technique of viewing
(f) -desis		6. surgical repair

Column A	Column B	Column C
(g) dys-	_____	7. cell that breaks down a matrix
(h) -genesis	_____	8. pertaining to destruction/breaking down
(i) -ic	_____	9. condition of softening
(j) inter-	_____	10. instrument to cut
(k) -itis	_____	11. inflammation of
(l) -lytic	_____	12. puncture to remove fluid
(m) -malacia	_____	13. producing/forming
(n) -oid	_____	14. pertaining to (i)
(o) -olisthesis	_____	15. pertaining to (ii)
(p) -oma	_____	16. instrument to view
(q) -plasty	_____	17. difficult/painful/bad
(r) -scope	_____	18. germ cell
(s) -scopy	_____	19. to bind together
(t) -tome	_____	20. between

Score

20

Test 14C

Combining forms of word roots

Match each combining form in Column A with a meaning in Column C by inserting the appropriate number in Column B.

Column A	Column B	Column C
(a) arthr/o	_____	1. bone
(b) burs/o	_____	2. marrow (of bone)
(c) calcin/o	_____	3. synovia/synovial membrane
(d) chondr/o	_____	4. pus
(e) cost/o	_____	5. joint
(f) disc/o	_____	6. vertebrae
(g) fibr/o	_____	7. bursa/sac of fluid
(h) kyph/o	_____	8. stone/rock
(i) lamin/o	_____	9. calcium
(j) lord/o	_____	10. meniscus/crescent-shaped
(k) menisc/o	_____	11. bend forward
(l) myel/o	_____	12. cartilage
(m) oste/o	_____	13. crooked
(n) petr/o	_____	14. fibre
(o) phyt/o	_____	15. hunchback
(p) por/o	_____	16. thin plate/lamina of vertebra
(q) py/o	_____	17. rib
(r) scoli/o	_____	18. passage/pore
(s) spondyl/o	_____	19. plant-like growth
(t) synovi/o	_____	20. intervertebral disc

Score

20

Test 14D

Write the meaning of:

(a) arthrochondritis _____

(b) bursolith _____

(c) spondylodesis _____

(d) chondroclast _____

(e) kyphotic _____

Score

5

Test 14E

Build words that mean:

(a) condition of pain in a joint _____

(b) inflammation of synovia
and adjacent bones _____

(c) condition of softening of
vertebrae _____

(d) disease of joints and bones _____

(e) germ cell of the synovial
membrane _____

Score

.
5

Check answers to Self-Assessment Tests on page 299.

Objectives

Once you have completed Unit 15 you should be able to:

- understand the meaning of medical words relating to the male reproductive system

- build medical words relating to the male reproductive system

- associate medical terms with their anatomical position

- understand medical abbreviations relating to the male reproductive system.

Exercise Guide

Use this list of word components and their meanings to complete the word exercises in this unit.

Prefixes

a-	without
crypt-	hidden
oligo-	deficiency/few
trans-	across/through

Roots/Combining forms

cyst/o	bladder
fer/o	to carry
posth/o	prepuce/foreskin
phren/o	diaphragm

Suffixes

-al	pertaining to
-algia	condition of pain
-cele	swelling/protrusion/hernia
-cide	something that kills/killing
-ectomy	removal of
-genesis	forming/capable of causing
-graphy	technique of recording/making an X-ray
-ia	condition of
-ic	pertaining to
-ism	process of
-itis	inflammation of
-lysis	breakdown/disintegration
-megaly	enlargement
-meter	measuring instrument
-oma	tumour/swelling
-ous	pertaining to/of the nature of
-pathia	condition of disease
-pathy	disease of
-pexy	surgical fixation/fix in place
-plasty	surgical repair/reconstruction
-rrhagia	condition of bursting forth/discharge of blood
-rrhaphy	suture/stitch/suturing
-rrhea (Am.)	excessive flow/discharge
-rrhoea	excessive flow/discharge
-sect(ion)	cut/cutting/excision
-stomy	opening into
-tomy	incision into
-uria	condition of urine

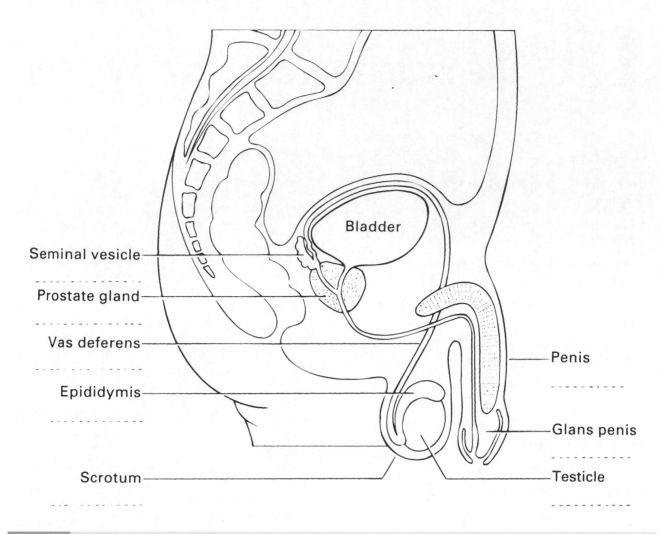

Seminal vesicle

Prostate gland

Vas deferens

Epididymis

Scrotum

Bladder

Penis

Glans penis

Testicle

Figure 75 The male reproductive system

ANATOMY EXERCISE

When you have finished Word Exercises 1–11, look at the word components listed below. Complete Figure 75 by writing the appropriate combining form on each dotted line. (You can check their meanings in the Quick Reference box on p. 188.)

Balan/o	Phall/o	Vas/o
Epididym/o	Prostat/o	Vesicul/o
Orchi/o	Scrot/o	

The male reproductive system

The male possesses paired reproductive organs known as the testes (synonymous with testicles). These are held in position outside the main cavities of the body by a sac known as the scrotum. Each testis produces millions of sperm cells (spermatozoa) that carry the male's genetic information. Once mature, sperms are mixed with glandular secretions to form a liquid known as semen.

Semen containing active swimming sperms is ejaculated from the penis during sexual intercourse. Sperms swim along the reproductive tract of the female to the oviducts where they may fuse with an egg in the process of fertilization.

Use the Exercise Guide at the beginning of this unit to complete Word Exercises 1–11 unless you are asked to work without it.

Root

Orch

*(From a Greek word **orchi**, meaning testis (or testicle), i.e. the male reproductive organ that produces spermatozoa.)*

Combining forms   **Orch/i/o, orchid/o**

WORD EXERCISE 1

Using your Exercise Guide, find the meaning of:

(a) **orchido**/pathy _____

(b) **orchio**/cele _____
(synonymous with scrotal hernia/scrotocele)

(c) crypt/**orch**/ism _____
(The testes should descend from the abdominal cavity approximately 2 months prior to birth. Failure to do this produces an undescended testis.)

(d) **orchio**/pexy (**orchido**/pexy) _____

Using your Exercise Guide, build words (using either **orch/i/o** or **orchid/o**) that mean:

(e) incision into a testicle _____

(f) surgical repair of a testicle _____

(g) removal of a testicle _____

(h) condition of pain in a testicle _____

Without using your Exercise Guide, write the meaning of:

(i) crypt/**orchido**/pexy _____
(synonymous with **orchido**/pexy)

Note.   The word testicle comes from the Latin *testiculus* meaning testis or male gonad (reproductive organ). The combining form **test/icul/o** is used in several common medical terms for example, **testo**sterone (-sterone meaning steroid hormone) and intra/**testicul**/ar (intra- meaning within, -ar meaning pertaining to).

Root

Scrot

*(From a Latin word **scrotum**. It refers to the scrotum, the pouch containing the testicles.)*

Combining forms   **Scrot/o**

WORD EXERCISE 2

Without using your Exercise Guide, build words that mean:

(a) removal of the scrotum _____

(b) plastic surgery/repair of the scrotum _____

(c) hernia/protrusion of the scrotum _____
(synonymous with **orchiocele**)

Using your Exercise Guide, find the meaning of:

(d) trans/**-scrot**/al _____

Two other conditions can result in a swelling of the testis:

> **Hydrocele**
> a swelling/protrusion/hernia due to an accumulation of fluid within the testis.
>
> **Varicocele**
> a swelling/protrusion/hernia of veins of the spermatic cords within the testis (from Latin *varicosus*, meaning varicose vein). Varicoceles need to be removed as they lead to pain and infertility.

Root

Phall

*(From a Greek word **phallos**, meaning the penis or male copulatory organ. It is also the male organ of urination.)*

Combining forms   **Phall/o**

WORD EXERCISE 3

Using your Exercise Guide, build words that mean:

(a) inflammation of the penis _____

(b) pertaining to the penis _____

Without using your Exercise Guide, build a word that means:

(c) removal of the penis _____

Penis is a Latin word referring to the male organ of copulation. **Pen**itis and **pen**ile are synonymous with

(a) and (b) above. An abnormally enlarged penis is known as a megalo**pen**is or megalo**phall**us.

Several abnormalities of the penis have been noted at birth. The urethra sometimes opens on to the dorsal (upper) surface of the penis. This is known as an **epispadia** (*epi-* meaning above, and *-spadia* condition of drawing out). Sometimes the urethra opens on to the posterior (lower) surface. This is a **hypospadia** (condition of drawing out below).

The swelling of the penis during erotic stimulation is known as tumescence (from Latin *tumescere*, meaning to swell). The subsidence of the swelling is known as detumescence (*de* meaning lack of). Once erect the penis can be inserted into the vagina in the act of sex. Words used synonymously with sex include:

> **Coitus**
> from Latin *coire*, meaning to come together.
>
> **Intercourse**
> from Latin *intercurrere*, meaning to run between.
>
> **Copulation**
> from Latin *copulare*, meaning to bind together.

The failure to produce an erection and perform the sexual act is known as impotence (from Latin *impotentia*, meaning inability). This condition is often due to psychological problems, but it can arise from lesions within the reproductive tract or nervous system.

> **Root** **Balan**
> *(From a Greek word **balanos**, meaning acorn. Here it refers to the sensitive, swollen end of the penis, known as the glans penis, which is covered with the prepuce of foreskin.)*
>
> *Combining forms* **Balan/o**

 WORD EXERCISE 4

Without using your Exercise Guide, build a word that means:

(a) inflammation of the glans penis _____

Using your Exercise Guide, find the meaning of:

(b) **balano**/rrhagia _____

(c) **balano**/posth/itis _____

The **prepuce**, or covering foreskin of the glans penis, sometimes needs to be cut, a process known as

preputiotomy. This is performed to relieve phimosis, a condition in which the foreskin is too tight and cannot retract.

The prepuce is removed in the process of circumcision (i.e. cutting around). This is often performed for religious rather than medical reasons.

> **Root** **Epididym**
> *(Derived from Greek words **epi** – on, **didymos** – twins/testicles. It refers to a coiled tube, the epididymis, which forms the first part of the duct system of each testis. The epididymes store sperm.)*
>
> *Combining forms* **Epididym/o**

 WORD EXERCISE 5

Without using your Exercise Guide, build words that mean:

(a) inflammation of the epididymis _____

(b) removal of the epididymis _____

Without using your Exercise Guide, write the meaning of:

(c) **epididymo**/-orch/itis _____

> **Root** **Vas**
> *(A Latin word meaning vessel or duct. Here it is used to mean vas deferens, the main secretory duct of the testis along which mature sperms move towards the penis.)*
>
> *Combining forms* **Vas/o**

 WORD EXERCISE 6

Without using your Exercise Guide, write the meaning of:

(a) **vas**/ectomy _____
(This operation (Fig. 76) is performed to sterilize the male, i.e. to make him incapable of reproduction. The cut ends of a section of the vas are tied off, a procedure known as bilateral ligation (from Latin *ligare*, meaning to bind). Following vasectomy, a reduced volume of semen is produced containing no sperm.)

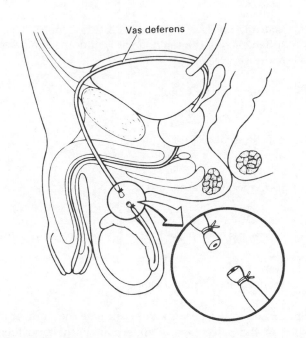
Vas deferens

Figure 76 Vasectomy

Using your Exercise Guide, find the meaning of:

(b) **vaso**/epididymo/stomy

(c) **vaso**/epididymo/graphy

(d) **vaso**/section

(e) **vaso**/rrhaphy

Without using your Exercise Guide, write the meaning of:

(f) **vaso**/-orchido/stomy

(g) **vaso**/**vaso**/stomy

(h) **vaso**/tomy

Root | **Vesicul**
*(From a Latin word **vesicula**, meaning vesicle/little bladder. It refers to the seminal vesicles, small pouches lying near the base of the bladder that secrete a nutrient fluid which becomes a component of semen.)*

Combining forms **Vesicul/o**

WORD EXERCISE 7

Without using your Exercise Guide, build words that mean:

(a) technique of making an X-ray of the seminal vesicles

(b) incision into a seminal vesicle

Without using your Exercise Guide, write the meaning of:

(c) vaso/**vesicul**/ectomy

Root | **Prostat**
*(From Greek **prostates**, meaning one who stands before. It is used to refer to the prostate gland surrounding the neck of the bladder and urethra in males. Secretions from the prostate gland are added to the semen during intercourse.)*

Combining forms **Prostat/o**

WORD EXERCISE 8

Using your Exercise Guide, find the meaning of:

(a) **prostato**/cysto/tomy

(b) **prostato**/megaly

Without using your Exercise Guide, write the meaning of:

(c) **prostat**/ectomy
(In elderly men there is a progressive enlargement of the prostate (prostatism) that obstructs the urethra, interfering with the passage of urine. Part or all of the gland can be removed by transurethral resection (TUR) to alleviate this condition (*trans*, meaning across, *resection*, meaning removal/excision). TUR involves inserting an endoscope into the urethra and using it to view and cut out pieces of prostate gland.)

(d) **prostato**/vesicul/ectomy

Root | **Semin**
*(From a Latin word **seminis**, meaning seed. It now refers to semen, the liquid secretion of the testicles, or to glands associated with the reproductive system.)*

Combining forms **Semin/i**

WORD EXERCISE 9

Using your Exercise Guide, find the meaning of:

(a) **semini**/fer/ous _____
(Spermatozoa flow along seminiferous tubules of the testis.)

(b) **semin**/uria _____

(c) **semin**/oma _____
(A malignancy of the testis. A change in size and shape of the testes is a symptom of this condition; their size can be measured with an **orchidometer**. When a testis is removed it can be replaced with a prosthesis.)

In**semina**tion refers to the deposition of semen in the female reproductive tract (from Latin *seminare*, meaning to sow).

Artificial insemination (AI) refers to the insertion of semen into the uterus via a cannula (tube) instead of by coitus. The sperm used in this procedure can be from two sources:

* AI by husband (AIH). In this procedure semen from the patient's husband is inseminated into the wife. It is used when there is difficulty in conceiving because of physical and/or psychological problems.

* AI by donor (AID). In this procedure semen from a male other than the female's partner is used. AID is used when the partner is sterile.

Root	Sperm
	(*From a Greek word* **sperma**, *meaning seed. It is used to mean sperm cells or spermatozoa (sing. spermatozoon). Sperm are ejaculated from the male during the peak of sexual excitement known as orgasm.*)
Combining forms	**Sperm/o, spermat/o** Also **sperm/i** (from New Latin **spermium**)

WORD EXERCISE 10

Using your Exercise Guide, find the meaning of:

(a) a/**sperm**/ia _____

(b) oligo/**sperm**/ia _____

(c) **spermi**/cide _____
(often used in conjunction with condoms and other contraceptives)

Using your Exercise Guide, build words using spermat/o that mean:

(d) condition of disease/ _____
abnormality of sperms

(e) formation of sperms _____

(f) breakdown/disintegration _____
of sperms

(g) flow of sperm _____
(abnormal, without orgasm)

Sperm counts are performed to estimate the number of sperms, the percentage of abnormal sperms and their mobility. The actual number of sperms is important in determining the fertility of the male. A sperm count of less than 60 million sperms per cm^3 of semen results in decreased fertility, even though only one sperm is required to fertilize an egg!

Semen containing sperms can be preserved at very low temperatures in a cryostat. Once thawed, the sperm are capable of fertilizing eggs and are used for artificial insemination.

Recently it has become possible to use sperm to fertilize eggs outside the body in laboratory glassware, a process known as in vitro fertilization (*vitro* meaning glass).

Medical equipment and clinical procedures

Revise the names of all instruments and procedures mentioned in this unit and then try Exercise 11.

WORD EXERCISE 11

Match each term in Column A with a description from Column C by placing an appropriate number in Column B.

Column A	Column B	Column C
(a) sperm count	_____	1. fusion of an egg and sperm in laboratory glassware
(b) transurethral resection	_____	2. material used to tie a cut vas

Column A	Column B	Column C
(c) vasectomy	_____	3. instrument to measure the size of a testicle
(d) orchidometer	_____	4. cutting of prostate through the urethra
(e) in vitro fertilization	_____	5. estimate of numbers of spermatozoa in 1 cm³ semen
(f) vasoligature	_____	6. the cutting and removal of a section of the spermduct

ANATOMY EXERCISE

Now complete the Anatomy Exercise on page 182.

CASE HISTORY 15

The object of this exercise is to understand words associated with a patient's medical history.

To complete the exercise:

- read through the passage on seminoma; unfamiliar words are underlined and you can find their meaning using the Word Help

- write the meaning of the medical terms shown in bold print.

Seminoma

Mr O, a 32-year-old father of two children, consulted his GP about a severe back pain. Although a regular football player he could not recall any recent injury that could account for his condition. During his consultation he mentioned that several months ago he had noticed his right testicle was swollen. It felt heavy and sometimes uncomfortable but he had ignored it assuming it would resolve. When his early medical record was checked it revealed a history of **cryptorchism** of the right testicle that had been rectified by **orchidopexy** at the age of 5 years.

Palpation showed the right testicle to be hard, smooth and swollen. It was easily separated from the epididymis and did not transilluminate. Mr O had not felt any pain and otherwise appeared in good health. There was no evidence of **orchitis**, epididymitis or torsion. He was counselled by his GP who referred him to the Urology department with suspected cancer of the testis.

Ultrasonography determined the presence of an **intratesticular** mass in the right testicle. A chest X-ray was negative for lung metastases, but a CT scan of his abdominopelvic region revealed retroperitoneal and para-aortic lymphadenopathy. He had elevated levels of the serum tumour markers βHCG and lactate dehydrogenase.

Mr O was advised of the need for surgical **orchidectomy** and the procedure was explained to him by the consultant.

Mr O's scrotal contents were examined and his right testicle removed through an inguinal approach with early clamping of the **spermatic** cord and its vessels. (Note, **trans-scrotal** biopsy is contra-indicated as a means of evaluating scrotal masses as it causes tumour cell shedding and spread of the tumour).

Histopathological analysis confirmed the presence of a malignant **seminoma** in the right testicle; the contralateral testis was biopsied at the same time and found to be normal.

Mr O's condition was assessed as Stage IIC and he was given chemotherapy with follow up chest X-ray, abdominopelvic CT scan and serum tumour marker determination every 3 months. At 6 months the residual retroperitoneal mass has shrunk and calcified, and he remains progression free.

WORD HELP

βHCG a serum tumour marker

calcified referring to deposition of calcium salts into a tissue

chemotherapy treatment using drugs (here cytotoxic drugs that destroy cancer cells)

contralateral pertaining to the opposite side

CT computed tomography

epididymis the first part of the duct system that leaves the testis and stores maturing sperm

epididymitis inflammation of the epididymis

GP general practitioner (family doctor)

histopathological pertaining to disease of a tissue

inguinal pertaining to the groin

lactate dehydrogenase a serum tumour marker

lymphadenopathy disease of lymph nodes (lymph glands)

malignant dangerous, capable of spreading

metastases parts of a tumour that have spread from one site to another

palpation act of feeling with the fingers using light pressure

para-aortic pertaining to beside the aorta

progression advancing, moving forward of a disease

retroperitoneal pertaining to behind the peritoneum

serum tumour marker certain chemicals are elevated to higher than normal levels in blood serum when tumours are present, they act as signs or markers of the presence of disease

WORD HELP (Contd.)

Stage IIC staging is a system of classifying malignant disease that will influence its treatment; this patient is at Stage IIC

torsion act of twisting/rotation

transilluminate shine a bright light through (note, a solid tumour will prevent transmission of light)

ultrasonography technique of recording (an image) using high frequency sound waves

urology study of the urinary tract (here department that diagnoses and treats disease and disorders of the urinary tract)

Now write the meaning of the following words from the case history without using your dictionary lists:

(a) cryptorchism _____

(b) orchidopexy _____

(c) orchitis _____

(d) intratesticular _____

(e) orchidectomy _____

(f) spermatic _____

(g) trans-scrotal _____

(h) seminoma _____

(Answers to the case history exercise are given in the Answers to Word Exercises beginning on page 275.)

Quick Reference

Combining forms relating to the reproductive system:

Balan/o	glans penis
Cyst/o	bladder
Epididym/o	epididymis
Orchi/o	testis
Phall/o	penis
Posth/o	prepuce/foreskin
Prostat/o	prostate
Scrot/o	scrotum
Semin/i	semen/testis
Sperm/i	spermatozoa/sperm
Varic/o	varicose vein
Vas/o	vas deferens/vessel
Vesicul/o	seminal vesicle

Abbreviations

Some common abbreviations related to the male reproductive system are listed below. Note, however, some are not standard and their meaning may vary from one health care setting to another. There is a more extensive list for reference on page 307.

AI	artificial insemination
AID	artificial insemination by donor
ICSH	interstitial cell stimulating hormone
pros	prostate
PSA	prostate specific antigen
SPP	suprapubic prostatectomy
STD	sexually transmitted disease
Syph	syphilis
TUR	transurethral resection
TURP	transurethral resection of prostate
VD	venereal disease
WR	Wasserman reaction test for syphilis

> ## NOW TRY THE WORD CHECK <

WORD CHECK

This self-check exercise lists all the word components used in this unit. First write down the meaning of as many word components as you can. Then check your answers using the Exercise Guide and Quick Reference box or the Glossary of Word Components (pp. 319–341).

Prefixes

a- *without*

crypt- *hidden*

epi- *above*

hypo- *below normal*

intra- *inside / within*

oligo- *deficiency / few*

trans- *across / through*

Combining forms of word roots

balan/o	glans penis
cyst/o	bladder
epididym/o	epididymis
fer/o	to carry
hydr/o	water
megal/o	enlargement
orchi/o	testicle / testis
phall/o	penis
posth/o	prepuce / foreskin
prostat/o	prostate gland
scrot/o	scrotum
semin/i	semen
sperm/i	sperm
varic/o	varicose vein
vas/o	vas deferens / vessel
vesicul/o	seminal vesicle

Suffixes

-al	pertaining to
-algia	condition of pain
-ar	pertaining to
-cele	hernia / swelling
-cide	to kill
-ectomy	removal of
-genesis	formation
-graphy	technique of x-raying
-ia	condition of
-ic	pertaining to
-ism	process of

-itis	inflammation of
-ligation	tie / tie
-lysis	breakdown / disintegration
-oma	tumour / swelling
-ous	pertaining to
-pathia	condition of disease
-pexy	surgical fixation
-plasty	surgical repair
-rrhagia	condition of bursting forth
-rrhaphy	suturing / stitching
-rrhoea (Am. -rrhea)	excessive flow / discharge
-sect(ion)	cut / excision
-spadia	condition of drawing out
-stomy	formation of an opening
-tomy	incision into
-uria	condition of urine

> **NOW TRY THE SELF-ASSESSMENT** <

SELF-ASSESSMENT

Test 15A

Below are some combining forms that refer to the anatomy of the male reproductive system. Indicate which part of the system they refer to by putting a number from the diagram (Fig. 77) next to each word.

(a)	scrot/o	3
(b)	orchid/o	7
(c)	phall/o	5
(d)	balan/o	6
(e)	vas/o	2

(f) prostat/o _____ 1

(g) vesicul/o _____ 4

(h) epididym/o _____ 8

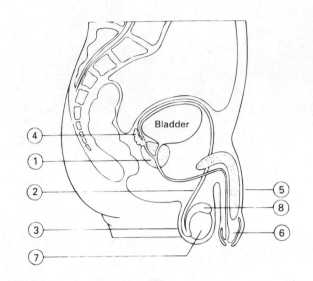

Figure 77   The male reproductive system

Score

8

8

Column A	Column B	Column C
(h) -ism	13	8. suturing
(i) oligo-	20	9. on/above/upon
(j) -ous	12/11	10. condition of bursting forth (of blood)
(k) -pexy	1	11. pertaining to (i)
(l) re-	7	12. pertaining to (ii)
(m) -rrhagia	10	13. process of
(n) -rrhaphy	8	14. excessive flow/discharge
(o) -rrhoea (Am. -rrhea)	14	15. producing/ forming
(p) -sect	19	16. hernia/protrusion/ swelling
(q) -spadia	2	17. condition of
(r) -stomy	5	18. to kill
(s) trans-	6	19. cut
(t) -uria	4	20. little/scanty/few

Score

20

Test 15B

Prefixes and suffixes

Match each prefix or suffix in Column A with a meaning in Column C by inserting the appropriate number in Column B.

Column A	Column B	Column C
(a) -cele	16	1. fixation
(b) -cide	18	2. condition of drawing out
(c) crypt-	3	3. hidden
(d) epi-	9	4. condition of urine/ urination
(e) -genesis	15	5. opening into
(f) -ia	17	6. across
(g) -ic	11/12	7. back

Test 15C

Combining forms of word roots

Match each combining form in Column A with a meaning in Column C by inserting the appropriate number in Column B.

Column A	Column B	Column C
(a) balan/o	4	1. to carry
(b) cyst/o	14	2. testis
(c) epididym/o	8	3. penis
(d) fer/o	1	4. glans penis

Column A   Column B   Column C

(e) hydr/o   12   5. prostate gland

(f) megal/o   15   6. prepuce

(g) orchid/o   2   7. semen

(h) phall/o   3   8. epididymis

(i) posth/o   6   9. varicose vein

(j) prostat/o   5   10. vessel

(k) scrot/o   13   11. vesicle (seminal)

(l) semin/i   7   12. water

(m) varic/o   9   13. scrotum

(n) vas/o   10   14. bladder

(o) vesicul/o   11   15. abnormal
                            enlargement

Score

15

Test 15E

Build words that mean:

(a) stitching/suturing of the testis _orchidorrhaphy_

(b) condition of pain in the prostate _prostatalgia_

(c) formation of an opening between the vas and epididymis _epididymovasostomy_

(d) inflammation of the scrotum _scrotitis_

(e) excessive flow/discharge from the prostate _prostatorrhoea_

Score

5

Check answers to Self-Assessment Tests on page 299.

Test 15D

Write the meaning of:

(a) orchidoepididymectomy _removal of the epididymes + testes_

(b) phallorrhoea (Am. phallorrhea) _excessive discharge from the penis_

(c) epididymovasectomy _removal of the vas deferens + epididymes_

(d) vasoligation _to tie off the vas deferens_

(e) spermaturia _condition of sperm in the urine_

Score

5

16 The female reproductive system

Objectives

Once you have completed Unit 16 you should be able to:

- understand the meaning of medical words relating to the female reproductive system

- build medical words relating to the female reproductive system

- associate medical terms with their anatomical position

- understand medical abbreviations relating to the female reproductive system.

Exercise Guide

Use this list of word components and their meanings to complete the word exercises in this unit.

Prefixes

a-	without
ante-	before
dys-	difficult/painful
endo-	within/inside
eu-	good
micro-	small
multi-	many
neo-	new
nulli-	none
oligo-	deficiency/little/few
peri-	around
pre-	before/in front of
primi-	first
pro-	before
secundi-	second

Roots/Combining forms

cyst/o	bladder (cyst)
cyt/e	cell
fer/o	to carry
haem/o	blood
hem/o (Am.)	blood
myc/o	fungus
perine/o	perineum
periton/e/o	peritoneum
phleb/o	vein
placent/o	placenta
rect/o	rectum
trachel/o	neck
vesic/o	bladder

Suffixes

-a	noun ending/a name e.g. of a condition
-agogue	agent that induces/promotes
-al	pertaining to
-algia	condition of pain
-arche	beginning
-blast	cell that forms … /immature germ cell
-cele	swelling/protrusion/hernia
-centesis	puncture
-dynia	condition of pain
-ectomy	removal of
-fuge	agent that suppresses/removes
-genesis	formation of
-genic	pertaining to formation
-gram	X-ray/tracing/recording
-graphy	making an X-ray/technique of recording
-ia	condition of
-ic	pertaining to
-ischia	condition of reducing/holding back
-itis	inflammation of
-lithiasis	abnormal condition of stones
-logy	study of
-malacia	condition of softening
-meter	measuring instrument
-metry	process of measuring
-oma	tumour/swelling
-osis	abnormal condition/disease of
-ous	pertaining to/of the nature of
-pathia	condition of disease
-pathy	disease of
-pause	stopping
-pexy	surgical fixation/fix in place
-plasty	surgical repair/reconstruction
-poiesis	formation
-ptosis	falling/displacement/prolapse
-rrhagic	pertaining to bursting forth (of blood)
-rrhaphy	suturing/stitching
-rrhexis	breaking/rupturing
-rrhea (Am.)	excessive discharge/flow
-rrhoea	excessive discharge/flow
-sclerosis	abnormal condition of hardening
-scope	viewing instrument
-scopy	visual examination/technique of viewing
-staxis	dripping
-stenosis	abnormal condition of narrowing
-stomy	formation of an opening/an opening
-tic	pertaining to
-tome	cutting instrument
-tomy	incision into
-toxic	pertaining to poisoning
-trophin	hormone that stimulates/nourishes
-tropic	pertaining to stimulating/affinity for
-tubal	pertaining to a tube

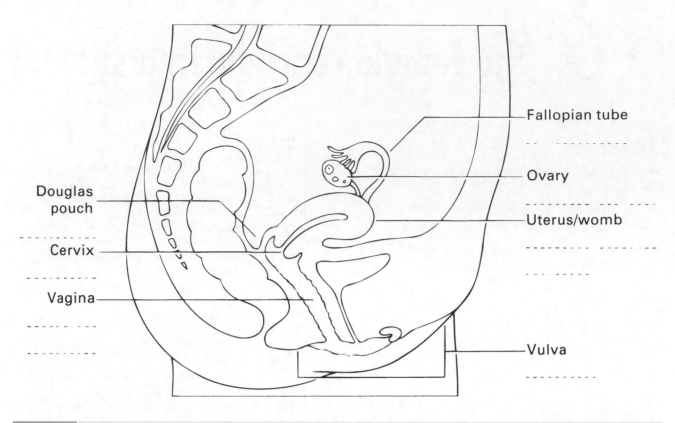

Figure 78   Section through female

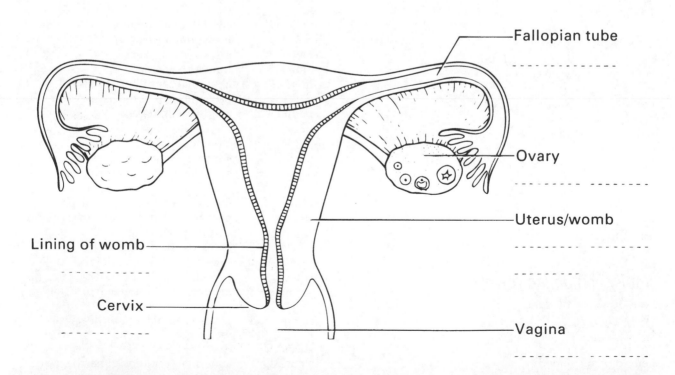

Figure 79   The female reproductive system

ANATOMY EXERCISE

When you have finished Word Exercises 1–14, look at the word components listed below. Complete Figures 78 and 79 by writing the appropriate combining form on each dotted line – more than one component may relate to the same position. (You can check their meanings in the Quick Reference box on p. 206.)

Cervic/o	Hyster/o	Salping/o
Colp/o	Metr/o	Uter/o
Culd/o	Oophor/o	Vagin/o
Endometr/i	Ovari/o	Vulv/o

The female reproductive system

The female possesses paired reproductive organs known as ovaries; these are located in the upper pelvic cavity on either side of the uterus. The function of the ovaries is to produce reproductive cells known as ova (eggs). The ovaries pass through a regular ovarian cycle in which one egg is released (ovulation) every 28 days. The egg passes into the oviduct where it may be fertilized by sperms ejaculated into the female reproductive tract by the male. Should an egg be fertilized, it will divide and grow into a new individual after implanting into the uterus. If the egg is not fertilized, it will disintegrate and may pass out of the body at menstruation.

Use the Exercise Guide at the beginning of this unit to complete Word Exercises 1–26 unless you are asked to work without it.

Root   **Oo**
(From a Greek word **oon***, meaning egg.)*

Combining forms   **Oo-**

WORD EXERCISE 1

Using your Exercise Guide, find the meaning of:

(a) **oo**/blast _____

(b) **oo**/cyte _____

(c) **oo**/genesis _____

Root   **Oophor**
(From a Greek word **oophoron***, derived from oion – egg, pherein – to bear. We use it to mean ovary, the egg-bearing gland.)*

Combining forms   **Oophor/o**

WORD EXERCISE 2

Using your Exercise Guide, build words that mean:

(a) removal of an ovary _____

(b) fixation of an ovary _____

(c) incision of an ovary _____

Using your Exercise Guide, find the meaning of:

(d) **oophoro**/cyst/ectomy _____
(Cyst refers to an ovarian cyst, a bladder-like growth in the ovary.)

(e) **oophoro**/stomy _____

Root   **Ovari**
(From a New Latin word **ovarium***, meaning ovary, derived from ova, meaning egg.)*

Combining forms   **Ovari/o**

WORD EXERCISE 3

Without using your Exercise Guide, build words that mean:

(a) removal of an ovary _____
(synonymous with oophorectomy)

(b) incision into an ovary _____
(often used to mean the removal of an ovarian cyst)

Using your Exercise Guide, find the meaning of:

(c) **ovario**/rrhexis _____

(d) **ovario**/tubal _____
   (The tube refers to an oviduct.)

(e) **ovario**/centesis _____

Approximately every 28 days an egg (or ovum) is released from one of the ovaries. This process is known as **ovulation**. Once released, the egg is picked up by the oviduct and it moves towards the uterus. An ovary that fails to release an egg is described as **anovular** (i.e. without eggs).

Root **Salping**
*(From Greek **salpingos**, meaning trumpet tube. Here it refers to the trumpet-shaped oviduct or Fallopian tube. This collects eggs ovulated from the ovary and passes them to the uterus.)*

Combining forms **Salping/o**

WORD EXERCISE 4

Without using your Exercise Guide, write the meaning of:

(a) **salpingo**/-oophor/ectomy _____

(b) ovario/**salping**/ectomy _____

(c) **salpingo**/pexy _____

Using your Exercise Guide, find the meaning of:

(d) **salpingo**/cele _____

(e) **salpingo**/-oophor/itis _____

Using your Exercise Guide, build words that mean:

(f) technique of making an _____
   X-ray of the oviduct
   (follows an injection of opaque dye)

(g) abnormal condition of _____
   calcareous stones/deposits
   in oviduct

(h) surgical repair of the _____
   oviduct

Root **Uter**
*(From a Latin word **uterus**, meaning womb. Here it is used to mean the uterus, the chamber in which a fertilized egg grows into a fetus and baby.)*

Combining forms **Uter/o**

WORD EXERCISE 5

Using your Exercise Guide, build words that mean:

(a) condition of pain in the _____
   uterus

(b) hardening of the uterus _____

Without using your Exercise Guide, write the meaning of:

(c) **utero**/tubal _____

(d) **utero**/salpingo/graphy _____

Using your Exercise Guide, find the meaning of:

(e) **utero**/vesic/al _____

(f) **utero**/rect/al _____

(g) **utero**/placent/al _____
   (The placenta is a disc-shaped structure that attaches the fetus to the lining of the uterus.)

Benign tumours of dense fibrous tissue and muscle called **fibroids** are frequently found in the uterus. They are removed by **fibroid/ectomy** or **myom/ectomy**. (**Myom** is from *myoma*, meaning muscle tumour.)

Root **Hyster**
*(From Greek word **hystera**, meaning womb. Here it is used to mean the uterus.)*

Combining forms **Hyster/o**

WORD EXERCISE 6

Using your Exercise Guide, build words that mean:

(a) instrument to view the womb _____

(b) abnormal condition of _____
   falling/displaced womb
   (also known as a prolapse)

(c) X-ray picture of the womb _____

Without using your Exercise Guide, write the meaning of:

(d) **hystero**/salpingo/graphy _____

(e) **hystero**/salpingo/stomy _____

(f) **hystero**/salpingo/-oophor/ _____
     ectomy

Using your Exercise Guide, find the meaning of:

(g) **hystero**/trachelo/rrhaphy _____

(h) **hystero**/trachelo/tomy _____

Root	Metr
	(From a Greek word **metra**, meaning womb. Here it is used to mean the uterus.)

Combining forms   **Metr/a/i/o**

WORD EXERCISE 7

Using your Exercise Guide, find the meaning of:

(a) **metro**/staxis _____

(b) **metro**/path/ia _____
     haemo/rrhag/ic/a
     (Am. metro/path/ia hemo/rrhag/ic/a)

(c) **metro**/periton/itis _____

(d) **metro**/phleb/itis _____

(e) **metro**/cyst/osis _____

(f) **metro**/ptosis _____

Using your Exercise Guide, build words that mean:

(g) condition of narrowed womb _____

(h) condition of softening of uterus _____

The endo**metrium** (meaning part within the womb) refers to the lining of the mucosa of the uterus. The endometrium grows during the 28-day menstrual cycle and disintegrates when it ends, producing the menstrual flow.

Using your Exercise Guide, find the meaning of:

(i) endo/**metr**/itis _____

(j) endo/**metri**/oma _____

Without using your Exercise Guide, write the meaning of:

(k) endo/**metri**/osis _____
     (refers to the endometrial
     tissue in abnormal locations)

Root	Men
	(From a Latin word **mensis**, meaning month. It refers to menstruation, that is, monthly bleeding from the womb. The bleeding arises from the disintegration of the endometrium.)

Combining forms   **Men/o**

WORD EXERCISE 8

Without using your Exercise Guide, write the meaning of:

(a) **meno**/staxis _____

Using your Exercise Guide, find the meaning of:

(b) **men**/arche _____

(c) **meno**/pause _____

(d) a/**meno**/rrhoea _____
     (Am. a/meno/rrhea)

(e) dys/**meno**/rrhoea _____
     (Am. dys/meno/rrhea)

(f) oligo/**meno**/rrhoea _____
     (Am. oligo/meno/rrhea)

(g) pre/**menstru**/al _____

Hysteroscopy and biopsy

In this procedure, a narrow endoscope known as a **hysteroscope** is inserted through the cervix to examine the uterus. Modern hysteroscopes are thin telescopes that fit through the cervix with minimal or no dilatation. The standard 4 mm hysteroscope gives a panoramic view of the cervical canal and uterine cavity and is suitable for most purposes. A diagnostic sheath around the main viewing telescope of the instrument allows saline or carbon dioxide to be pumped in, thereby inflating the uterus and improving the field of view.

Hysteroscopy is a simple, inexpensive diagnostic technique used to investigate women with abnormal uterine bleeding. It has been particularly valuable in the investigation of post menopausal bleeding to exclude endometrial cancer. Once positioned, the hysteroscope is used to observe fibroids, polyps and adhesions, and to biopsy the endometrium (i.e. remove living suspicious tissue for examination). Benign polyps are usually removed and examined as they are difficult to differentiate from malignant lesions.

A more complex instrument the **microcolpohystero-scope** has different levels of magnification (1–150×) as well as diagnostic and operative sheaths. It can produce a panoramic view of the endocervix and uterine cavity or be used at close range to examine the cellular and vascular structure of the endometrium. During **operative hysteroscopy** various instruments including biopsy or grasping forceps, scissors, diathermy probes and laser fibres are passed into the body through the operative sheath. The surgeon controls the instruments whilst viewing the uterine cavity through the telescope component of the device.

Another instrument called a **resectoscope** used over many years for prostate and bladder surgery, has been modified for use as an operative hysteroscope. It has a built in wire loop that uses a high frequency electric current to cut and coagulate the tissues of the endometrium. The resectoscope is used for transcervical resection of the endometrium (TCRE), a technique of ablating (cutting away) the endometrium in women with dysfunctional uterine bleeding (menorrhagia). It can also remove small to medium submucous fibroids and provide biopsy specimens for histological analysis.

Flexible endoscopy using a 3–5 mm directional endoscope with an insufflating channel (to blow in gas or fluid) is also proving useful in hysteroscopy and salpingoscopy. The larger endoscopes also have a channel wide enough to accommodate surgical instruments.

Biopsy specimens removed by any of these instruments are sent to the pathology laboratory for processing and histological analysis. (The word biopsy is formed from *bio-* meaning life and *-opsy* meaning process of viewing. A biopsy is the removal and examination of tissue from a living body.)

 Root   **Cervic**
*(From a Latin word **cervix**, meaning the neck of the uterus, the cervix uteri.)*

Combining forms   **Cervic/o**

 WORD EXERCISE 9

Without using your Exercise Guide, build words that mean:

(a) inflammation of the cervix   _____

(b) removal of the cervix   _____

Adult women are advised to have periodic cervical smears. This procedure involves taking a sample of cells from the cervix and subjecting them to cytological examination (Pap test, named after cytologist G. Papanicolaou). Neoplastic cells can be removed in their early stages of growth, thereby preventing cervical cancer. The risk of developing cervical cancer is related to the number of sexual partners and is the result of transmission of a virus (HPV – human papilloma virus).

Root   **Colp**
*(From a Greek word **colpos**, meaning hollow. It is now used to mean vagina, a hollow chamber that receives the penis during copulation and through which the baby will pass at birth.)*

Combining forms   **Colp/o**

WORD EXERCISE 10

Using your Exercise Guide, find the meaning of:

(a) **colpo**/scopy   _____

(b) **colpo**/micro/scope
(used in situ, i.e. to examine the vagina directly)

Without using your Exercise Guide, write the meaning of:

(c) **colpo**/gram   _____

(d) **colpo**/perineo/rrhaphy   _____

The perineum is the region between the thighs bounded by the anus and vulva in the female. Perineotomy is used synonymously with episio/tomy (*episi* – meaning pubic region). This incision is made during the birth of a child when the vaginal orifice does not stretch sufficiently to allow an easy birth.

(e) **colpo**/hyster/ectomy   _____

(f) metro/**colpo**/cele _____

(g) cervico/**colp**/itis _____

Without using your Exercise Guide, build words that mean:

(h) surgical repair of the
    perineum and vagina _____

(i) surgical fixation of the vagina _____

Root Vagin
(From a Latin word **vagina**, *meaning sheath. It refers to the vagina, the musculo-membranous passage extending from the cervix uteri to the vulva. Synonymous with colpos.)*

Combining forms **Vagin/o**

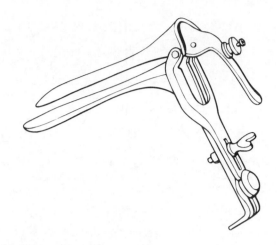

Figure 80 Vaginal speculum

WORD EXERCISE 12

Without using your Exercise Guide, write the meaning of:

(a) **vulvo**/vagin/itis _____

(b) **vulvo**/vagino/plasty _____

Root Culd
(From a French word **cul-de-sac**, *meaning bottom of the bag or sack. Here it is used to mean the blindly ending Douglas cavity or rectouterine pouch, which lies above the posterior vaginal fornix.)*

Combining forms **Culd/o**

WORD EXERCISE 11

Without using your Exercise Guide, write the meaning of:

(a) **vagino**/perineo/tomy _____

(b) **vagino**/perineo/rrhaphy _____

(c) **vagino**/vesic/al _____

Using your Exercise Guide, build words that mean:

(d) abnormal condition of fungal
    infection of the vagina _____

(e) disease of the vagina _____

Investigations of disorders of the vagina and cervix usually require the use of a vaginal speculum to hold the walls of the vagina apart. There are many types of vaginal specula, one of which is shown in Figure 80.

Two small glands situated on either side of the external orifice of the vagina are known as the **greater vestibular glands** or **Bartholin's glands** (after C. Bartholin, a Danish anatomist). They produce mucus to lubricate the vagina. Sometimes the glands become inflamed, a condition known as **bartholin**itis.

WORD EXERCISE 13

Without using your Exercise Guide, write the meaning of:

(a) **culdo**/scope _____
    (This allows examination of the uterus, oviducts, ovaries and peritoneal cavity; Fig. 81)

(b) **culdo**/scopy _____

(c) **culdo**/centesis _____

Root Vulv
(From a Latin word **vulva**, *meaning womb. It is used to mean vulva, pudendum femina or external genitalia.)*

Combining forms **Vulv/o**

Root Gynaec
(From a Greek word **gyne**, *meaning woman. Here it refers to the female reproductive system.)*

Combining forms **Gynaec/o Gynec/o**

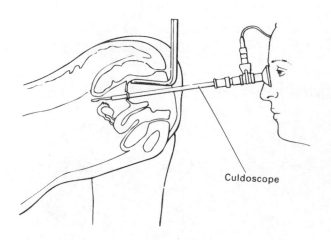

Culdoscope

Figure 81 Culdoscopy

WORD EXERCISE 14

Using your Exercise Guide, find the meaning of:

(a) **gynaeco**/logy _____
(Am. gyneco/logy; refers to diseases peculiar to women, i.e. of the female reproductive tract)

(b) **gynaeco**/genic _____
(Am. gyneco/genic)

ANATOMY EXERCISE

Now complete the Anatomy Exercise on page 195.

Abbreviations

You should learn common abbreviations related to the female reproductive system. Note, however, some are not standard and their meaning may vary from one health care setting to another. There is a more extensive list for reference on page 307.

CACX	cancer of the cervix
DUB	dysfunctional uterine bleeding
Gyn	gynaecology (Am. gynecology)
in utero	within the uterus
IUCD	intrauterine contraceptive device

Abbreviations (Contd.)

IUFB	intrauterine foreign body
LMP	last menstrual period
Pap	Papanicolaou smear test
PMB	post-menopausal bleeding
PMS	premenstrual syndrome
PV	per vagina
VE	vaginal examination

Terms relating to pregnancy, birth and lactation

After approximately 9 months (**the period of gestation**) a baby is expelled from the mother's body by muscular contractions of the uterus. The onset of uterine contractions is termed labour (or **parturition**). The period immediately following birth is known as the **puerperium**, in which time the reproductive organs tend to revert to their original state. The terms **antepartum** and **postpartum** are also used to indicate the periods before and after birth. **Ante** is usually used to mean up to 3 months before birth.

Occasionally, fertilized eggs grow outside the uterus (extrauterine development). When these implant and grow they are known as **ectopic** pregnancies. The most common ectopic site is the Fallopian tube; rupture of this by a pregnancy constitutes a surgical emergency.

The successful entry of a sperm into an egg at fertilization is known as **conception** and it is this event that creates a new individual. The fertilized egg then divides and forms into a ball of cells (the blastocyst) that must implant into the lining (endometrium) of the uterus to complete its development. **Pregnancy** begins when implantation is complete.

Following implantation, a structure known as the **placenta** (from Latin meaning cake) forms. This is a vascular structure, developed about the third month of pregnancy and attached to the wall of the uterus. Through the placenta the fetus is supplied with oxygen and nutrients and wastes are removed. The placenta is expelled as the afterbirth, usually within 1 hour of birth.

Root | **Gravida**
(A Latin word meaning heavy or pregnant. It is used to describe a woman in relation to her pregnancies. e.g. first pregnancy.)

Combining forms   **-gravida**

WORD EXERCISE 15

Using your Exercise Guide, find the meaning of:

(a) primi/**gravida** _____
(gravida I)

(b) secundi/**gravida** _____
(gravida II)

(c) multi/**gravida** _____
(more than twice)

(d) pro/**gravid** _____

Root | **Para**
(From a Latin word **parere**, meaning to bear/bring forth. It is used to refer to a woman and the number of her previous pregnancies.)

Combining forms | **-para**

WORD EXERCISE 16

Without using your Exercise Guide, write the meaning of:

(a) primi/**para** _____
(Primi/para can be used synonymously with uni/para (*uni* – one).)

(b) secundi/**para** _____

(c) multi/**para** _____

(d) nulli/**para** _____

Another word that refers to pregnancy is **cyesis** (from Greek *kyesis*, meaning conception). **Pseudocyesis** refers to a false pregnancy, i.e. signs and symptoms of early pregnancy, a result of an overwhelming desire to have a child.

Root | **Fet**
(From a Latin word **fetus**, i.e. an unborn baby. A human embryo becomes a fetus 8 weeks after fertilization, i.e. when the organ systems have been laid down.)

Combining forms | **Fet/o**

Note. Foetus is an alternative spelling of fetus. Once the usual spelling in British English, it is becoming less common.

WORD EXERCISE 17

Without using your Exercise Guide, write the meaning of:

(a) **feto**/logy _____

(b) **feto**/scope _____

(c) **feto**/placent/al _____

Using your Exercise Guide, build words that mean:

(d) pertaining to poisoning _____
of the fetus

(e) measurement of the fetus _____

The part of the fetus that lies in the lower part of the uterus is known as the presenting part. In a normal birth the vertex of the skull forms the presenting part and it enters the birth canal first. If other parts enter first, e.g. the buttocks, they are known as **malpresentations**.

Various manoeuvres can be made to turn or change the position of the fetus in the uterus. The term **version** (from Latin *vertere*, meaning to turn) is used for these manoeuvres. Many types have been described, e.g.:

Cephalic version
changes the position of the fetus from breech (buttocks first) to cephalic (head first) towards the birth canal.

External version
changes the position of the fetus by manipulation through the abdominal wall.

Internal version
changes the position of the fetus by hand within the uterus.

Root | **Amni**
(From a Greek word **amnia**, meaning the bowl in which blood was caught. It is now used to mean the amnion, the fetal membrane that retains the amniotic fluid surrounding a developing fetus.)

Combining forms | **Amni/o**

WORD EXERCISE 18

Using your Exercise Guide, find the meaning of:

(a) **amnio**/tome _____

(b) feto/**amnio**/tic _____

Without using your Exercise Guide, build words that mean:

(c) technique of cutting the amnion _____

(d) an instrument to visually examine the amnion (see Fig. 82) _____

Without using your Exercise Guide, write the meaning of:

(e) **amnio**/graphy _____

(f) **amnio**/gram _____

(g) **amnio**/centesis _____

Figure 82 shows the developing amnion and Figure 83 the position of the needle used to withdraw amniotic fluid during amniocentesis.

This procedure is used to remove amniotic fluid for analysis, to inject solutions that will induce abortion or infuse dyes for radiographic studies. Various fetal abnormalities can be detected by analysing the amniotic fluid, e.g. spina bifida. In this condition the vertebral arches fail to surround the spinal cord, exposing the cord and meninges which may protrude through the defective vertebrae. The disorder can be detected before birth by the presence of increased levels of alpha-fetoprotein (AFP) in the amniotic fluid. AFP is also raised when the fetus is anencephalic.

Genetic disorders can also be identified by analysing the chromosomes present in cells sloughed off the developing fetus into the amniotic fluid, e.g. Down's

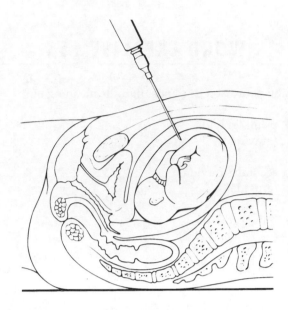

syndrome (mongolism). In this condition 47 chromosomes are present instead of the normal 46. Parents can use the information from amniocentesis to decide to continue a pregnancy or abort a defective fetus.

The outermost of the fetal membranes is known as the **chorion** (from Greek, meaning outer membrane). It develops extensions, known as villi, that become part of the placenta. The combining form **chori/o** is used to mean chorion (see Fig. 82).

Without using your Exercise Guide, write the meaning of:

(h) chorio/**amnion**/ic _____

(i) chorio/**amnion**/itis _____

Root Obstetric
*(From a Latin word **obstetrix**, meaning midwife.)*

Combining forms **Obstetr/ic-**

Obstetric- is mainly used in:

Obstetrics
The science dealing with the care of the pregnant woman during all stages of pregnancy and the period following birth.

Obstetrician
A person who specializes in obstetrics (*-ician* meaning person associated with …). Often doctors specialize in obstetrics and gynaecology.

Obstetrical forceps
Large forceps consisting of two flat blades connected to a handle. They are used to pull on a fetal head or rotate it to facilitate vaginal delivery (Figs 84 and 85) (*-ical* means pertaining to).

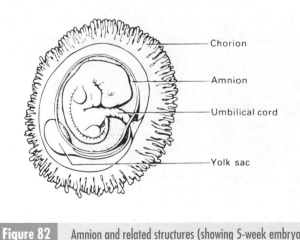

Figure 82 Amnion and related structures (showing 5-week embryo)

Chorion

Amnion

Umbilical cord

Yolk sac

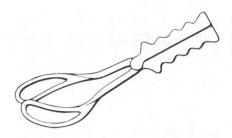

Figure 84   Obstetrical forceps

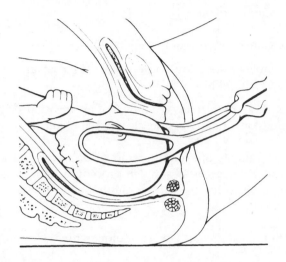

Figure 85   Obstetrical forceps in use

Another device used by obstetricians to assist delivery is the **vacuum extractor**. This suction device is attached to the head as it presents through the birth canal and is used to pull the baby out.

Root   **Placent**
*(From a Latin word **plakoenta**, meaning a flat cake. Here it is used to mean placenta).*

Combining forms   **Placent/o**

WORD EXERCISE 19

Without using your Exercise Guide, build words that mean:

(a) technique of making an
     X-ray of the placenta   _____

(b) any disease of the placenta   _____

Many abnormalities of the placenta have been noted. Two common disorders are:

Adherent placenta
   This placenta is fused to the uterine wall so that separation is slow and delivery of the placenta is delayed. When the placenta is not expelled it is known as a retained placenta.

Placenta praevia (Am. placenta previa)
   This placenta forms abnormally in the lower part of the uterus over the internal opening of the cervix. The condition gives rise to haemorrhage (Am. hemorrhage) during pregnancy and threatens the life of the fetus.

Root   **Toc**
            *(From a Greek word **tokos**, meaning birth/labour.)*

Combining forms   **Toc/o, tok/o**

WORD EXERCISE 20

Without using your Exercise Guide, write the meaning of:

(a) dys/**toc**/ia   _____

(b) **toco**/logy   _____
     (synonymous with obstetrics)

Using your Exercise Guide, find the meaning of:

(c) eu/**toc**/ia   _____

Labour can be monitored by recording uterine contractions using a device called a **tocograph**; the procedure is known as **tocography**. When the fetal heart is monitored with the uterine contractions during delivery, it is known as **cardiotocography**.

If labour is late or slow, the uterus can be induced to produce forcible contractions by the administration of **oxytocin**, a hormone that is produced naturally by the pituitary gland. Various compounds with oxytocin-like activity are available for this purpose.

The 6–8 weeks following birth is known as the **puerperium** (from Latin *puerperus*, meaning child-bearing). This is the time when the reproductive system involutes (reverts) to its state before pregnancy. Puerperal sepsis is a serious infection of the genital tract occurring within 21 days of abortion or childbirth.

Other problems can arise following birth, e.g.:

Postpartum haemorrhage
   (Am. postpartum hemorrhage) excessive bleeding from birth canal.

Eclampsia
   sudden convulsion due to toxaemia of pregnancy. The signs of pre-eclampsia in pregnancy include albuminuria, hypertension and oedema.

Root — **Nat**
(From a Latin word **natalis**, *meaning birth.)*

Combining forms **Nat/o**

 ## WORD EXERCISE 21

Using your Exercise Guide, find the meaning of:

(a) neo/**nat**/al _____

(b) ante/**nat**/al _____

(c) peri/**nat**/al _____

Without using your Exercise Guide, write the meaning of:

(d) pre/**nat**/al _____

(e) neo/**nato**/logy _____
(A neonate is a newborn baby up to 1 month old.)

Root — **Mamm**
(From a Latin word **mamma**, *meaning breast. It refers to the mammary glands (breasts) that secrete milk during lactation following birth.)*

Combining forms **Mamm/o**

WORD EXERCISE 22

Without using your Exercise Guide, write the meaning of:

(a) **mammo**/graphy _____

(b) **mammo**/plasty _____
(sometimes performed to increase or decrease the size of breasts)

Using your Exercise Guide, find the meaning of:

(c) **mammo**/tropic _____

Root — **Mast**
(From a Greek word **mastos**, *meaning breast.)*

Combining forms **Mast/o**

 ## WORD EXERCISE 23

Without using your Exercise Guide, build words that mean:

(a) technique of making X-ray of breast _____

(b) surgical repair of breast _____

(c) removal of breast _____

There are two forms of this operation:

• Simple mastectomy – removal of the breast and overlying skin

• Radical mastectomy – removal of the breast, overlying skin, underlying muscle and lymphatic tissue.

Some patients opt for the removal of a breast cancer (mastadenoma) by a simpler procedure known as a lumpectomy. In this just the mass of abnormal cells is removed.

Without using your Exercise Guide, write the meaning of:

(d) **gynaeco**/mast/ia _____
(Am. gyneco/mast/ia; seen in males)

Root — **Lact**
(From a Latin word **lactis**, *meaning milk.)*

Combining forms **Lact/i/o**

 ## WORD EXERCISE 24

Using your Exercise Guide, find the meaning of:

(a) **lact**/agogue _____

(b) **lacti**/fer/ous _____

(c) **lacto**/meter _____
(for specific gravity)

(d) **lacto**/trophin _____
(a hormone synonymous with prolactin)

(e) pro/**lactin** _____
(hormone acts on breasts)

(f) **lacti**/fuge _____

Without using your Exercise Guide, write the meaning of:

(g) **lacto**/genic _____

Root	Galact

Galact
(From a Greek word **galaktos**, *meaning milk.)*

Combining forms   **Galact/o**

WORD EXERCISE 25

Without using your Exercise Guide, write the meaning of:

(a) **galact**/agogue _____

(b) **galacto**/rrhoea _____
(Am. galacto/rrhea; an abnormal condition)

(c) **galact**/ischia _____

(d) **galacto**/poiesis _____

Medical equipment and clinical procedures

Revise the names of all instruments and procedures introduced in this unit before completing Exercise 26.

WORD EXERCISE 26

Match each term in Column A with a description from Column C by placing the appropriate number in Column B.

Column A	Column B	Column C
(a) vaginal speculum	_____	1. technique of recording uterine contractions
(b) colposcope	_____	2. instrument used to view the uterus
(c) Pap test	_____	3. technique of examining peritoneal cavity via vaginal fornix and rectouterine pouch
(d) culdoscopy	_____	4. instrument used to cut amnion
(e) fetoscope	_____	5. instrument used to view the vagina and cervix
(f) hysteroscope	_____	6. instrument used to measure the specific gravity of milk
(g) amniotome	_____	7. technique of examining cells from a cervical smear
(h) lactometer	_____	8. instrument to assist passage of a baby through the birth canal
(i) obstetrical forceps	_____	9. instrument to hold walls of the vagina apart
(j) tocography	_____	10. instrument inserted into amniotic cavity to visually examine a fetus

CASE HISTORY 16

The object of this exercise is to understand words associated with a patient's medical history.

To complete the exercise:

• read through the passage on pregnancy associated hypertension; unfamiliar words are underlined and you can find their meaning using the Word Help

• write the meaning of the medical terms shown in bold print.

Pregnancy associated hypertension

Mrs P, a **primigravida** aged 25, presented to her <u>GP</u> with 12 weeks of **amenorrhoea** (Am. amenorrhea); examination confirmed the dates of <u>gestation</u>. Her <u>BP</u> was at 120/80, her urine was sterile and showed no protein on <u>dipstick testing</u>.

Mrs P's pregnancy progressed normally until 35 weeks of gestation when her BP rose to 150/95 mm Hg. She was admitted to the <u>Obs-Gyn</u> Unit for rest and observation. Serial <u>ultrasound cephalometry</u> was commenced and twice weekly 24 hour urine collection for <u>oestrogen</u> excretion estimation.

In addition, daily fetal **cardiotocography** was performed. All these tests were normal and her BP fell to 124/80 within 2 days of admission. After 5 days she was allowed home with instructions to rest and was seen weekly at **antenatal** clinic.

Antenatal investigations continued to be normal with evidence of good fetal growth until 3 days before term when her blood pressure increased to 155/95 and her urine was protein ++ . Over the next 24 hours her blood pressure was maintained and she had <u>proteinuria</u> of 3 g/24 hours. Vaginal examination showed a long cervix that was not dilated.

Mrs P had developed pregnancy associated <u>hypertension</u> or <u>pre-eclamptic</u> <u>toxaemia</u>, increasing the risk of **perinatal** <u>mortality</u>. The **obstetrician** considered performing a lower section Caesarean section (LSCS) since the risk becomes minimal after 24 hours of **puerperium**. Instead, the decision was taken to induce labour. Her cervix was dilated with a catheter left in place for 24 hours and partially ripened by local application of <u>prostaglandin</u>. Labour was induced by artificial rupture of the **amniotic** membranes and an infusion of <u>oxytocin</u>. After 8 hours she gave birth to a healthy male and her recovery was uneventful.

WORD HELP

BP blood pressure

dipstick testing tests using paper sticks coated with indicators that change colour when protein is present

gestation period of pregnancy

GP general practitioner (family doctor)

hypertension high blood pressure

mortality death rate

Obs-Gyn obstetrics and gynaecology (Am. gynecology)

oestrogen female sex hormone

oxytocin hormone that stimulates uterine contractions (to induce birth)

pre-eclamptic condition before or leading to eclampsia, (due to toxaemia (Am. toxemia))

prostaglandin agent that stimulates uterine contractions

proteinuria condition of protein in the urine

toxaemia the word means condition of poisoned blood, but refers to the toxic effects of eclampsia: high blood pressure, proteinuria etc. There is a risk of convulsion and toxic effects on the baby

ultrasound cephalometry using ultrasound images to measure the size of the head

Now write the meaning of the following words from the case history without using your dictionary lists:

(a) primigravida

(b) amenorrhoea (Am. amenorrhea)

(c) cardiotocography

(d) antenatal

(e) perinatal

(f) obstetrician

(g) puerperium

(h) amniotic

(Answers to the case history exercise are given in the Answers to Word Exercises beginning on page 275.)

Quick Reference

Combining forms relating to the female reproductive system:

Amni/o	amnion
Bartholin/o	greater vestibular glands/ Bartholin's glands of the vagina
Cervic/o	cervix
Chori/o	chorion/outer fetal membrane
Colp/o	vagina
Culd/o	Douglas cavity/ rectouterine pouch
Endometr/i	endometrium/lining of womb/uterus
Fet/o (Am.)	fetus
Galact/o	milk
-gravida	pregnancy/pregnant woman
Gynaec/o	female
Gynec/o (Am.)	female
Hyster/o	uterus
Lact/o/i	milk
Mamm/o	breast
Mast/o	breast
Men/o	menses/menstruation/ monthly flow
Metr/o	uterus/womb
Nat/o	birth
Obstetric	pertaining to midwifery
Oo-	egg
Oophor/o	ovary
Ovari/o	ovary
-para	to bear/bring forth offspring
Perine/o	perineum
Placent/o	placenta
Salping/o	Fallopian tube
Toc/o	labour/birth
Trachel/o	neck
Uter/o	uterus
Vagin/o	vagina
Vulv/o	vulva

Abbreviations

Some common abbreviations related to obstetrics are listed below. Note, however, some are not standard and their meaning may vary from one health care setting to another. There is a more extensive list for reference on page 307.

AB, ab, abor	abortion
AFP	alpha-fetoprotein
APH	antepartum haemorrhage (Am. hemorrhage)
BBA	born before arrival
C-Sect	caesarean section (Am. cesarean)
FDIU	fetal death in utero
GI and GII	gravida I and gravida II
IUD	intrauterine death
LCCS	low cervical caesarean section (Am. cesarean)
LGA	large for gestational age
NFTD	normal full-term delivery
Obs-Gyn	obstetrics and gynaecology (Am. gynecology)

> ## NOW TRY THE WORD CHECK <

WORD CHECK

This self-check exercise lists all the word components used in this unit. First write down the meaning of as many word components as you can. Then check your answers using the Exercise Guide and Quick Reference box or the Glossary of Word Components (pp. 319–341).

Prefixes

a-

ante-

dys-

endo-

eu-

extra-

micro-

multi-

neo-

nulli-

oligo-

peri-

post-

pre-

primi-

pro-

pseudo-

secundi-

Combining forms of word roots

amni/o

bartholin/o

cardi/o

cervic/o

chori/o

colp/o

culd/o

cyst/o

cyt/o

fer/o

fet/o

fibr/o

galact/o

gravida

gynaec/o
(Am. gynec/o)

haem/o
(Am. hem/o)

hyster/o

lact/o

mamm/o

mast/o

men/o

metr/o

myc/o

nat/o

obstetric-

oo-

oophor/o

ovari/o

-para

perine/o

peritone/o

phleb/o

placent/o

rect/o

salping/o

sten/o

toc/o

trachel/o

uter/o

vagin/o

vesic/o

vulv/o

Suffixes

-a

-agogue

-al

-algia

-arche

-blast

-cele

-centesis

-dynia

-ectomy

-fuge

-genesis

-genic

-gram

-graphy

-ia

-ic

-ischia

-itis

-lithiasis

-logy

-malacia

-meter

-metry

-natal

-osis

-ous

-pathia

-pathy

-pause

-pexy

-plasty

-poiesis

-ptosis

-rrhagic

-rrhaphy

-rrhexis

-rrhoea
(Am. -rrhea)

-sclerosis _____

-scope _____

-scopy _____

-staxis _____

-stenosis _____

-stomy _____

-tome _____

-tomy _____

-toxic _____

-trophic _____

-tropic _____

-tubal _____

> **NOW TRY THE SELF-ASSESSMENT** <

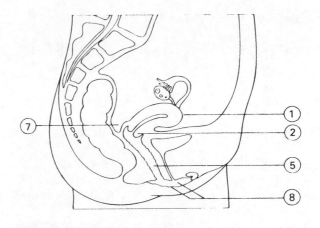

Figure 86 Section through female

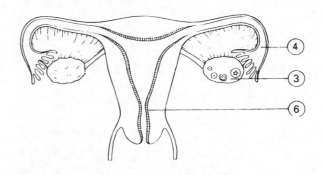

Figure 87 The female reproductive system

SELF-ASSESSMENT

Test 16A

Below are some combining forms that refer to the anatomy of the female reproductive system. Indicate which part of the system they refer to by putting a number from the diagrams (Figs 86 and 87) next to each word.

(a) oophor/o _____

(b) salping/o _____

(c) hyster/o _____

(d) endometr/o _____

(e) cervic/o _____

(f) colp/o _____

(g) vulv/o _____

(h) culd/o _____

Score

8

Test 16B

Prefixes and suffixes

Match each prefix and suffix in Column A with a meaning in Column C by inserting the appropriate number in Column B.

Column A	Column B	Column C
(a) -agogue	_____	1. to drip (blood)
(b) ante-	_____	2. pertaining to birth
(c) eu-	_____	3. stop/pause
(d) -ischia	_____	4. new
(e) multi-	_____	5. stimulate/induce
(f) -natal	_____	6. after
(g) neo-	_____	7. few/little
(h) nulli-	_____	8. condition of bursting forth (of blood)

Column A	Column B	Column C
(i) oligo-	_____	9. pertaining to tube/oviduct
(j) -ous	_____	10. before (i)
(k) -pause	_____	11. before (ii)
(l) -pexy	_____	12. good
(m) post-	_____	13. fixation by surgery
(n) pre-	_____	14. pertaining to stimulating
(o) primi-	_____	15. pertaining to
(p) -rrhagia	_____	16. second
(q) secundi-	_____	17. none
(r) -staxis	_____	18. first
(s) -tropic	_____	19. condition of blocking/holding back
(t) -tubal	_____	20. many

Score

20

Test 16C

Combining forms of word roots

Match each combining form in Column A with a meaning in Column C by inserting the appropriate number in Column B.

Column A	Column B	Column C
(a) cervic/o	_____	1. woman
(b) colp/o	_____	2. breast (i)
(c) culd/o	_____	3. breast (ii)
(d) gravida	_____	4. menstruation/monthly

Column A	Column B	Column C
(e) gynaec/o (Am. gynec/o)	_____	5. birth
(f) hyster/o	_____	6. vulva (external genitalia)
(g) lact/o	_____	7. placenta
(h) mamm/o	_____	8. pregnant heavy/pregnant woman
(i) mast/o	_____	9. perineum/area between anus and vulva
(j) men/o	_____	10. pertaining to midwifery and childbirth
(k) metr/o	_____	11. to bear/bring forth baby
(l) nat/o	_____	12. uterus (i)
(m) obstetric-	_____	13. uterus (ii)
(n) oo-	_____	14. uterus (iii)
(o) oophor/o	_____	15. neck (of womb)
(p) ovari/o	_____	16. Douglas pouch/rectouterine cavity
(q) -para	_____	17. vagina (i)
(r) perine/o	_____	18. vagina (ii)
(s) placent/o	_____	19. egg
(t) salping/o	_____	20. ovary (i)
(u) trachel/o	_____	21. ovary (ii)
(v) uter/o	_____	22. cervix uteri
(w) vagin/o	_____	23. Fallopian tube
(x) vesic/o	_____	24. milk
(y) vulv/o	_____	25. bladder

Score

25

Test 16D

Write the meaning of:

(a) tocometer   _____

(b) oophorohysterectomy   _____

(c) mastopexy   _____

(d) hysterorrhexis   _____

(e) metropathy   _____

Score

5

Test 16E

Build words that mean:

(a) surgical repair of the Douglas   _____
     pouch/rectouterine pouch

(b) formation of an opening   _____
     into a Fallopian tube

(c) rupture of the amnion   _____

(d) displacement/prolapse of   _____
     the vagina (use colp/o)

(e) study of cells of the vagina   _____
     (use colp/o)

Score

5

Check answers to Self-Assessment Tests on page 299.

17 The endocrine system

Objectives

Once you have completed Unit 17 you should be able to:

- understand the meaning of medical words relating to the endocrine system

- build medical words relating to the endocrine system

- associate medical terms with their anatomical position

- understand medical abbreviations relating to the endocrine system.

Exercise Guide

Use this list of word components and their meanings to complete the word exercises in this unit.

Prefixes

acro-	extremities/point
hyper-	above normal/excessive
hypo-	below normal/deficient
para-	beside/near

Roots/Combining forms

aden/o	gland
blast/o	germ cell/cell that forms ...
chondr/o	cartilage
gloss/o	tongue
-gyne	woman
kal/i	potassium
natr/i	sodium

Suffixes

-aemia	condition of blood
-al	pertaining to
-ectomy	removal of
-emia (Am.)	condition of blood
-genesis	formation of
-genic	pertaining to formation/ originating in
-globulin	protein
-ia	condition of
-ic	pertaining to
-ism	process of/state or condition
-itis	inflammation of
-megaly	enlargement
-micria	condition of small size
-oma	tumour/swelling
-osis	abnormal condition/disease of
-plasia	condition of growth/formation of (cells)
-ptosis	falling/displacement/prolapse
-static	pertaining to stopping/controlling
-tomy	incision into
-toxic	pertaining to poisoning
-trophic	pertaining to nourishment
-tropic	pertaining to affinity for/stimulating
-uresis	excrete in urine/urinate
-uria	condition of urine

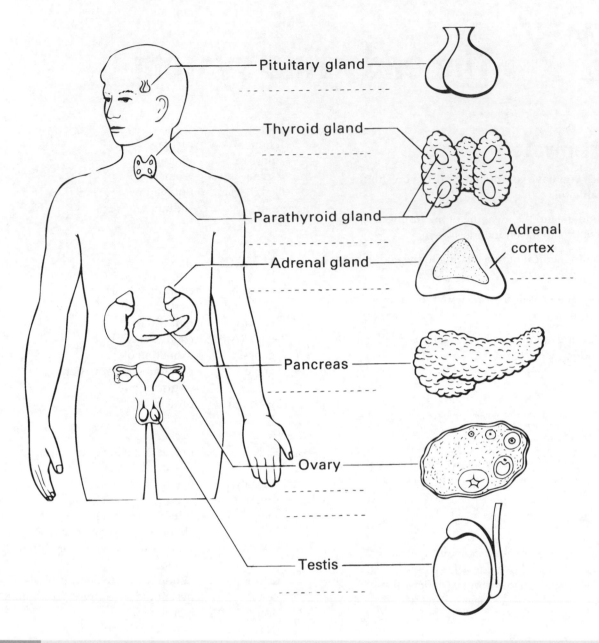

Figure 88 The endocrine system

ANATOMY EXERCISE

When you have finished Word Exercises 1–6, look at the word components listed below. Complete Figure 88 by writing the appropriate combining form on each dotted line – more than one component may relate to the same position. (You can check their meanings in the Quick Reference box on p. 220.)

Adren/o	Orchid/o	Parathyroid/o
Adrenocortic/o	Ovari/o	Pituitar-
Hypophys-	Pancreat/o	Thyr/o
Oophor/o		

The endocrine system

The endocrine system is composed of a diverse group of glands that secrete hormones directly into the bloodstream. Once released, hormones travel in the blood to all parts of the body. Low concentrations of hormones in the blood stimulate specific target tissues and exert a regulatory effect on their cellular processes.

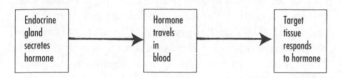

The concentration of hormones that circulate in the blood is precisely regulated by the brain and the endocrine glands. Many endocrine disorders are brought about by changes in the output of hormones. Abnormal levels of hormones produce symptoms that range from minor to severely disabling disease and death.

In this unit we will examine terms associated with each endocrine gland.

Use the Exercise Guide at the beginning of this unit to complete Word Exercises 1–6 unless you are asked to work without it.

The pituitary gland

Root	Pituitar
	*(From a Latin word **pituita**, meaning slime/phlegm. It refers to the pituitary, a small gland that grows from the base of the brain on a stalk. It is commonly called the 'master' gland of the endocrine system because it releases tropic hormones that regulate other endocrine glands.)*
Combining forms	**-pituitar-** *(-**pituitar**ism is used when referring to the process of pituitary secretion.)*

WORD EXERCISE 1

Using your Exercise Guide, find the meaning of:

(a) hypo/**pituitar**/ism _____

(b) hyper/**pituitar**/ism _____

One of the hormones produced by the pituitary gland is somatotrophin or human growth hormone (HGH). Underproduction of this results in **acromicria** and **dwarfism**. Overproduction of growth hormone produces **acromegaly** and **giantism**.

(c) acro/micria _____

(d) acro/megaly _____

Once it was realized that the pituitary gland is not the source of spit and phlegm, scientists renamed the gland the **hypophysis** (*hypo* – below, *physis* – growth, i.e. growth below the brain). Pituitary and hypophysis are now used synonymously. The hypophysis consists of a downgrowth from the brain, known as the neurohypophysis, and attached to it a glandular part, known as the adenohypophysis.

Removal of the hypophysis is known as **hypophys/ectomy**.

The thyroid gland

Root	Thyr
	*(From a Greek word **thyreoidos**, meaning resembling a shield. It refers to the shield-shaped thyroid gland that lies above the trachea. It secretes the thyroid hormones tri-iodothyronine, T_3 and thyroxine, T_4, which control the metabolic rate of all cells.)*
Combining forms	**Thyr/o -thyroid-**

WORD EXERCISE 2

Using your Exercise Guide, find the meaning of:

(a) **thyro**/gloss/al_ _____

(b) **thyro**/aden/itis _____

(c) **thyro**/globulin _____

(d) **thyro**/chondro/tomy _____

(e) **thyro**/toxic/osis _____
(Graves' disease, generally replaced by the term hyper/thyroid/ism)

A symptom of this disorder is **exophthalmos**, protruding eyes. The extent of this can be measured using a technique known as **exophthalmometry**.

(f) para**thyroid** _____
(This refers to endocrine glands called the parathyroids that lie beside the thyroid gland. The parathyroids consists of four small glands that secrete parathyroid hormone.)

(g) **parathyroid**/ectomy _____

Without using your Exercise Guide, write the meaning of:

(h) hyper/**parathyroid**/ism _____
(leads to excess calcium in blood, hyper/calc/aemia; Am. hyper/calc/emia)

(i) **thyro**/megaly _____

Without using your Exercise Guide, build words that mean:

(j) process of secreting above normal levels of thyroid hormone _____

(k) process of secreting below normal levels of thyroid hormone _____

In infants this results in poor growth and mental retardation and is known as **congenital hypothyroidism** (formerly cretinism). In adults the condition is known as **hypothyroidism** (also myxoedema (Am. myxedema) a term that refers to the accumulation of mucopolysaccarides under the skin). It gives rise to 'puffy' swollen skin, dry hair, weight gain, bradycardia, sensitivity to cold and lethargy.

Using your Exercise Guide, build words that mean:

(l) downward displacement of the thyroid _____

(m) pertaining to affinity for the thyroid gland _____

(n) pertaining to originating in the thyroid gland _____

Any enlargement of the thyroid gland is also known as a **goitre** and it is a feature of many thyroid diseases. Goitres have been grouped in different ways and a simple classification is shown here:

> **Simple**
> Goitres that are not producing the signs and symptoms of hyperthyroidism.
>
> **Toxic**
> Goitres that are producing the signs and symptoms of hyperthyroidism. Also known as hyperthyroiditis, exophthalmic goitre and Graves' disease).
>
> **Malignant**
> Goitres that are the seat of new, malignant growth (carcinomas of the thyroid).

Thyroid goitres are investigated by the administration of radioactive iodine. The iodine is taken up by the thyroid gland which becomes slightly radioactive. The presence of radioactivity in the gland is detected with a scanner that outlines the gland and generates an image. We will look at this in more detail in Unit 18.

The pancreas

We have already examined the role of the pancreas in digestion in Unit 2; here we examine its role as an endocrine gland. Among the cells in the pancreas that produce digestive enzymes, are small patches of tissue called the **Islets of Langerhan's**. The Islets secrete the hormones **insulin** and **glucagon** directly into the blood. These play a major role in the regulation of blood glucose concentration.

Root	**Pancreat**
	(Derived from Greek **pankreas**, *pan – all, kreas – flesh. Here it is used to mean the pancreas.)*
Combining forms	**Pancreat/o**

WORD EXERCISE 3

Without using your Exercise Guide, write the meaning of:

(a) **pancreato**/tropic _____
(Some of the pituitary hormones have such an action.)

Insulin (named after Latin *insula*, meaning island) is secreted by the Islets of Langerhans. Once in the bloodstream, it stimulates the uptake of sugar by tissue cells. Its overall effect is to lower blood sugar levels in the body following the intake of glucose in the diet. The combining forms derived from this are **insulin/o** (meaning insulin or Islets of Langerhans).

Using your Exercise Guide, find the meaning of:

(b) **insulino**/genesis _____

(c) **insulin**/oma _____

Without using your Exercise Guide, write the meaning of:

(d) **insulin**/itis _____

(e) hyper/**insulin**/ism _____

If the body fails to produce insulin, blood sugar levels rise and glucose appears in the urine; this abnormal condition is known as **diabetes mellitus**. The name diabetes is derived from two Greek words, one meaning a siphon and the other meaning to pass through. The name reflects the most obvious symptoms; excessive thirst (**polydipsia**) followed by drinking and excessive urination (**polyuria**), just like the passing of water through a siphon. The second name mellitus is a Latin word meaning honey/sugar. Diabetes mellitus therefore refers to the passing of large quantities of water containing sugar through the body.

(**Polydipsia** is formed from *poly* – meaning too much, *dips/o* – thirst and *-ia* condition of).

There are two main types of diabetes mellitus:

Type 1
early onset diabetes, seen in young subjects, due to hereditary factors and/or autoimmune disease. It is also known as insulin-dependent diabetes mellitus (IDDM). These patients require insulin injections to remain alive.

Type 2
late onset diabetes mellitus. This is also known as non-insulin-dependent diabetes mellitus (NIDDM). Dietary factors are involved and it can be controlled by a change in diet and/or drugs that lower blood sugar levels.

Complications of diabetes mellitus include a tendency to develop cataracts, retinopathy and neuropathy. It is diagnosed by blood glucose estimation and glucose tolerance tests. The latter test involves administering a known quantity of glucose and measuring the amounts that appear in the blood and urine in a set time.

Below are terms that can be used to describe sugar levels in blood and urine. The combining form **glyc/o** is used to mean sugar (from Greek *glykys*, meaning sweet).

Using your Exercise Guide, find the meaning of:

(f) hypo/**glyc**/aemia _____
    (Am. hypo/glyc/emia)

(g) hyper/**glyc**/aemia _____
    (Am. hyper/glyc/emia)

(h) **glycos**/uria _____
    (Patients can estimate the state of their own blood sugar level from the amount present in their urine. Glucose oxidase papers are used to test for glucose in the urine; they change colour in the presence of glucose.)

(i) **glyco**/static _____

Untreated diabetes results in the tissue cells using fatty acids as a source of energy instead of sugar. This leads to the release of chemicals known as ketones into the blood and urine. Ketones such as acetone have a toxic effect on the body that is known as **ketosis**. The ketones are strong acids and their accumulation causes a

progressive increase in the acidity of the blood called **ketoacidosis**; this may be fatal in uncontrolled diabetes.

The adrenal gland

Root

Adren
*(From Latin **ad** – to/near, **renes** – kidneys. It refers to the adrenal gland, a small triangle-shaped gland that lies above each kidney. The inner part of the gland called the medulla, secretes adrenalin, the outer part called the cortex, secretes steroid hormones.)*

Combining forms   **Adren/o**

WORD EXERCISE 4

Without using your Exercise Guide, build words that mean:

(a) enlarged adrenal gland _____

(b) pertaining to poisonous
    to the adrenal _____

(c) pertaining to stimulating/
    acting on the adrenal _____

The adrenal cortex forms the outer layer of the adrenal gland; it produces a variety of steroid hormones (**steroidogenesis**). There are three main types:

Androgens
types of male sex hormone.

Glucocorticoids
hormones that control glucose, protein and lipid metabolism.

Mineralocorticoids
hormones that regulate fluid and electrolyte balance.

Aldosterone is an example of a mineralocorticoid. It enables the body to retain sodium and excrete potassium. Abnormal aldosterone production results in the disturbances of sodium and potassium levels named in (d), (e) and (f) below.

Using your Exercise Guide, find the meaning of:

(d) hyper/natr/aemia _____
    (Am. hyper/natr/emia)

(e) hypo/kal/aemia _____
    (Am. hypo/kal/emia)

(f) natri/uresis _____

The combining form **adrenocortic/o** is used when referring to the adrenal cortex itself. Corticosteroid refers to the steroid hormones of the adrenal cortex.

(g) **adrenocortico/**trophic _____
(Some of the hormones of the pituitary have this effect.)

(h) **adrenocortico/**hyper/plasia _____

Major disorders of hormone production by the adrenal cortex include:

Hyperfunction

> **Cushing's syndrome**
> A condition, in which over-production of adrenocorticotrophic hormone (ACTH) by the pituitary stimulates the adrenal cortex to release steroid hormones; these raise blood pressure, increase sodium retention and bring about hyperglycaemia (Am. hyperglycemia).
>
> **Adrenogenital syndrome**
> A condition in which over-production of male sex hormones leads to virilization (masculinization) in women and precocity (premature sexual maturity) in boys.

Hypofunction

> **Addison's disease**
> A condition due to the failure of the adrenal cortex to produce sufficient glucocorticoids and mineralocorticoids. It results in loss of sodium and water, and a fall in blood pressure. Patients will die within 4–14 days unless given specific hormone replacement therapy.

The ovary and testis

The ovary and the testis are endocrine organs as well as reproductive organs. In their endocrine role they produce sex hormones that function to control the development of the reproductive system and maintain its activity. Note that we have already used the combining forms for the ovary (oophor/o and ovari/o) and testis (orchid/o).

First, let's examine the endocrine role of the testis. This gland secretes male sex hormones called **androgens** that stimulate the development of the male reproductive tract and secondary sexual characteristics such as beard growth, a deep voice and the male physique. The main androgen produced by the testis is **testosterone**; it is also produced in small quantities by the adrenal cortex of both men and women. In women excess secretion leads to masculinization, one obvious effect being the growth of facial hair (hirsutism).

Root **Andr**
*(From a Greek word **andros**, meaning man/male.)*

Combining forms **Andr/o**

WORD EXERCISE 5

Using your Exercise Guide, find the meaning of:

(a) **andro**/gyne _____
(actually a female hermaphrodite)

(b) **andro**/blast/oma _____

The ovary is also an endocrine gland secreting several types of sex hormone, for example:

> **Oestrogens (Am. estrogens)**
> Steroid hormones that regulate the development of the female reproductive tract, menstrual cycle and secondary sexual characteristics, such as the growth of pubic hair and the female body form. Compounds that have oestrogen-like actions on the body are described as **oestrogenic** (Am. estrogenic).
>
> **Progestogens**
> Steroid hormones that maintain the receptivity of the uterus to fertilized eggs and stimulate the growth of the uterus during pregnancy.

Medical equipment and clinical procedures

Revise the names of medical equipment and procedures mentioned in this unit and then try Exercise 6. Some imaging procedures used for examining the endocrine system will be studied in Unit 18 as the techniques involved are similar to those used for other systems.

WORD EXERCISE 6

Match each term in Column A with a description from Column C by placing an appropriate number in Column B.

Column A	Column B	Column C
(a) adrenal function test	_____	1. imaging of the thyroid gland following administration of radioactive iodine

Column A	Column B	Column C

(b) glucose tolerance test _____ 2. test for hypothyroidism by measuring concentration of iodine in blood

(c) protein bound iodine test (PBI) _____ 3. a test used to diagnose diabetes mellitus

(d) glucose oxidase paper strip test (Clinistix) _____ 4. measurement of 24-hour output of corticosteroids

(e) thyroid scan _____ 5. indicates the relative amount of glucose in urine

ANATOMY EXERCISE

Now complete the Anatomy Exercise on page 214.

CASE HISTORY 17

The object of this exercise is to understand words associated with a patient's medical history.

To complete the exercise:

• read through the passage on diabetes mellitus; unfamiliar words are underlined and you can find their meaning using the Word Help

• write the meaning of the medical terms shown in bold print.

Diabetes mellitus

W, a 14-year-old boy on holiday in the locality, was brought into Accident and Emergency by his worried parents. Prior to admission he had complained of tiredness and insomnia, and his mother had noticed that despite a good appetite he had become thinner. On the morning of admission he suffered abdominal pain, nausea and vomiting, his breathing had become irregular and at times he appeared semiconscious. Further questioning of the parents indicated the patient had recently developed polydipsia and **polyuria**.

On admission he was conscious and hyperventilating; he was dehydrated and his breath had the fruity odour of ketones. Blood and urine samples were analysed

and quickly indicated clinically significant levels of **glycosuria**, **hyperglycaemia** and **ketonaemia**. W's condition was diagnosed as diabetic **ketoacidosis** and emergency treatment was commenced.

Vital signs on admission

Pulse	Oral temp	BP 110/70
98 per minute	36.0°C	
Blood glucose	Urine 3+	Hyperventilating
28 mmol/litre	ketones	

He was given an initial intravenous infusion of 6 units of soluble insulin followed by 6 units hourly. His fluid and electrolyte loss were replaced by an intravenous saline infusion. His blood glucose was monitored hourly and electrolytes 2 hourly in the initial phase of treatment. When his blood glucose reached its normal value, he was given a saline infusion of 5% Dextrose containing 20 mmol KCL litre^{-1}. The dose of insulin was adjusted according to the hourly blood glucose results.

W's parents were informed their son was suffering from Type 1 diabetes mellitus also known as insulin-dependent diabetes mellitus (IDDM), a chronic incurable condition brought on by a failure of the **pancreatic islets** to produce insulin.

Once recovered from his acute attack he was referred to the diabetic clinician for advice on insulin therapy and his GP was informed. He responded well to advice, and now self-administers two daily injections of insulin. His regimen was adjusted to avoid **hypoglycaemia** and give good **glycaemic** control. Both injections consist of a mixture of short and intermediate-acting insulins, the first before breakfast and the second before his evening meal.

WORD HELP

clinician expert on treating and advising patients

chronic lasting/lingering for a long time

electrolyte the ionized salts in the blood (e.g sodium and potassium ions)

GP general practitioner (family doctor)

hyperventilating above normal ventilation rate of the lungs (rapid deep breathing)

insomnia condition of inability to sleep

insulin a hormone secreted by the pancreas that lowers blood sugar

islets small islands of cells that secrete insulin in the pancreas (Islets of Langerhan's)

ketones ketone bodies (chemicals formed in diabetes from breakdown of fat)

polydipsia condition of too much/excessive thirst

regimen regulated scheme (e.g. of taking drugs/medication)

Now write the meaning of the following words from the case history without using your dictionary lists:

(a) polyuria — *cond. of passing too much urine.*

(b) glycosuria — *cond. of glucose in the urine.*

(c) hyperglycaemia (Am. hyperglycemia) — *cond. of above normal levels of glucose in the blood.*

(d) ketonaemia (Am. ketonemia) — *cond. of ketones in the blood*

(e) ketoacidosis — *ab. cond. of acidity caused by ketones*

(f) pancreatic — *pert. to the pancreas.*

(g) hypoglycaemia (Am. hypoglycemia) — *cond. of below normal levels of sugar in the blood*

(h) glycaemic (Am. glycemic) — *pert. to glucose in the blood*

(Answers to the case history exercise are given in the Answers to Word Exercises beginning on page 275.)

Abbreviations

Some common abbreviations related to the endocrine system are listed below. Note, however, some are not standard and their meaning may vary from one health care setting to another. There is a more extensive list for reference on page 307.

ACTH	adrenocorticotrophic hormone
BSS	blood sugar series
FSH	follicle-stimulating hormone
HGH	human growth hormone
HRT	hormone replacement therapy
IDDM	Insulin-dependent diabetes mellitus
LH	luteinizing hormone
NIDDM	non-insulin-dependent diabetes mellitus
OGTT	oral glucose tolerance test
PRL	prolactin
T_3, T_4	tri-iodothyronine, tetraiodothyronine (thyroxine)
TSH	thyroid stimulating hormone

Quick Reference

Combining forms relating to the endocrine system:

Aden/o	gland
Adren/o	adrenal gland
Adrenocortic/o	adrenal cortex
Andr/o	male
Cortic/o	cortex
Estr/o (Am.)	estrogen
-globulin	protein
Glyc/o	sugar
Hypophys-	hypophysis/ pituitary gland
Insulin/o	insulin
Kal/i	potassium
Ket/o	ketones
Natr/i	sodium
Oestr/o	oestrogen
Oophor/o	ovary
Orchid/o	testis
Ovari/o	ovary
Pancreat/o	pancreas
Parathyroid/o	parathyroid gland
Pituitar-	pituitary
Progest/o	progesterone
Thyr/o	thyroid gland

> ## NOW TRY THE WORD CHECK <

WORD CHECK

This self-check exercise lists all the word components used in this unit. First write down the meaning of as many word components as you can. Then check your answers using the Exercise Guide and Quick Reference box or the Glossary of Word Components (pp. 319–341).

Prefixes

acro- — *extremities*

hyper- — *above normal*

hypo- — *below normal.*

para- — *beside/near.*

poly- — *many.*

Combining forms of word roots

acid/o — *acid.*

aden/o	gland	-ic	pertaining to
adren/o	adrenal gland	-ism	process of
andr/o	male	-itis	inflammation of
blast/o	immature germ cell	-megaly	enlargement of
chondr/o	cartilage	-micria	condition of small size
cortic/o	cortex	-oid	resembling
dips/o	thirst	-oma	tumour/swelling
globulin	protein	-osis	abnormal condition of
gloss/o	tongue	-plasia	condition of growth
-gyne	woman	-ptosis	downward displacement of
insulin/o	insulin	-static	pert. to stopping/controlling
kal/i	potassium	-tomy	incision into
ket/o/n	ketones	-toxic	pert. to poisonous
natr/i	sodium	-trophic	pert. to nourishing
oestr/o (Am. estr/o)	oestrogen	-tropic	pert. to stimulating
		-uresis	excrete in urine
pancreat/o	pancreas	-uria	cond. of urine
physis	growth		
pituitar-	pituitary gland		
progest/o	progesterone		
thyr/o	thyroid gland		

> **NOW TRY THE SELF-ASSESSMENT** <

Suffixes

-aemia (Am. -emia)	condition of blood
-al	pertaining to
-ectomy	removal of
-genesis	formation
-genic	pertaining to formation
-ia	condition of

SELF-ASSESSMENT

Test 17A

Below are some combining forms that refer to the anatomy of the endocrine system. Indicate which part of the system they refer to by putting a number from the diagram (Fig. 89) next to each word.

(a) adren/o	4
(b) parathyroid/o	3
(c) andr/o	7

(d) thyroid/o _____2_____

(e) insulin/o _____5_____

(f) oestr/o _____6_____
(Am. estr/o)

(g) pituitar- _____1_____

(h) adrenocortic/o _____8_____

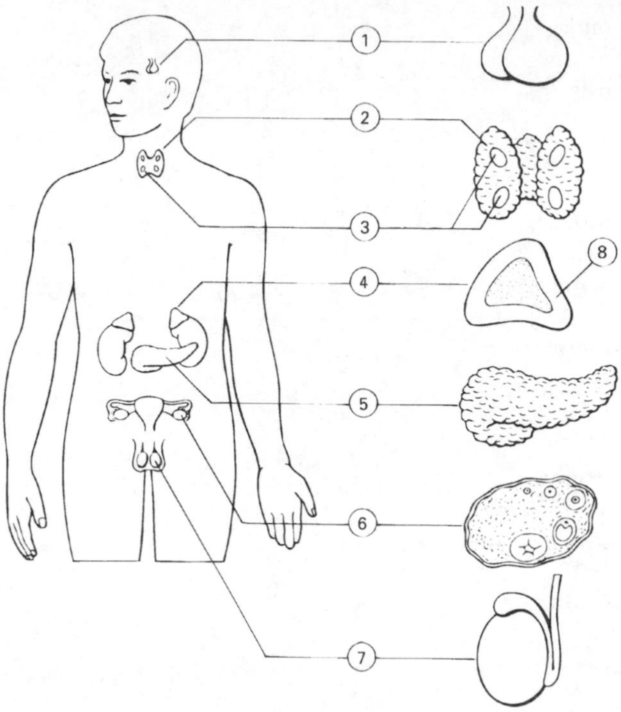

Column A	Column B	Column C
(c) andr/o	20	3. pancreas
(d) blast/o	1	4. progesterone
(e) -globin	19	5. pertaining to constant/ unchanging/ controlling
(f) glyc/o	8	6. condition of growth (increase of cells)
(g) hyper-	18	7. oestrogen (Am. estrogen)
(h) hypo-	10	8. sugar
(i) insulin/o	15	9. hypophysis
(j) micr/o	2	10. below
(k) oestr/o (Am. estr/o)	7	11. gland
(l) pancreat/o	3	12. thyroid
(m) para-	17	13. pertaining to affinity for/ acting on
(n) -plasia	6	14. pertaining to nourishment
(o) pituitar-	9	15. insulin/islets of Langerhans
(p) progest/o	4	16. extremity/point
(q) -static	5	17. beside/near
(r) thyr/o	12	18. above
(s) -trophic	14	19. protein
(t) -tropic	13	20. man/male

Figure 89 The endocrine system

Score

8

Test 17B

Prefixes, suffixes and combining forms of word roots

Match a word component from Column A with a meaning in Column C by inserting the appropriate number in Column B.

Score

20

Column A	Column B	Column C
(a) acro-	16	1. germ cell
(b) aden/o	11	2. small

Test 17C

Write the meaning of:

(a) thyroparathyroidectomy — *removal of the parathyroid + thyroid gland.*

(b) pituicyte — *pituitary cell.*

(c) adrenomegaly — *enlargement of the adrenal gland.*

(d) glycotropic — *pert. to affinity for glucose.*

(e) hyperketonaemia (Am. hyperketonemia) — *cond. of above normal levels of ketones in the blood.*

Score

5

Test 17D

Build words that mean:

(a) process of producing too much insulin — *hyperinsulinism*

(b) condition of too little sodium in the blood — *hyponatraemia*

(c) pertaining to nourishing the thyroid gland (use thyr/o) — *thyrotrophic*

(d) pertaining to acting on/ stimulating the adrenal — *adrenotropic*

(e) process of producing too little parathyroid hormone — *hypoparathyroidism*

Score

5

Check answers to Self-Assessment Tests on page 299.

18 Radiology and nuclear medicine

Objectives

Once you have completed Unit 18 you should be able to:

- understand the meaning of medical words relating to radiology and nuclear medicine

- build medical words relating to radiology and nuclear medicine

- understand medical abbreviations relating to radiology and nuclear medicine.

Exercise Guide

Use this list of word components and their meanings to complete the word exercises in this unit.

Prefixes

ultra-	beyond

Roots/Combining forms

angi/o	vessel
cardi/o	heart
encephal/o	brain
esophag/o (Am.)	esophagus/gullet
oesophag/o	oesophagus/gullet

Suffixes

-er	one who
-genic	pertaining to formation/ originating in
-gram	X-ray picture/tracing/recording
-graph	usually an instrument that records/an X-ray picture
-graphy	technique of recording/making an X-ray
-ist	specialist
-logist	specialist who studies
-logy	study of
-scope	viewing instrument
-therapist	specialist who treats (disease)
-therapy	treatment

Radiology

Radiology is the study of the diagnosis of disease by the use of radiant energy (radiation). In the past this meant the use of X-rays to make an image of the internal components of the body. Today many other forms of radiation are used to aid both diagnosis and treatment of disease. Developments in physics and technology are bringing rapid changes to this branch of medicine.

Before completing the first exercise, review the terms below:

> **-gram**
> recording/picture/tracing/X-ray.
>
> **-graph**
> usually refers to an instrument that records by making a picture or tracing but it is also used here to mean a recording or X-ray picture.
>
> **-graphy**
> technique of making a recording, i.e. a picture, X-ray, tracing or writing.

Use the Exercise Guide at the beginning of this unit to complete Word Exercises 1–10 unless you are asked to work without it.

Root   **Radi**
(From a Latin word **radius**, meaning a ray. Here it is used to mean X-rays, the invisible rays produced by an X-ray machine. Also used to mean radiation/radioactivity.)

Combining forms   **Radi/o**

WORD EXERCISE 1

Using your Exercise Guide, find the meaning of:

(a) **radio**/logist _____
(a physician, i.e. medically qualified)

(b) **radio**/graph _____
(refers to an X-ray picture)

(c) **radio**/graphy _____

(d) **radio**/graph/er _____
(refers to a technician who is not medically qualified)

(e) **radio**/therapist _____

Some radiographic procedures require the use of a contrast medium or agent to improve the quality of the image. Contrast agents are required because there is little difference in the density of the soft parts of the body and X-rays pass through them without producing a distinct image of individual organs. The contrast medium is administered to the patient, filling a cavity such as the stomach. The X-ray is taken and the outline of the cavity recorded on the radiograph.

An example of a contrast medium is barium sulphate, a radio-opaque substance that absorbs X-rays. It shows up on X-ray film as a white area that has not allowed X-rays to pass. This property of barium sulphate makes it particularly useful for outlining the digestive tract where it is administered as:

> **A barium 'meal' (swallow)**
> To outline the upper parts of the digestive system the barium is given as a drink.
>
> **A barium enema**
> To outline the lower parts of the digestive system. In this procedure barium is injected via the anus into the rectum and colon. Sometimes air is also administered with the barium to increase contrast; this is known as a **double contrast radiograph**.

Iodine is another contrast agent that can be added to make various fluids radio-opaque. It is often the contrast agent used in angiocardiography, arteriography and venography.

Root   **Roentgen**
(From the name of Wilhelm K. **Roentgen**, a German physicist who discovered X-rays. It is used to mean X-rays.)

Combining forms   **Roentgen/o**

WORD EXERCISE 2

Without using your Exercise Guide, write the meaning of:

(a) **roentgeno**/graphy _____

(b) **roentgeno**/logist _____
(synonymous with radiologist)

Using your Exercise Guide, find the meaning of:

(c) **roentgeno**/gram _____
(synonymous with radiograph, but as this German name is difficult to pronounce, radiograph is more commonly used)

(d) **roentgeno**/cardio/gram _____

The movement of internal parts of the body can be observed using a technique known as fluoroscopy. In this procedure X-rays pass through the body on to a phosphor screen (a fluorescent screen, i.e. one from which light flows). As the X-rays strike the screen, the phosphor emits light, producing an image which is viewed as it is generated. Fluoroscopy is useful for observing movement of the oesophagus (Am. esophagus), stomach and heart. If necessary, a recording/ picture can be made of the light image from the screen. (**Fluor** is from Latin *fluere*, meaning to flow. It is used to mean something that is luminous, i.e. emitting light.)

Using your Exercise Guide, build a word that means:

(e) instrument used for the _____ direct X-ray examination of the body (fluoroscopy)

Without using your Exercise Guide, build a word that means:

(f) technique of recording a _____ radiographic image produced by fluoroscopy

Root	Cine
	*(From a Greek word **kinein**, meaning movement. Here the combining forms are used to mean a moving film, i.e. a motion picture on film or video.)*

Combining forms   **Cine, cinemat/o**

WORD EXERCISE 3

Without using your Exercise Guide, write the meaning of:

(a) **cine**/radio/graph _____

(b) roentgeno/**cinemato**/graphy _____

Using your Exercise Guide, find the meaning of:

(c) **cine**/angio/cardio/graphy _____

(d) **cine**/oesophago/gram _____ (Am. cine-esophago/gram)

Root	Tom
	*(From a Greek word **tomos**, meaning a slice or section.)*

Combining forms   **Tom/o**

A **tomograph** is an instrument that uses X-rays to obtain images of sections through the body. It uses a thin beam of X-rays that rotates around the patient. X-ray photons emitted from the patient are detected and converted into an image by a computer. The images produced by this device show more detail than a simple X-ray.

WORD EXERCISE 4

Without using your Exercise Guide, write the meaning of:

(a) **tomo**/gram _____

(b) **tomo**/graphy _____ (This procedure is usually called computed tomography (CT), but it is also known as CT scanning, computerized axial tomography (CAT) and CAT scanning).

Nuclear medicine

This branch of medicine uses **radioisotopes** (also called **radionuclides**) to diagnose and treat disease. In some texts it is called nuclear radiology. Terms used for diagnostic radiology include nuclear imaging and radionuclide imaging.

Radioisotopes

Radioisotopes are elements that exhibit the property of spontaneous decay, emitting radiation in the process. The radiation is in the form of high-speed particles and energy-containing rays. Elements that emit alpha, beta or gamma radiation are used as diagnostic labels to trace the route and uptake of chemicals administered into the body. The radioisotope behaves like a transmitter, passing radiation from inside to the outside of the body. Ideally, radioisotopes should give off gamma radiation as alpha and beta particles can damage cells. Many different diagnostic techniques have been devised that use radioisotopes; one procedure is described below.

First the specific isotope or tracer is given to the patient. Once in the body it continues to emit radiation and is absorbed or excluded from the tissues and organs under investigation. Next a Geigy–Muller tube or gamma camera is passed over the surface of the body to detect gamma rays emitted by the isotope; this is also known as a **radioisotope scan**. Finally an image is constructed showing the distributon of radioactivity within the tissues and organs. **Radioisotope scans** are used to image the heart, liver, biliary tract, bone, thyroid and kidney.

Here are some examples of the use of specific radioisotopes:

> **99MTc (technetium)**
> 99MTc is administered to the patient in trace quantities. It is excluded from normal brain tissue but accumulates in some brain tumours. A tumour can be detected by locating the gamma rays emitted from it.
>
> **123I (iodine)**
> 123I is rapidly taken up by the thyroid gland. A radioisotope scan of the gland will outline the now radioactive gland and information from this will aid the diagnosis of various thyroid disorders, e.g. thyrotoxicosis.
>
> **57Co (cobalt)**
> 57Co is used to trace the uptake of vitamin B_{12} by the body and from this a diagnosis of megaloblastic anaemia can be made.

Scintigraphy

Scintigraphy is the technique of producing a radioisotope scan. A radioisotope with an affinity for a particular organ or tissue is injected into the body and the distribution of the radioactivity is followed using an instrument called a **scintillation counter (scintiscanner)**. This device contains a **scintillator**, a substance that emits light in contact with ionizing radiation. There is a flash of light for each ionizing event and the number of flashes (or counts) is related to the radioactivity present in the area being scanned. Scintillation counters can be moved over the outer surface of the body to locate radioisotopes within particular organs and build an image (scintigram/scintiscan) of their distribution. The **gamma camera** mentioned earlier is a scintillation counter.

Root	Scint
	*(From a Latin word **scintilla**, meaning spark/emitting sparks/light.)*
Combining forms	**Scint/i, scintill/a**

WORD EXERCISE 5

Without using your Exercise Guide, write the meaning of:

(a) **scinti**/gram _____

(b) **scinti**/graphy _____

Positron Emission Tomography (PET)

This is another imaging technique that traces the distribution of radioisotopes within the body. **Positron emission tomography** (PET scanning) uses radioisotopes (radionuclides) that emit short-lived particles called positrons (β +radiation). The isotopes, which are injected intravenously, are taken up by particular tissues, for example 11C-2-deoxy-D-glucose can penetrate the blood–brain barrier and is used by brain cells as a source of energy. Once inside brain cells the isotope decays emitting positrons; the more active the cells, the more labelled glucose is taken up and the more positrons are emitted.

The positrons immediately collide with electrons, yielding gamma ray photons that have sufficient energy to leave the body. These photons are detected by a large array of scintillation detectors that surround the patient. The position of the emerging photons is determined and used to construct a cross sectional computerized image that shows the distribution of the radioisotopes in the tissues.

PET is used to investigate physiological processes such as the blood perfusion of organs and metabolism and has found particular application in the study of the brain in patients with neurological deficits caused by strokes and epilepsy.

The half-life of radionuclides used in PET is short-lived so they cannot be stored and used when required. The technique is dependent on the immediate production of radionuclides in a complex and expensive device called a **cyclotron** and the services of **radiochemical** and **radiopharmaceutical** laboratories. These restrictions have limited its use to special centres with appropriate facilities. Recently, mini cyclotrons have been designed for on site production of radionuclides and these are leading to increased use of this imaging technique.

Radiotherapy

Radiotherapy is the treatment of disease by X-rays and other forms of radiation. In particular the radiation is used to destroy malignant cancer cells by exposing them to a lethal dose of radiation.

Teletherapy (External beam therapy)

This is the administration of radiation from an external source at a distance from the body (*tele*- meaning far away/operating at a distance). Radiotherapy machines generate the radiation used in this form of treatment and there has been a move towards ever more powerful devices. To maximize the therapeutic advantages of radiotherapy, it is necessary to give a tumouricidal (Am. tumoricidal) dose of radiation to a planned target volume and minimize the dose to surrounding tissue.

(Here *tumour-* means a mass of cancer cells, *-cidal* pertaining to killing).

The first high energy beams were produced by the decay of radioactive sources. The cobalt sixty (^{60}Co) radiotherapy machine still in use produces radiation at energies of between 1 and 4 MeV (mega-electron-volts, 1 MeV = 1 million electronvolts). At its centre is a cobalt sixty high energy radiation source that emits gamma(γ)-ray photons which are directed at the patient through an opening called a collimator. This machine has been particularly useful for treating tumours of the head, neck and metastatic spread to lymph nodes.

Cobalt sixty machines have been largely superseded by linear accelerators that generate X-ray photons or electron beams at very high energy levels (3–35 MeV) and contain no radioactive sources. In electron mode these complex machines accelerate a beam of electrons to near the speed of light and direct them on to superficial lesions near the surface of the body. In photon mode the beam of electrons is made to collide with a metal target generating high energy X-ray photons that can be used to destroy tumours deep within the body.

Brachytherapy

The term **brachytherapy** (*brachy-* meaning short) means the administration of radiation in close proximity to a tumour. It is accomplished by the implantation of radioactive sources into the body. The sealed source has been used to deliver radiation in three main ways: into the surface of the skin, into a cavity (intracavity) and directly into a tissue or tumour (interstitial).

Needles containing radium (^{226}Ra) and emitting gamma ray photons at 0.2–2.4 MeV were first used. A needle consists of a platinum or alloy tube with a sharp (trocar) point at one end and an eyelet for a thread at the other. The radioactive material is loaded into the needle in cells (this minimizes spillage if damaged) and they are sealed in with gold solder. The needle is inserted directly into a tumour and left for a fixed time before being withdrawn. Caesium (^{137}Cs) (Am. Cesium) has been used as a radium substitute for intracavity and interstitial brachytherapy.

Tubes and seeds are similar to needles, but they have no sharp points; instead they fit into an applicator for insertion into a body cavity. Radon gas seeds (^{222}Rn) were used as a substitute for radium, and these have been superseded by gold (^{198}Au) seeds for interstitial implants. Typically they have a length of 5 mm and a diameter of 1.35 mm, small enough to be inserted into a tumour and left forming harmless foreign bodies once their radioactivity has decayed to a negligible value (half-life 3.8 days)

Other sources include: Caesium (^{137}Cs) needles, Gold (^{198}Au) grains and tubes, and iridium (^{192}Ir) wires, hairpins, seeds and ribbons.

In the 1930s brachytherapy needles were inserted into the patient manually; this exposed medical and nursing staff to high doses of radiation. The afterloading technique has been developed to reduce the handling times of radioactive sources. In this procedure, non-radioactive needles, tubing and applicators are precisely positioned in the patient before the introduction of the radioactive sources. The sources are only introduced when they can be quickly loaded into the appropriate points in the patient, thereby reducing exposure to medical staff. Improved afterloading machines are now available that further reduce unwanted exposure. This, with the development of new radionuclides, has made brachytherapy a much safer form of treatment.

Radionuclides are also administered to patients in unsealed forms, for example, Iodine (^{131}I) emits beta radiation and is used as a treatment for thyrotoxicosis. The iodine is available as an injection, drink or capsule, the latter being safer as it reduces the risk of spillage. Once absorbed, the iodine is preferentially absorbed by the thyroid gland delivering a therapeutic dose of radiation. This causes the gland to atrophy and reduce its output of thyroid hormones.

WORD EXERCISE 6

Without using your Exercise Guide, write the meaning of:

(a) **radio**/therapy _____

(b) **radio**/therapist _____
(a physician, medically qualified)

Ultrasonography

When high-frequency sound waves are directed at the body, internal organs and masses reflect the sound to a different extent. They are said to have different echo textures. These internal echoes are detected and converted into an image. The size and shape of easily recognized organs can be investigated using this technique and it is widely used for examining a fetus in utero.

Root	Son
	*(From a Latin word **sonus**, meaning sound.)*
Combining forms	**Son/o**

Note the next exercise refers to techniques using **ultrasound**, high-frequency sounds beyond human hearing.

WORD EXERCISE 7

Using your Exercise Guide, find the meaning of:

(a) ultra/**sono**/gram _____
    (a picture/tracing)

Without using your Exercise Guide, write the meaning of:

(b) ultra/**sono**/graphy _____

(c) ultra/**sono**/graph _____
    (an instrument)

Root	Echo
	(A Greek word meaning the repetition of sounds owing to reflection by an obstacle. Here it is used to mean ultrasound echoes.)
Combining forms	**Echo-**

WORD EXERCISE 8

Using your Exercise Guide, find the meaning of:

(a) **echo**/encephalo/gram _____

Using your Exercise Guide, build a word that means:

(b) pertaining to forming/ _____
    generating an echo

Without using your Exercise Guide, build words that mean:

(c) recording/picture of echo _____
    (synonymous with ultrasonogram)

(d) instrument that records _____
    echoes from the brain

(e) recording/picture of _____
    heart echoes

(f) technique of making _____
    a picture/tracing using echoes

Thermography

Thermography is the technique of recording temperature differences throughout the body on film.

Our bodies radiate a range of infrared waves at different frequencies. The frequency of the radiation depends on the temperature of the body. Thermography uses electronic equipment to convert infrared radiation into visible light which is used to form an image. Thermography has proved of great benefit in the detection of breast and testicular tumours. Tumours contain abnormally active cells and so tend to be warmer than surrounding areas.

Root	Therm
	*(From a Greek word **therme** meaning heat.)*
Combining forms	**Therm/o**

WORD EXERCISE 9

Without using your Exercise Guide, write the meaning of:

(a) **thermo**/gram _____

(b) scrotal **thermo**/graphy _____

Medical equipment and clinical procedures

Revise the names of all instruments and techniques used in this unit before trying Exercise 10.

WORD EXERCISE 10

Match each term in Column A with a description in Column C by placing an appropriate number in Column B.

Column A	Column B	Column C
(a) radiography	_____	1. instrument that detects gamma rays from radioisotopes
(b) fluoroscopy	_____	2. technique of using ultrasound echoes to image the heart
(c) thermography	_____	3. chemical used to improve detail of an X-ray
(d) ultrasonograph	_____	4. technique of making an X-ray

Column A	Column B	Column C
(e) computerized tomograph	_____	5. instrument that makes tracing/picture using reflected sound
(f) radiotherapy	_____	6. instrument that uses X-rays to image a slice through the body
(g) cineradiography	_____	7. direct observation of X-ray picture using a fluorescent screen
(h) gamma camera	_____	8. technique of recording body heat on film
(i) echocardiography	_____	9. treatment of disorders using radiation
(j) contrast medium	_____	10. technique of using X-rays to make a moving picture

CASE HISTORY 18

The object of this exercise is to understand words associated with a patient's medical history.

To complete the exercise:

- read through the passage on cancer of the larynx; unfamiliar words are underlined and you can find their meaning using the Word Help

- write the meaning of the medical terms shown in bold print.

Cancer of the larynx

Mr R, aged 42, was referred to the ENT clinic with suspected cancer of the larynx. He had been a 15 per day cigarette smoker for 22 years. His main symptom was hoarseness (dysphonia) which had been present for about 2 months; otherwise, he seemed to be in good health. He was admitted to have his larynx formally assessed.

Direct laryngoscopy under anaesthesia confirmed the presence of a glottic tumour affecting both vocal cords. Following biopsy, histological analysis classified the tumour as a squamous cell carcinoma.

A chest **radiograph** excluded the presence of metastatic deposits and bronchial carcinoma. Computed **tomography** excluded lymph node and cartilage involvement with no spread into the hypopharynx.

Following discussion at a joint clinic, the ENT surgeon and **radiotherapist** staged Mr R's tumour at T1b N0 with

no metastatic involvement. He was prescribed a course of radical **radiotherapy** to try to conserve his larynx.

Immobilization of Mr R's neck was achieved by a well-fitting perspex shell reaching from the angle of the jaw down to just below the clavicle. The radiotherapist placed him in the supine position (without a mouthbite) with his neck straight to prevent the spinal cord curving anteriorly. The tumour was localized using CT scanning and the dose distribution outlined on the **tomogram** centering on the proposed target volume.

Mr R was placed in the same perspex shell and position for radiotherapy. The aim of his treatment was to administer a **tumouricidal** dose of radiation centred on his vocal cords. As he had a short neck, two anterior, oblique beams were used to irradiate the whole larynx. The wedged beams were angled at 90° to give a homogeneous dose to the target volume and to reduce the dose to the skin and spinal cord. He was administered 60 Gy in twenty-five fractions in 5 weeks (4–6 MeV) from a **linear accelerator**.

Mr R was advised of the possibility of side-effects such as difficulty in swallowing, exacerbated hoarseness, desquamation and rarely oedema (Am. edema) leading to obstruction. These often peak around the twelfth treatment with resolution of the tumour in approximately 2 months.

Mr R made an uneventful recovery, his only complaints being difficulty in swallowing and a sore throat. Recent follow-up examinations by the ENT surgeon and diagnostic **ultrasonography** showed no evidence of tumour recurrence. He appears well, and his voice is showing signs of recovery.

WORD HELP

anterior front/from the front of the body

biopsy removal and examination of living tissue

carcinoma malignant growth from epidermal cells

clavicle collar bone

desquamation the shedding of cells from the epidermis

dysphonia condition of difficulty/pain on speaking

ENT ear, nose and throat

glottic pertaining to the glottis (vocal apparatus of the larynx)

Gy gray (SI unit of absorbed radiation dose)

histological pertaining to histology (here histological analysis for classification and signs of malignancy)

hoarseness rough, grating, discordant voice making speech difficult

homogeneous uniform quality in all parts

hypopharynx the laryngeal part of the pharynx

laryngoscopy technique of viewing the larynx

localized here refers to determination of the position of the target volume in relation to the patient's anatomy and skin reference points

WORD HELP (Contd.)

metastatic pertaining to metastases (parts of a tumour that have spread from one site to another)

MeV mega-electronvolt

oblique slanting

oedema (Am. edema) accumulation of fluid in a tissue

squamous pertaining to scale-like/from squamous epithelium

supine lying on the back so the face is upward

target volume tumour volume

radical direct to the root or cause (treatment to eliminate disease) extensive

resolution abatement of a pathological process and the return of affected tissues to normal

T1b N0 staging symbols   T – tumour   N – node
T1b – tumour at stage 1b   N0–no node involvement

wedge wedge-shaped devices that act as filters to absorb radiation. They are used to adjust the dose received on either side of the body

Now write the meaning of the following words from the case history without using your dictionary lists:

(a) radiograph _____

(b) tomography _____

(c) radiotherapist _____

(d) radiotherapy _____

(e) tomogram _____

(f) tumouricidal
(Am. tumoricidal) _____

(g) linear accelerator _____

(h) ultrasonography _____

(Answers to the case history exercise are given in the Answers to Word Exercises beginning on page 275.)

Quick Reference

Combining forms relating to radiology and nuclear medicine:

Cine/o	movement/motion (picture)
Ech/o	reflected sound
Fluor/o	fluorescent/luminous/ flow
Radi/o	radiation/X-ray
Roentgen/o	X-ray
Scint/i	spark/flash of light
Son/o	sound
Therm/o	heat
Tom/o	slice/section
Ultrason/o	ultrasound

Abbreviations

Some common abbreviations related to radiation and nuclear medicine are listed below. Note, however, some are not standard and their meaning may vary from one health care setting to another. There is a more extensive list for reference on page 307.

AXR	abdominal X-ray
Ba	barium
CAT	computerized axial tomography
CXR	chest X-ray
DSA	digital subtraction angiography
DXT	deep X-ray therapy
EUA	examination under anaesthesia (Am. anesthesia)
MRI	magnetic resonance imaging
NMR	nuclear magnetic resonance
PET	positron emission tomography
US	ultrasound/ultrasonography
XR	X-ray

NOW TRY THE WORD CHECK

WORD CHECK

This self-check exercise lists all the word components used in this unit. First write down the meaning of as many word components as you can. Then check your answers using the Exercise Guide and Quick Reference box or the Glossary of Word Components (pp. 319–341).

Prefixes

ultra- _____

Combining forms of word roots

angi/o _____

cardi/o _____

cine/o _____

ech/o _____

encephal/o _____

fluor/o _____

oesophag/o _____
(Am. esophag/o)

radi/o _____

roentgen/o _____

scint/o _____

son/o _____

therm/o _____

tom/o _____

Suffixes

-cidal _____

-er _____

-genic _____

-gram _____

-graph _____

-graphy _____

-ist _____

-logy _____

-scope _____

-scopy _____

-therapy _____

> **NOW TRY THE SELF-ASSESSMENT** <

SELF-ASSESSMENT

Test 18A

Prefixes, suffixes and combining forms of word roots

Match each word component in Column A with a meaning in Column C by inserting the appropriate number in Column B.

Column A	Column B	Column C
(a) angi/o	_____	1. X-ray/radiation
(b) cinemat/o	_____	2. X-rays
(c) ech/o	_____	3. specialist
(d) -er	_____	4. treatment
(e) fluor/o	_____	5. beyond/excess
(f) -genic	_____	6. slice/section/cut
(g) -gram	_____	7. sound
(h) -graph	_____	8. heat
(i) -graphy	_____	9. technique of recording/making picture
(j) -ist	_____	10. technique of visual examination
(k) radi/o	_____	11. vessel
(l) roentgen/o	_____	12. picture/tracing/X-ray picture
(m) scint/i	_____	13. movement/motion picture
(n) -scope	_____	14. pertaining to formation/originating in
(o) -scopy	_____	15. reflected sound
(p) son/o	_____	16. instrument to view
(q) -therapy	_____	17. luminous (to flow)
(r) -therm/o	_____	18. spark (flash or light)
(s) tom/o	_____	19. instrument that records/tracing or picture, or the picture/tracing/ X-ray itself
(t) ultra-	_____	20. one who

Score

20

Test 18B

Write the meaning of:

(a) roentgenotherapy _____

(b) sonologist _____

(c) thermoradiotherapy _____

(d) radiocinematograph _____

(e) ultrasonotomography _____

Score

5

Test 18C

Build words that mean:

(a) treatment using ultrasound _____

(b) pertaining to examination
    by a fluoroscope _____

(c) technique of making a
    picture of vessels using
    sparks/flashes of light _____

(d) instrument used to detect
    and image heat from the body _____

(e) technique of imaging the brain
    using echoes (use ech/o) _____

Score

5

Check answers to Self-Assessment Tests on page 299.

19 Oncology

Objectives

Once you have completed Unit 19 you should be able to:

- understand the meaning of medical words relating to oncology
- build medical words relating to oncology
- understand medical abbreviations relating to oncology.

Exercise guide

Use this list of word components and their meanings to complete the word exercises in this unit.

Roots/Combining forms

angi/o	vessel
chondr/o	cartilage
haem/o	blood
hem/o (Am.)	blood
leiomy/o	smooth muscle
mening/i	meninges (membranes of CNS)
rhabdomy/o	striated muscle

Suffixes

-eal	pertaining to
-genesis	formation of
-genic	pertaining to formation/ originating in
-ia	condition of
-ic	pertaining to
-ist	specialist
-logist	specialist who studies
-logy	study of
-lysis	breakdown/disintegration
-oma	tumour/swelling
-osis	abnormal condition/disease/ abnormal increase
-static	pertaining to stopping/controlling
-tropic	pertaining to stimulating/affinity for

Oncology

This branch of medicine deals with the study and treatment of malignant tumours (Am. tumors) commonly called cancers. A tumour is a mass or swelling forming from dividing cells which appear to be out of control. Benign tumours remain localized and do not threaten life but malignant tumours spread and may lead to death. Tumours spread when they release cells into the blood and lymph; the tumour cells multiply in new sites forming secondary growths or **metastases** (from Greek *meta + histanai*, *meta* meaning changed in form, *histanai* to place/set, i.e. a growth in a different position).

As tumours grow they consume nutrients, depriving normal cells of essential metabolic components. A clinical feature called **cachexia** is seen in advanced stages of disease (from Greek *kakos* meaning bad and *hexis* meaning state). The body appears to suffer from malnutrition and becomes thin and 'wastes' away.

In this unit we will examine terms that relate to common types of tumour.

Use the Exercise Guide at the beginning of this unit to complete Word Exercises 1–3 unless you are asked to work without it.

Root	Onc
	*(From a Greek word **onkos**, meaning bulk. Here it is used to mean a tumour (Am. tumor).)*

Combining forms   **Onc/o**

WORD EXERCISE 1

Using your Exercise Guide, find the meaning of:

(a) **onc**/osis   _____

(b) **onco**/genesis   _____

(c) **onco**/tropic   _____

Using your Exercise Guide, build words that mean:

(d) pertaining to formation of a tumour   _____

(e) destruction/disintegration of a tumour   _____

(f) person who specializes in the study and treatment of tumours   _____

The process of tumour formation is also known as **neoplasia** (*neo-* meaning new, *-plas-* forming/growing and *-ia* condition of) and the tumour itself as a **neoplasm**. Neoplastic, derived in the same way, is also used to mean pertaining to a new growth (synonymous with oncogenic).

Before we study the next word root, we need to examine the use of the suffix *-oma*. Used by itself in combination with a tissue type, it indicates a benign tumour, e.g. oste**oma** – a benign bone tumour.

Malignant tumours may also be designated by *-oma* but they are usually preceded by the word **malignant**, e.g. **malignant melanoma**, a malignant tumour of the pigment cells and **malignant lymphoma**, a malignant tumour of lymphatic tissue.

The suffix *-oma* is also used in **blastoma**, meaning a tumour that forms from embryonic (germ) cells of an organ. Examples include: **glioblastoma**, a tumour that contains neuroglia (a type of brain cell or gliacyte) and **retinoblastoma** a tumour that grows from embryonic cells in the retina of the eye.

(To confuse matters, *-oma* is occasionally used for a non-neoplastic condition such as **haematoma** (Am. **hematoma**), that refers to a swelling filled with blood and is not a new growth of cells.)

Two terms that are widely used when referring to malignant tumours are:

> **Carcinoma**
> a malignant tumour of epithelial origin. Remember epithelia cover organs and line cavities and form membranes and glands.
>
> **Sarcoma**
> a malignant tumour of supporting tissues, including connective tissues and muscle.

These terms are studied in the exercises that follow:

Root	Carcin
	*(From a Greek word **karkinos**, meaning crab. It is used to mean a malignant tumour/cancer.)*

Combining forms   **Carcin/o**

A **carcin**oma is a tumour of an epithelium and there are numerous types. They are usually named by using the word carcinoma preceded by the histological type and followed by the organ of origin, for example:

> **Squamous cell carcinoma of the lung**
> originates in non-glandular epithelium.
>
> **Adenocarcinoma of the breast**
> originates in a glandular epithelium within the breast.

Often carcinomas are more simply named, e.g. as carcinoma of the colon or carcinoma of the urinary bladder.

Note. A substance that stimulates the formation of a malignant tumour is known as a **carcinogen**.

WORD EXERCISE 2

Without using your Exercise Guide, write the meaning of:

(a) **carcino**/genic _____

(b) **carcino**/lysis _____

Using your Exercise Guide, find the meaning of:

(c) **carcino**/static _____

Also from this root we have the word cancer, which is imprecisely used to mean carcinoma or cancer in situ. It is sometimes preceded by words that indicate the cause of a cancer, e.g.:

• radiologist's cancer

• smoker's cancer

• asbestos cancer.

Root	**Sarc**
	*(From a Greek word **sarkoma**, meaning a fleshy growth. Here it is used to mean a malignant tumour.)*

Combining forms   **Sarc/o**

Sarcomas are malignant tumours that are less common than carcinomas. They are derived from cells that have developed from the supporting tissues of the body, such as the connective tissues, i.e. bone, cartilage, blood and lymph, and from muscle tissue. The word **sarcoma** is preceded by the tissue type as in osteo**sarcoma**, a malignant bone tumour. (**Sarcomat/o** is the combining form of sarcoma).

WORD EXERCISE 3

Using your Exercise Guide, find the meaning of:

(a) chondro/**sarcoma** _____

(b) leiomyo/**sarcoma** _____

(c) rhabdomyo/**sarcoma** _____

(d) mening/eal **sarcoma** _____

(e) haem/angio/**sarcoma** _____
   (Am. hem/angio/sarcoma)

Without using your Exercise Guide, write the meaning of:

(f) **sarcomat**/osis _____

Most malignant tumours arise from epithelial tissues. When a malignant tumour no longer resembles its tissue of origin and its cells are disordered, it is described as **anaplastic** (*ana-* meaning backward, *-plast* growth and *-ic* pertaining to).

Another form of malignant tumour is the mixed tissue tumour. These contain cells that resemble both epithelial and connective tissue cells.

Diagnosis of malignant tumours

Precise classification of malignant tumours is essential for determining their likely growth characteristics. Once a tumour has been classified, appropriate treatment can be planned and the patient can be given a prognosis (forecast of the probable course of their disease).

Attempts to develop an international language for describing the extent of malignant disease have been made. One of these is in widespread use and is known as the **TNM** system.

T – tumour
   categorizes the primary tumour and its size.

N – nodes
   defines the number of lymph nodes that have been invaded.

M – metastases
   indicates the presence or absence of metastases.

The extent of malignant disease defined by these categories is termed **staging**. Staging defines the size of tumour, its growth and progression at any one point.

Many different staging systems are in use for different cancers. It is not possible to study them here, but we have included a basic system which is outlined below.

T

T_0	no primary tumour
T_1	primary tumour limited to site of origin
T_{2-4}	progressive increase in size of primary tumour
T_x	primary tumour cannot be assessed
T_{is}	primary tumour in situ

N

N_0	no evidence of spread to nodes
N_1	spread to nodes in immediate area
N_{2-4}	increasing number of lymph nodes invaded
N_x	lymph nodes cannot be assessed

M

M_0	no evidence of metastases
M_{1-3}	ascending degrees of metastases

Using the above system, we can see the principle of how a cancer is staged. For example, if a tumour was classified at T_2 N_1 M_0, this stage would indicate that the primary tumour is large and has spread to deeper structures (T_2). It has spread to one lymph node draining the area (N_1) and there is no evidence of a distant metastasis (M_0).

Staging is not an exact description of a tumour's progress but it is a useful way to estimate the course of the disease when planning treatment (therapy).

Medical equipment and clinical procedures

We have already described the main instruments and procedures that are used in the diagnosis and treatment of cancers in Unit 18. Tumours can be detected using radiography, computerized tomography, thermography, magnetic resonance imaging, positron emission tomography etc.

The main types of treatments are:

- radiotherapy: the use of radiation/X-rays by medically qualified radiotherapists (-*ist* meaning specialist) to destroy tumour cells

- chemotherapy: the use of chemicals i.e. cytotoxic drugs to poison tumour cells

- excision surgery: the use of surgery to remove a mass of tumour cells.

CASE HISTORY 19

The object of this exercise is to understand words associated with a patient's medical history.

To complete the exercise:

- read through the passage on glioblastoma multiforme; unfamiliar words are underlined and you can find their meaning using the Word Help

- write the meaning of the medical terms shown in bold print.

Glioblastoma multiforme

Mr S, a 59-year-old male senior office worker noticed a loss of verbal fluency and had difficulty in recalling the names of common objects and friends. He was reprimanded by his employer over a decline in his previously high standard of written work. His condition worsened, and he was persuaded by his colleagues to seek medical advice. He was referred to the neurology unit by his GP.

On examination by the neurologist he appeared alert and intelligent but made several mistakes when asked to name common objects and spell simple words. He could not remember a simple name and address after 5 minutes.

His optic discs were normal, but there was no venous pulsation. Vision was restricted in the upper temporal visual field in the right eye and upper nasal field in the left eye. There was a mild lower facial weakness and a slight increase in reflexes of the right arm and leg. The right plantar reflex was extensor.

The presence of dysphasia, memory loss, right homonymous field restriction and mild pyramidal signs suggested a lesion affecting the upper temporal lobe of the left cerebral hemisphere.

A CXR excluded a bronchial **neoplasm** which is the commonest cause of cerebral **metastases** in a smoker. A CT scan demonstrated a mixed, high and low density intracranial lesion in the left temporal region and excluded **meningioma**. EEG demonstrated a wave abnormality in the left temporal region and a left carotid arteriogram indicated displacement of cerebral branches by a temporal **mass**. The commonest cause of lesions presenting in this way is malignant **glioma**.

A case conference was arranged with the **oncologist** to disclose the prognosis to Mr S and his family and to outline the options for treatment. The **radiotherapist** required histological confirmation of the diagnosis before commencing treatment. Mr S was administered dexamethasone to reduce the oedema (Am. edema) around the tumour and improve the symptoms of raised intracranial pressure. A brain biopsy confirmed glioblastoma multiforme.

Mr S underwent neurosurgery, part of the temporal lobe was removed to provide an internal decompression and the tumour was sucked out. Unfortunately, malignant gliomas infiltrate into brain tissue and are difficult to remove completely. Surgery was followed by a radical course of cobalt sixty radiotherapy in combination with **chemotherapy** and small doses of <u>steroids</u>. His speech defect and writing improved considerably for many months following surgery. Now, a year later, he shows signs of deterioration with a right <u>hemiparesis</u>, dysphasia and occasional <u>grand mal seizures</u>.

WORD HELP

arteriogram tracing/X-ray picture of arteries

biopsy removal and examination of living tissue

carotid the carotid artery in the neck

cerebral hemisphere lateral half of the cerebrum

cobalt sixty (⁶⁰Co) isotope of cobalt that emits gamma rays that can destroy cancer cells

CT computed tomography

CXR chest X-ray

decompression relief of pressure

dysphasia condition of difficulty in speaking

EEG electroencephalogram/electroencephalography

extensor straightening (here refers to the Babinski reflex, a response in which the toes curl upwards or dorsiflex when the sole of the foot is stroked, instead of the normal plantar flexion in which the toes curl down)

glioblastoma tumour of embryonic/germ cells that contains neuroglia (a type of brain cell)

GP general practitioner (family doctor)

grand mal seizure form of epileptic fit in which consciousness is lost

hemiparesis partial or slight paralysis, weakness of a limb

histological pertaining to histology (here histological analysis for classification and signs of malignancy)

intracranial pertaining to within the cranium

homonymous corresponding halves

lesion pathological change in a tissue

malignant dangerous, capable of spreading

multiforme having many forms (here referring to the fact that the tumour may be derived from different types of cells)

oedema (Am. edema) accumulation of fluid in a tissue

plantar pertaining to the sole of the foot

prognosis forecast of the probable outcome and course of a disease

pyramidal referring to the pyramidal tract in the brain, an area that initiates voluntary skilled movements of skeletal muscles, especially the fingers

radical direct to the root or cause (treatment to eliminate disease), extensive

steroid drugs used to suppress inflammation and reduce oedema

temporal pertaining to the temple/temporal bone (the temple is the flat region on either side of the head)

Now write the meaning of the following words from the case history without using your dictionary lists:

(a) neoplasm _____

(b) metastases _____

(c) meningioma _____

(d) mass _____

(e) glioma _____

(f) oncologist _____

(g) radiotherapist _____

(h) chemotherapy _____

(Answers to the case history exercise are given in the Answers to Word Exercises beginning on page 275.)

Quick Reference

Combining forms relating to oncology:

Aden/o	gland
Blast/o	embryonic/germ cell
Cancer/o	cancer
Carcin/o	cancerous/malignant
Melan/o	pigment
Onc/o	tumour
Sarc/o	fleshy/connective tissue
Sarcomat/o	sarcoma/malignant tumour

Abbreviations

Some common abbreviations related to oncology are listed below. Note, however, some are not standard and their meaning may vary from one health care setting to another. There is a more extensive list for reference on page 307.

BCC	basal cell carcinoma
BT	bone tumour
BX or Bx	biopsy
CA or Ca	cancer/carcinoma
CACX	cancer of the cervix
CF	cancer free
MEN	multiple endocrine neoplasia
Metas	metastasis
N & V	nausea and vomiting
SA	sarcoma
T	tumour
t	terminal

 NOW TRY THE WORD CHECK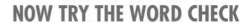

WORD CHECK

This self-check exercise lists all the word components used in this unit. First write down the meaning of as many word components as you can. Then check your answers using the Exercise Guide and Quick Reference box or the Glossary of Word Components (pp. 319–341).

Prefixes

ana- _____

meta- _____

neo- _____

Combining forms of word roots

aden/o _____

angi/o _____

blast/o _____

cancer/o _____

carcin/o _____

chem/o _____

chondr/o _____

cyt/o _____

gli/a/o _____

haem/o
(Am. hem/o) _____

leiomy/o _____

melan/o _____

meningi/o _____

onc/o _____

rhabdomy/o _____

sarc/o _____

sarcomat/o _____

Suffixes

-genic _____

-genesis _____

-ia _____

-ic _____

-ist _____

-logy _____

-lysis _____

-oma _____

-osis _____

-plasia _____

-plastic _____

-static _____

-therapy _____

-toxic _____

-tropic _____

 ▷ **NOW TRY THE SELF-ASSESSMENT** ◁

 ## SELF-ASSESSMENT

Test 19A

Prefixes, suffixes and combining forms of word roots

Match each word component in Column A with a meaning in Column C by inserting the appropriate number in Column B.

Column A	Column B	Column C
(a) aden/o	_____	1. pertaining to
(b) ana-	_____	2. change position or form

Column A	Column B	Column C
(c) cancer/o	_____	3. pertaining to formation/originating in
(d) carcinoma	_____	4. membranes of CNS
(e) chondr/o	_____	5. striated muscle
(f) -genic	_____	6. condition of growth (increase of cells)
(g) -ic	_____	7. pertaining to stopping/controlling
(h) -ist	_____	8. pertaining to affinity for/acting on
(i) leiomy/o	_____	9. gland
(j) melan/o	_____	10. cancer (general term)
(k) meningi/o	_____	11. cancer/tumour (medical term)
(l) meta-	_____	12. cartilage
(m) neo-	_____	13. tumour/swelling (benign or malignant)
(n) -oma	_____	14. malignant tumour of epithelium
(o) onc/o	_____	15. malignant tumour of supporting tissue
(p) -plasia	_____	16. specialist
(q) rhabdomy/o	_____	17. smooth muscle
(r) sarcomat/o	_____	18. pigment
(s) -static	_____	19. new
(t) -tropic	_____	20. backward

Score

20

Test 19B

Write the meaning of:

(a) fibrosarcoma
(fibr/o – fibre/fibrous)   _____

(b) gastric adenocarcinoma
(gastr/o – stomach)   _____

(c) hepatocellular carcinoma
(hepat/o – liver)   _____

(d) anaplastic thyroid carcinoma
(thyr/o – thyroid)   _____

(e) bronchogenic carcinoma
(bronch/o – bronchus)   _____

Score

5

Test 19C

Build words that mean:

(a) malignant tumour of lymph
(use sarc/o)   _____

(b) benign tumour of cartilage   _____

(c) a malignant tumour originating
in bone (use sarc/o)   _____

(d) condition of a new growth of cells   _____

(e) the treatment of tumours   _____

Score

5

Check answers to Self-Assessment Tests on page 299.

20 Anatomical position

Objectives

Once you have completed Unit 20 you should be able to:

- understand the meaning of medical words relating to the anatomical position

- build medical words relating to regions and positions in the body

- associate medical terms with their anatomical position

- understand medical abbreviations relating to anatomical positions

- visualize and name the planes of the body.

Exercise Guide

Use this list of word components and their meanings to complete the word exercises in this unit.

Prefixes

epi-	above/upon/on
hypo-	below/under

Roots/Combining forms

bucc/o	cheek
cardi/o	heart
cephal/o	head
chondr/o	cartilage
cost/o	rib
crani/o	cranium/skull
derm/o	skin
faci/o	face
-ganglion	ganglion
gastr/o	stomach
hepat/o	liver
ili/o	hip/ilium/flank
mamm/o	breast/mammary gland
nas/o	nose
or/o	mouth
ot/o	ear
placent/o	placenta
stern/o	sternum
ven/o	vein
vertebr/o	vertebra/spine

Suffixes

-ac	pertaining to
-al	pertaining to
-ary	pertaining to
-iac	pertaining to
-ic	pertaining to
-ous	pertaining to/of the nature of
-ver(ted)	turned

Anatomical position

In this unit we will examine a selection of terms that refer to the position of organs and tissues within the body. Many of these terms are also used to indicate the position of injuries, pain, disease and surgical operations.

The **anatomical position** of the body (Fig. 90) is a reference system that all doctors and medical texts use when describing body components. We always refer to position in the patient's body as if he/she were standing upright with arms at the sides and palms of the hands facing forward, head erect and eyes looking forward.

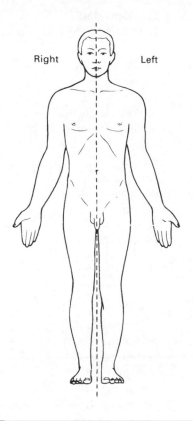

Figure 90	The anatomical position

With the body in the anatomical position we can draw an imaginary line down the middle of the body (Fig. 90). This is called the **midline** or **median line** and it bisects the body into right and left sides. Note that right and left refer to the sides of the patient in the anatomical position, not those of the observer.

Directions

We can now see how the imaginary midline can be used to indicate directions when a body is in the anatomical position. Parts that lie nearer to the median line of the body than other parts are described as **medial** to that part. Any part that lies further away is said to be **lateral** to the first part (Fig. 91). To summarize:

Medial	pertaining to towards the median line (or midline)
Lateral	pertaining to away from the median line (or midline)

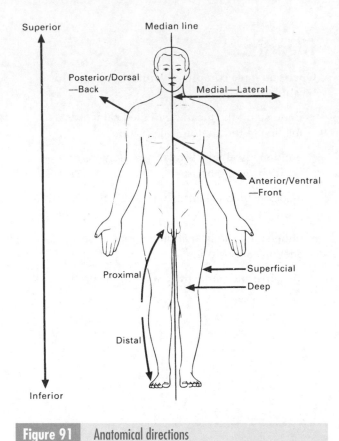

Figure 91	Anatomical directions

Other directions can also be seen in Figure 91.

Superior towards the head, upper
Inferior away from the head, lower
Anterior (ventral) front
Posterior (dorsal) back
Proximal pertaining to near point of attachment or point of origin
Distal pertaining to further from point of attachment or origin
Superficial pertaining to near the surface of the body
Deep away from the surface of the body

WORD EXERCISE 1

Using the information in Figure 91, complete the following sentences by deleting the incorrect word:

(a) The eyes are superior/inferior to the mouth.

(b) The mouth is superior/inferior to the nose.

(c) The ear is medial/lateral to the eye

(d) The nostril is medial/lateral to the eye.

(e) The umbilicus lies on the anterior/posterior surface of the abdomen.

(f) The vertebrae lie close to the dorsal/ventral surface of the body.

(g) The wrist is proximal/distal to the elbow.

(h) The ankles are proximal/distal to the toes.

(i) The ribs are superficial/deep to the lungs.

These terms can also be applied to organ systems and tissues within the body. They too are described as if they are in the anatomical position, e.g. the digestive system (Fig. 92).

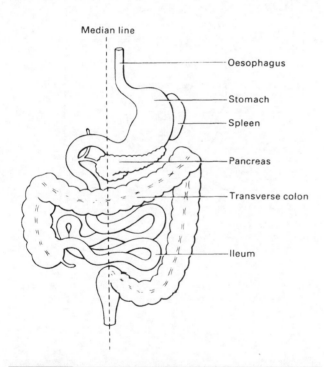

Median line

Oesophagus

Stomach

Spleen

Pancreas

Transverse colon

Ileum

Figure 92   Digestive system position

WORD EXERCISE 2

Using information from Figure 92, complete the following sentences by deleting the incorrect word:

(a) The pancreas is superior/inferior to the stomach.

(b) The oesophagus is superior/inferior to the stomach.

(c) The stomach is medial/lateral to the spleen.

(d) The oesophagus is proximal/distal to the stomach.

(e) The transverse colon is anterior/posterior to the ileum.

(f) The ileum is dorsal/ventral to the transverse colon.

Regions

With the body in the anatomical position, it can be divided into the cephalic, thoracic, abdominal and pelvic regions (Fig. 93).

Each of these regions can be subdivided; the simplest example is perhaps the division of the abdominopelvic region into quadrants (Fig. 94).

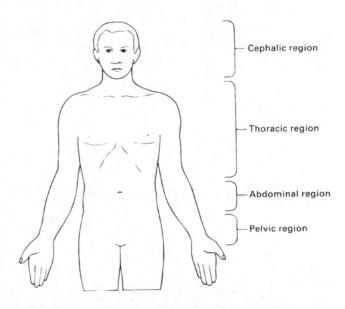

Cephalic region

Thoracic region

Abdominal region

Pelvic region

Figure 93   Regions of the trunk and head

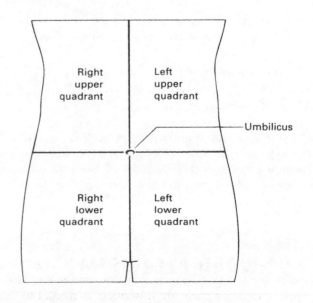

Right upper quadrant

Left upper quadrant

Umbilicus

Right lower quadrant

Left lower quadrant

Figure 94   Abdominopelvic region (quadrants)

Doctors and health personnel often use this simple system to describe the position of abdominopelvic pain. The quadrants are formed by imaginary vertical and horizontal lines through the umbilicus. A more complex method is to divide the abdominopelvic region into nine regions (Fig. 95).

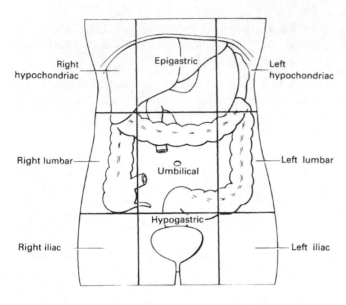

Column A	Number
(a) cephalic region	
(b) cranial region	
(c) facial region	
(d) otic region	
(e) oral region	
(f) mammary region	
(g) nasal region	
(h) buccal region	

Figure 95 Abdominopelvic region (nine regions)

   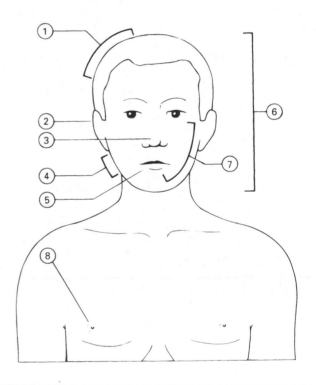

WORD EXERCISE 3

Using your Exercise Guide, find the meaning of:

(a) hypo/chondr/iac region _____
(The word refers to the cartilage of the rib-cage.)

(b) epi/gastr/ic region _____

(c) ili/ac region _____

The cephalic regions and the upper and lower extremities can also be subdivided into regions. These are examined in the next two exercises. Use your Exercise Guide to find the meaning of unfamiliar words.

WORD EXERCISE 4

Examine Figure 96 and match the regions listed in Column A with a number from the diagram:

Figure 96 Regions of the head and thorax

WORD EXERCISE 5

Look at Figures 97 and 98 and label the regions of each limb by selecting an appropriate region from the list below. The first region has been labelled for you.

hallux region   great toe

crural region   leg

pedal region	foot
digital/phalangeal region	toes
patellar region	knee
femoral region	thigh
tarsal region	ankle
axillary region	armpit
palmar/volar region	palm
antebrachial region	forearm
digital/phalangeal region	fingers
brachial region	arm
pollex region	thumb
carpal region	wrist

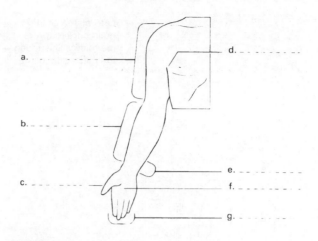

Figure 98 Arm regions

left halves. The flat surfaces formed in each cut half illustrate the **median** or **midsagittal plane**. Figure 99 shows the direction of the cut that forms the midsagittal plane. Figure 100 shows a midsagittal section through the brain when cut in this plane and viewed from the side.

Any plane parallel to the midsagittal or median plane is called a **parasagittal** or **paramedian plane** (*para* meaning besides) (Fig. 101).

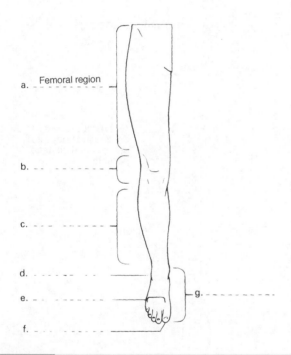

Figure 97 Leg regions

Planes

Planes are imaginary flat surfaces that form a reference system indicating the direction in which organs have been cut, drawn or photographed. When a body structure is studied, it is often viewed in section and the section is formed from a cut made in relation to one of the planes.

Imagine a vertical cut made along the midline from the front of the body to the back dividing it into right and

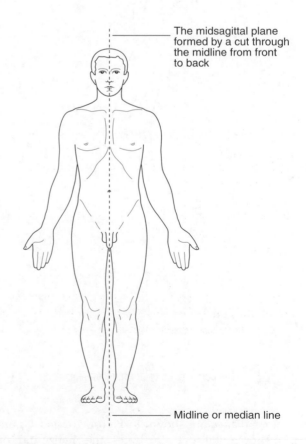

The midsagittal plane formed by a cut through the midline from front to back

Midline or median line

Figure 99 The midsagittal or median plane

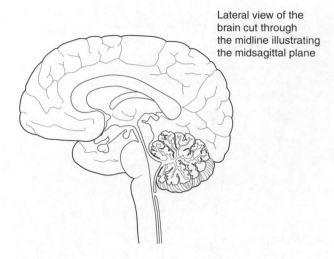

Lateral view of the brain cut through the midline illustrating the midsagittal plane

Figure 100   A midsagittal section through the brain

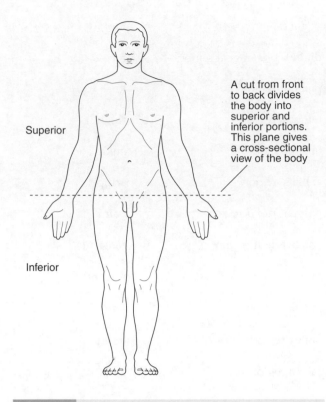

A cut from front to back divides the body into superior and inferior portions. This plane gives a cross-sectional view of the body

Superior

Inferior

Figure 102   The horizontal or transverse plane

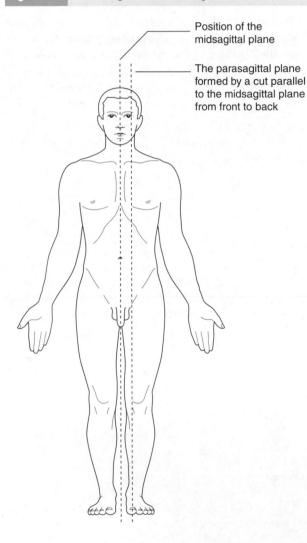

Position of the midsagittal plane

The parasagittal plane formed by a cut parallel to the midsagittal plane from front to back

Figure 101   The parasagittal or paramedian plane

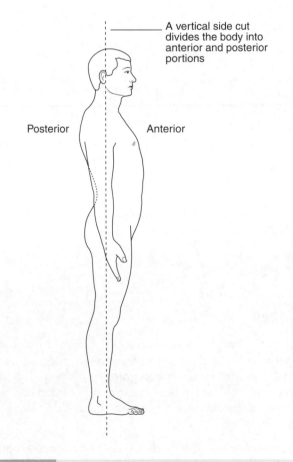

A vertical side cut divides the body into anterior and posterior portions

Posterior   Anterior

Figure 103   The frontal or coronal plane

Two other planes are shown in Figure 102 and Figure 103. A horizontal cut illustrates the **horizontal** or **transverse plane** (Fig. 102). This is the equivalent of a cross-section through the body dividing it into superior and inferior portions.

A vertical side cut divides the body into anterior and posterior portions at right angles to the sagittal plane and illustrates the **frontal** or **coronal plane** (Fig. 103).

Figure 104 summarizes the three main planes of the body.

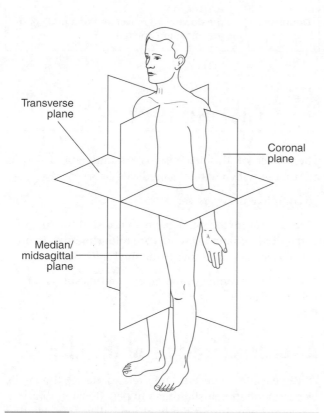

Transverse plane

Coronal plane

Median/ midsagittal plane

Figure 104   The planes of the body

WORD EXERCISE 6

Match a plane in Column A to a description in Column C by inserting a number in Column B.

Column A	Column B	Column C
(a) midsagittal plane		1. divides the body into superior and inferior portions
(b) transverse plane		2. a plane parallel to the median plane
(c) frontal plane		3. divides the body into right and left halves
(d) parasagittal plane		4. divides the body into anterior and posterior portions

Locating parts of the body

There are a large number of locative prefixes that act as prepositions when placed in front of word roots. These tell us about the position of structures within the body. Use the list of locative prefixes below to complete the next two exercises.

Locative prefixes

Above	epi-, hyper-, super-, supra-
Across	trans-
After	post-
Against	anti, contra-
Around	circum-, peri-
Away	ab-, apo-, ef-
Back	dorsi-, dorso-, post-, re-, retro-
Backward	opistho-, retro (also means back/behind)
Before/front	ante-, pre-, pro-, ventri
Below	hypo-, infra-, sub-
Behind/after	dorsi-, dorso-, post-
Beside	para-
Between	inter-
Down	de-
Front/in front	pro-, ventr-
In/inside	em-, en-, endo-, in-, intra-
Left	laevo- (Am. levo-)
Middle	medi-, meso-
Out/outside	ec-, ect-, ef-, exo-, extra-
Right	dextro-
Side	later-
Through	dia-, per-
To/towards/near	ad-, af-
Under	infra-, sub-
Upon	epi-
Within	intra-

WORD EXERCISE 7

Use the locative prefix list to fill in each blank with an appropriate prefix:

(a) The region beside the nose _____ nasal region

(b) Disc between vertebrae _____ vertebral disc

(c) Region upon the stomach _____ gastric region

(d) Pertaining to after a ganglion _____ ganglionic

(e) Condition of right _____ cardia
  displacement of heart

(f) Nerve below orbit of eye _____ orbital nerve

WORD EXERCISE 8

Use your Exercise Guide and the locative prefix list to find the meaning of:

(a) peri/cardi/al _____

(b) intra/ven/ous _____

(c) inter/cost/al _____

(d) retro/verted uterus _____

(e) supra/hepat/ic _____

(f) infra/stern/al _____

(g) pre/ganglion/ic _____

(h) extra/placent/al _____

(i) sub/epiderm/al _____

Some of the locative prefixes we have listed are incorporated into words that indicate the direction of movement of parts of the body. Before noting some examples we need to describe the main actions of muscles.

Muscles that bend limbs by decreasing the angles between articulating bones are called **flexors** and those that increase the angles after they have flexed are called **extensors**. The action of flexors is known as **flexion** and that of extensors, **extension**. Examples of prefixes that indicate direction of movements at joints are shown in bold:

Dorsiflexion	the movement that bends the foot back (upwards) from the anatomical position (*dorsi-* meaning back)
Plantar flexion	the movement that bends the foot downwards from the anatomical position (*plantar* meaning pertaining to the sole of the foot)
Abduction	the movement of a part away from the midline (*ab-* meaning away from).
Adduction	the movement of a part towards the midline (*ad-* meaning to)
Inversion	the movement of the sole inward so the soles face each other (*in-* meaning in/inward)
Eversion	the movement of the sole in the outwards, so the soles face away from each other (*e-* meaning out from)

Circumduction	the movement in which the distal ends of a bone move in a circle (*circum-* meaning around)
Protraction	the movement of a part forward/in front e.g. the jaw (*pro-* meaning in front/before)
Retraction	the movement of a protracted part back (*re-* meaning back /contrary)
Elevation	the upward movement of a body part e.g. the jaw
Depression	the downward movement of a body part (*de-* meaning down/from)

CASE HISTORY 20

The object of this exercise is to understand words associated with a patient's medical history.

To complete the exercise:

- read through the passage on an unusual fracture of the tibia; unfamiliar words are underlined and you can find their meaning using the Word Help

- write the meaning of the medical terms shown in bold print.

An unusual fracture of the tibia

A 13-year-old male was referred to the Orthopaedic Department after sustaining a hyperextension injury to his right knee during a school football match. He had immediate onset of pain and swelling during the first few hours following the injury. On admission he could not bear weight on the knee and flexion and extension exacerbated the pain. His medical record indicated no previous injury to his right lower extremity and he appeared to be in good health.

Examination of the right lower extremity revealed a knee effusion with soft tissue swelling and diffuse tenderness over the **proximal** tibial growth plate. There were **superficial** skin lacerations on the **anterior** and **medial** surface of his right thigh. He could not **dorsiflex** or evert his foot and sensation in the **lateral** calf and foot was reduced. Vascular insufficiency in the injured extremity was assessed; the popliteal, dorsalis pedis and posterior tibial pulses were palpable with good **distal** refilling.

Lateral and **anteroposterior** radiographs demonstrated a proximal tibial fracture classified as a Salter-Harris type III. The intra-articular fracture extended along the articular surface into the medial and lateral plateaus. The epiphyseal plate was anteriorly displaced on the metaphysis.

He underwent open reduction and internal fixation with a 3 mm Steinmann pin; recovery was uneventful and his articular surface was preserved.

WORD HELP

calf fleshy back part of leg below the knee

dorsalis pedis pulse pulse on the dorsal foot (the upper part of the foot)

effusion a fluid discharge into a part/escape of fluid into an enclosed space

flexion decreasing the angle between two bones (here bending the leg)

epiphyseal pertaining to the epiphysis, the end of a long bone separated from the main shaft by a cartilage plate

evert turn the sole of the foot outward at the ankle joint

extension increasing the angle between two bones (here straightening the leg)

exacerbated increased severity of symptoms

hyperextension forcible over-extending of a limb (here extending the knee joint so far that the lower leg bends forwards)

intra-articular within a joint or inside the cavity of a joint

laceration a tear in a tissue

lower extremity a leg (hip, thigh, leg, ankle and foot taken as one structure)

metaphysis the wider part at the end of the main shaft of a long bone adjacent to the epiphysis

open reduction an operation that exposes bones for restoration of displaced tissue

orthopaedic pertaining to orthopaedics (study of the locomotor/movement system)

palpable able to be felt using light pressure with the fingers

plateau flat region (here the expanded end of the tibia that articulates with the femur)

popliteal pulse pertaining to the pulse behind the knee

posterior tibial pulse in the foot posterior to the lower end of the tibia

radiograph here meaning an X-ray picture/recording

Salter-Harris type III classification system for growth plate injuries

tibial pertaining to the tibia

vascular pertaining to blood vessels

Now write the meaning of the following words from the case history without using your dictionary lists:

(a) proximal

(b) superficial

(c) anterior

(d) medial

(e) dorsiflex

(f) lateral

(g) distal

(h) anteroposterior

(Answers to the case history exercise are given in the Answers to Word Exercises beginning on page 275.)

Quick Reference

Combining forms relating to anatomical parts and positions of the body:

Anter/o	front/anterior
Axill/o	armpit
Brachi/o	arm
Bucc/o	cheek
Carp/o	carpal/wrist bones
Cephal/o	head
Crani/o	cranium
Crur/o	leg
Digit/o	finger/toe
Faci/o	face
Femor/o	femur/thigh
Hallux	great toe
Ili/o	ilium/flank
Infer/o	towards the feet/inferior
Later/o	side
Mamm/o	breast/mammary gland
Nas/o	nose
Or/o	mouth
Ot/o	ear
Palm/o	palm
Patell/o	patella/knee cap
Ped/o	foot
Phalang/o	phalange/finger/toe
Pollex	thumb
Poster/o	back/posterior
Super/o	towards the head/superior
Tars/o	tarsus/ankle
Vol/o	palm

Abbreviations

Some common abbreviations related to anatomical position are listed below. Note, however, some are not standard and their meaning may vary from one health care setting to another. There is a more extensive list for reference on page 307.

ant	anterior
inf	inferior

Abbreviations (Contd.)

lat	lateral
LLQ	left lower quadrant
LUQ	left upper quadrant
med	medial
pos	position
post	posterior
prox	proximal
RLQ	right lower quadant
RUQ	right upper quadrant
sup	superior

NOW TRY THE WORD CHECK

WORD CHECK

This self-check exercise lists all the word components used in this unit. First write down the meaning of as many word components as you can. Then check your answers using the Exercise Guide and Quick Reference box or the Glossary of Word Components (pp. 319–341).

Prefixes

ab- _____

ad- _____

af- _____

ante _____

anti- _____

apo- _____

circum- _____

contra- _____

dextro- _____

dia- _____

dorso- _____

ec- _____

ect- _____

ef- _____

em- _____

en- _____

endo- _____

exo- _____

extra- _____

in- _____

infra- _____

inter- _____

intra- _____

laevo-
(Am. levo-) _____

medi- _____

meso- _____

opistho- _____

para- _____

per- _____

peri- _____

pre- _____

pro- _____

retro- _____

super- _____

supra- _____

trans- _____

ventro- _____

Combining forms of word roots

anter/o _____

axill/o _____

brachi/o _____

bucc/o _____

cardi/o _____

carp/o _____

cephal/o _____

chondr/o _____

cost/o _____

crani/o _____

crur/o _____

derm/o _____

digit/o _____

faci/o _____

femor/o _____

-ganglion _____

gastr/o _____

hallux _____

hepat/o _____

ili/o _____

infer/o _____

later/o _____

mamm/o _____

nas/o _____

or/o _____

ot/o _____

palm/o _____

patell/o _____

ped/o _____

phalang/o _____

placent/o _____

pollex _____

poster/o _____

stern/o _____

super/o _____

ven/o _____

tars/o _____

verteb/o _____

vol/o _____

Suffixes

-ac _____

-al _____

-ary _____

-ia _____

-iac _____

-ic _____

-ous _____

-ver(ted) _____

> **NOW TRY THE SELF-ASSESSMENT** <

SELF-ASSESSMENT

Test 20A

Combining forms relating to parts of body

Match each combining form in Column A with a meaning in Column C by inserting the appropriate number in Column B.

Column A	Column B	Column C
(a) abdomin/o	_____	1. head
(b) axill/o	_____	2. leg
(c) brachi/o	_____	3. great toe
(d) carp/o	_____	4. ankle/tarsus
(e) cephal/o	_____	5. palm (i)

Column A	Column B	Column C	Column A	Column B	Column C
(f) crani/o	_____	6. palm (ii)	(f) ec-	_____	6. side
(g) crur/o	_____	7. knee	(g) en-	_____	7. around (i)
(h) digit/o	_____	8. finger/toe (i)	(h) epi-	_____	8. around (ii)
(i) femor/o	_____	9. finger/toe (ii)	(i) infra-	_____	9. away
(j) hallux	_____	10. pelvis	(j) inter-	_____	10. before/in front of
(k) ili/o	_____	11. thumb	(k) laevo- (Am. levo-)	_____	11. beside
(l) palm/o	_____	12. thigh/femur	(l) later-	_____	12. towards
(m) patell/o	_____	13. abdomen	(m) para-	_____	13. after/behind
(n) ped/o	_____	14. skull/cranium	(n) per-	_____	14. right
(o) pelv/i	_____	15. thorax	(o) peri-	_____	15. upon
(p) phalang/o	_____	16. foot	(p) post-	_____	16. in
(q) pollex	_____	17. arm	(q) pre-	_____	17. above
(r) tars/o	_____	18. armpit	(r) retro-	_____	18. left
(s) thorac/o	_____	19. ilium/flank	(s) supra-	_____	19. below
(t) vol/o	_____	20. wrist	(t) trans-	_____	20. out

Score

20

Score

20

Test 20B

Locative prefixes

Match each locative prefix from Column A with a meaning in Column C by inserting the appropriate number in Column B.

Column A	Column B	Column C
(a) ab-	_____	1. through (i)
(b) ad-	_____	2. through (ii)
(c) circum-	_____	3. backward/behind
(d) dextro-	_____	4. across
(e) dia-	_____	5. between

Test 20C

Write the meaning of:

(a) interphalangeal _____

(b) dextroversion _____

(c) retrobuccal _____

(d) supracostal _____

(e) intranasal _____

Score

5

Test 20D

Build words that mean:

(a) pertaining to the side   _____

(b) a turning towards the left   _____

(c) pertaining to after a ganglion   _____

(d) pertaining to below the liver   _____

(e) pertaining to across the skin   _____

Score

5

Check answers to Self-Assessment Tests on page 299.

Pharmacology and microbiology

Objectives

Once you have completed Unit 21 you should be able to:

- understand the meaning of medical words relating to pharmacology and microbiology

- deduce the use or action of drugs from their classification

- understand medical abbreviations associated with pharmacology and microbiology.

Exercise Guide

Use this list of word components and their meanings to complete the word exercises in this unit.

Prefixes

a-	without
an-	without
anti-	against
dia-	through
neo-	new
oxy-	quick
retro-	back/backward

Roots/Combining forms

acid/o	acid
aem-	blood
aesthet/o	sensation/sensitivity
anxi/o	anxiety
alges/i/o	sense of pain
bacill/o	bacillus/bacilli
bacteri/o	bacterium/bacteria
bi/o	life/living
bronch/i/o	bronchus/bronchial tubes
cocc/o	coccus/cocci
cycl/o	ciliary body
cyt/o	cell
dynam/o	force/power (of movement)
epilept/o	epilepsy
esthet/o (Am.)	sensation/sensitivity
fibrin/o	fibrin (a protein that forms the fibres of blood clots)
fung/i/o	fungus
gonad/o	gonads/reproductive organs
haem/o	blood
hem/o (Am.)	blood
helmint/h/o	worms
hypn/o	sleep
immun/o	immune/immunity
kerat/o	epidermis/cornea

kinet/o	motion/movement
lact/i/o	milk
muc/o	mucus
oestr/o (Am. estr/o)	oestrogen (a female sex-hormone)/oestrus
pharmac/o	drug
plas/m/o	growth
prurit/o	itching
psych/o	mind
(r)rhythm/o	rhythm
septic/o	sepsis/infection
staphylococc/o	staphylococcus/staphylococci
spasm/o/d	spasm
spirill/o	spirillum/spirilla
streptococc/o	streptococcus/streptococci
thyroid/o	thyroid
toc/o	labour/birth
tox/ic/o	poison/poisonous to
troph/o	nourish/stimulate
tuss/i	cough
ur/o	urine
vir/o	virus/virion

Suffixes

-aemia	condition of blood
-al	pertaining to/type of drug
-ase	an enzyme
-cidal	pertaining to killing
-cide	agent that kills/killing
-form	having the form/structure of
-gen	precursor/agent that produces
-genic	pertaining to formation
-gnosy	process of judgment/knowledge
-ia	condition of
-ic	type of drug/pertaining to
-in	non-specific suffix indicating a chemical
-ine	substance thought to be derived from ammonia
-ist	specialist
-ite	end-product
-ity	state/condition
-ive	pertaining to/type of drug
-logist	specialist who studies
-logy	study of
-lytic	drug that breaks down .../pertaining to breakdown
-oid	resembling
-ose	carbohydrate/sugar/starch
-osis	abnormal condition/disease of
-plegic	drug that paralyses/condition of paralysis
-rrhea (Am.)	excessive discharge/flow
-rrhoea	excessive discharge/flow
-static	pertaining to stopping/agent that stops
-tic	pertaining to
-uria	condition of urine
-y	process/condition

Pharmacology

Pharmacology is the science that deals with the study of drugs. By drugs we mean medicinal substances that can be used to treat, prevent or diagnose disease and illness. Research into the properties and potential use of substances showing physiological activity has enabled the pharmaceutical industry to market new and more effective drugs.

Root

Pharmac
(From a Greek word **pharmakon** *meaning drug.)*

Combining forms **Pharmac/o**

WORD EXERCISE 1

Without using your Exercise Guide write the meaning of:

(a) **pharmaco**/logy _____

(b) **pharmaco**/logist _____

(c) **pharmaco**/psych/osis _____

There are several specialisms related to pharmacology that are not completely understood from their name:

Pharmacognosy
the study of (*gnos-* knowledge of) crude drugs of vegetable and animal origin.

Pharmacokinetics
the study of the way drugs are absorbed, metabolized and excreted, i.e. what the body does to the drug and how it moves through the body.

Pharmacodynamics
the study of the action of drugs, i.e. what the drug does to the body.

Pharmacy
the study of the process of preparing and dispensing medicinal drugs or a place where drugs are compounded or dispensed.

Therapeutics
the branch of medicine that deals with the treatment of disease. Treatment can be **palliative** i.e. alleviates symptoms or **curative**. In common usage, therapeutics refers mainly to the use of drugs to treat disease.

Chemotherapy
the treatment of disease using chemical agents (a main type of treatment for cancer).

Toxicology
the study of poisons and other toxic substances and their effect on the body.

Naming drugs

Drugs are known by several different names.

The brand, trade or propriety name
Following extensive research and development, pharmaceutical companies assign brand names to their products for marketing purposes. Each drug and its name is the exclusive property of the company with patent rights to its manufacture. The patent will expire after a fixed time (usually 17 years) allowing time for development costs to be recouped. When the patent has expired the drug may be manufactured by other companies under different brand names or under the drug's generic name.

The generic name
Each drug has an official non-propriety or generic name. This name is assigned to it in its early stage of development and is often a description of its chemical composition or class. A generic drug may be manufactured by any number of companies under different brand names once the patent has expired.

A recent EEC directive requires the use of a recommended International Non-propriety Name (rINN) for medicinal substances. Many British Approved Names (BANs) have been changed or modified to comply with the rINN directive.

The chemical name
This name indicates a drug formula. It is used by a manufacturer or pharmacist when making up a formulation.

Authoritative information about the use, structure, manufacture and the dosage of medicinal drugs is documented in large reference texts known as a *pharmacopoeia*.

WORD EXERCISE 2

In pharmacology certain suffixes are used to denote types of substance:

Suffix	Meaning	Examples
-ose	a type of sugar	glu**cose**/mal**tose**
-ase	indicates an enzyme	amyl**ase**/sucr**ase**

Suffix	Meaning	Examples
-ine	substance derived from ammonia	am**ine**/alan**ine**
-ite	end product	metabol**ite**
-gen	precursor/agent that produces	trypsino**gen**
-in	non-specific suffix denoting a chemical agent	trister**in**
-ic	denotes a type of medicinal drug	mucoly**tic**

Match a biochemical name from Column A with a description in Column C by inserting the appropriate number in Column B.

Column A	Column B	Column C
(a) lip/ase	_____	1. a sugar
(b) rib/ose	_____	2. chemical that produces an action
(c) ser/ine	_____	3. an enzyme
(d) progesto/gen	_____	4. medicinal agent that dilates the pupil
(e) mydria/t/ic	_____	5. chemical related to ammonia

Drug classification

Drugs can be classified by their therapeutic use or action. Exercises 3–14 list the classifications of drugs used to treat disorders associated with the body systems we have studied in this book.

Note. The suffixes -al, -ic and -ive are all used to mean *pertaining to* but they can all be used in pharmacology to indicate a type of drug.

The action of a drug can often be deduced from its classification. To do this we split the word classification into its components, find their meaning and then try to deduce an action or use. The technique can be practised in Word Exercises 3–14.

 ## WORD EXERCISE 3

Many classifications have the prefix **anti-** meaning against. Using your Exercise Guide write the meaning of:

(a) **anti**/bacteri/al _____

(b) **anti**/bio/tic _____

(c) **anti**/fung/al _____

(d) **anti**/vir/al _____

(e) **anti**/prurit/ic _____

In the following examples the *i* of the prefix *anti-* is dropped for roots beginning with a vowel or the letter h.

(f) **ant**/acid _____

(g) **ant**/helmint/ic _____

 ## WORD EXERCISE 4

Several drug classifications have the prefix **an-** meaning without. Using your Exercise Guide write the meaning of:

(a) **an**/alges/ic _____

(b) **an**/aesthe/tic (Am. an/esthe/tic) _____

Word Exercises 5–14 list many types of drug associated with systems studied in this book.

Drug classifications associated with the digestive system

WORD EXERCISE 5

Without using your Exercise Guide write the meaning of:

(a) anti/diarrhoe/al _____

(b) anti/spasmod/ic (acts on intestines) _____

Others include:

---

laxatives
    promote evacuation of the bowels

H₂–receptor antagonists
    prevent the secretion of acid by the gastric mucosa (lining of the stomach) and promote the healing of ulcers

---

Drug classifications associated with the breathing system

WORD EXERCISE 6

Using your Exercise Guide write the meaning of:

(a) muco/lytic _____

(b) anti/tuss/ive _____

(c) broncho/dilator _____
(dilate means to widen, not listed in the Exercise
Guide)

Others include:

antihistamines
used to counteract the effects of histamine, a chemical
released during allergic reactions such as asthma.

corticosteroids
used to reduce inflammation. Here they are used for
prophylaxis in the treatment of asthma by reducing
inflammation in the bronchial mucosa (lining).

decongestants
reduce the feeling of congestion in the nose.

diuretics
used to promote the excretion of urine, thereby
relieving the oedema (Am. edema) of heart failure.

inotropics
used to increase or decrease the force of contraction of
heart muscle (myocardium).

sympathomimetics
these drugs mimic the action of the sympathetic
nervous system and are used to raise blood pressure.

Drug classifications associated with the urinary system

anti-diruretic hormone
a hormone that acts on the kidney stimulating
reabsorption of water thereby reducing the formation
of urine.

diuretics
promote the excretion of urine.

uricosurics
used to increase the excretion of uric acid in urine
thereby relieving the symptoms of gout.

xanthine-oxidase inhibitors
used for the palliative treatment of gout.

Drug classifications associated with the cardiovascular system and blood

WORD EXERCISE 7

Using your Exercise Guide write the meaning of:

(a) fibrino/lytic _____

(b) anti/fibrino/lytic _____

(c) anti/-a/rrhythm/ic _____

(d) haemo/static _____
(Am. hemo/static)

Others include:

anticoagulants
used to prevent clotting/coagulation of blood.

antiplatelet drugs
decrease platelet aggregation in arteries, thereby
inhibiting clot formation.

antihypertensives
used to treat hypertension (high blood pressure).

Drug classifications associated with the nervous system

WORD EXERCISE 8

Using your Exercise Guide write the meaning of:

(a) hypno/tic _____

(b) anxio/lytic _____

(c) anti/epilep/tic _____

(d) anti/psycho/tic _____

Others include:

antidepressants
used to prevent or relieve depression.

CNS stimulants
drugs that have limited use for treating narcolepsy
(a recurrent, uncontrollable desire to sleep).

anti-emetics
used to prevent vomiting (emesis).

opioid analgesics
    used to relieve moderate to severe pain particularly of visceral origin (opioid – refers to a synthetic narcotic resembling but not derived from opium).

Drug classifications associated with the eye

WORD EXERCISE 9

Using your Exercise Guide write the meaning of:

(a) cyclo/plegic _____

Others include:

eye lotions
    for irrigation of the eye.

topical anti-infective preparations
    antibacterials, antifungals and antivirals applied directly to the eye.

topical corticosteroids
    anti-inflammatory steroids applied directly to the eye.

mydriatics
    used to dilate the pupil.

local anaesthetics (Am. anesthetics)
    used to reduce sensation in the eye.

miotics
    drugs used to treat glaucoma that narrow the pupil.

Drug classifications associated with the ear

topical astringents
    drugs used to treat inflammation and dry up secretion of fluid.

topical anti-infective preparations
    antibacterials and antifungals applied directly to the external ear for treatment of otitis externa.

Drug classifications associated with the mouth and nose

oral antihistamines
    drugs that reduce the symptoms of histamine, here used for treatment of nasal allergy.

systemic nasal decongestants
    drugs used for symptomatic relief in chronic nasal obstruction.

topical decongestants
    drugs applied directly to the nose as drops or spray to relieve congestion.

Drug classifications associated with the skin

WORD EXERCISE 10

Using your Exercise Guide write the meaning of:

(a) anti/prurit/ic _____

(b) kerato/lytic _____

Others include:

vehicles
    inert substances added to drugs to give a suitable consistency for transfer into the body; vehicles do not possess therapeutic properties.

emollients
    agents that soften or soothe the skin.

desloughing agents
    agents that remove dead tissue from a wound.

Drug classifications associated with the musculoskeletal system

non-steroidal anti-inflammatory drugs (NSAIDs)
    In full doses these have analgesic and anti-inflammatory effects. They are used to treat painful inflammatory conditions such as rheumatic disease; aspirin is a familiar example.

relaxants
    drugs that block the neuromuscular junction and produce relaxation of muscles, they are widely used in anaesthesia.

uricosurics
    drugs that promote the excretion of uric acid in the urine thereby relieving the symptoms of gout.

Drug classifications associated with the reproductive system

WORD EXERCISE 11

Using your Exercise Guide write the meaning of:

(a) oxy/toc/ic _____

(b) gonado/troph/in _____

Without using your Exercise Guide write the meaning of:

(c) anti/-oestro/gen _____
    (Am. anti/estro/gen)

Others include:

---

contraceptives
used to prevent conception i.e. the fertilization of an egg by a sperm. `Family planning pills contain sex hormones that inhibit the release of eggs from the ovary thereby preventing a pregnancy.

prostaglandins
used to induce abortion, augment labour and to minimize blood loss from the placental site.

sex hormones
used for hormone replacement therapy (HRT). For example, menopausal symptoms are relieved by small doses of the female sex hormone oestrogen. The male sex hormones called androgens are used for replacement therapy in castrated males.

Drug classifications associated with the endocrine system

(This section deals with examples of drug classifications other than those that act on the reproductive system.)

 WORD EXERCISE 12

Without using your Exercise Guide write the meaning of:

(a) anti/thyroid _____

Others include:

---

antidiabetics
used for non-insulin dependent diabetes, act against diabetes by increasing insulin secretion.

insulins
insulin is a hormone that lowers blood glucose in patients with diabetes mellitus. Many different forms of insulin e.g. short, intermediate and long-acting are available for injection.

corticosteroids
steroids produced by the adrenal cortex or their synthetic equivalents used for replacement therapy when secretion by the adrenal glands is insufficient.

human growth hormones
growth hormone of human origin (somatotrophin) has been used to stimulate growth in patients of short stature. This has been replaced by somatotropin, a biosynthetic human growth hormone which has a similar effect.

Drug classifications associated with oncology

Drugs used in oncology aim to prevent the replication of cancer cells and destroy them by interfering with their metabolism. The process of using drugs in this way to destroy tumours is called **chemotherapy**.

 WORD EXERCISE 13

Using your Exercise Guide write the meaning of:

(a) cyto/tox/ic _____

(b) anti/neo/plas/tic _____

Others include:

---

alkylating drugs
damage DNA (genes) and interfere with the replication of cancer cells.

antimetabolites
drugs that combine with and inhibit vital cell enzymes.

vinca alkaloids
drugs originally derived from the plant species *Vinca* that have the ability to directly interrupt the process of cell division.

Drug classifications associated with the immune system

These drugs are used to suppress rejection of transplanted organs in their recipients and treat autoimmune diseases (*auto-* meaning self, **autoimmunity** is an abnormal response of the immune system to the body's own tissues).

 WORD EXERCISE 14

Without using your Exercise Guide write the meaning of:

(a) immuno/suppressant _____
(suppress means prevent/stop)

(b) cyto/tox/ic immuno/suppressant _____

Abbreviations

Some common abbreviations related to drug administration are listed below. Note, however, some are not standard and their meaning may vary from one health care setting to another. There is a more extensive list for reference on page 307.

bid.	twice a day
cap.	capsule
disp.	dispense
im.	intramuscular
iv.	intravenous
od	every day
OTC	over the counter (non-prescription drugs)
po	per os, by mouth, orally
prn	when required
qid.	four times a day
tab.	tablet
tid.	three times a day

Microbiology

Microbiology is the study of small organisms (*micro* – small, *bio* – life, *logy* – study of). In the field of health, pathogenic microorganisms such as bacteria, protozoa, fungi and viruses are responsible for infectious disease. Swabs, fluids and tissues taken from patients suspected of having an infection are sent to the microbiology laboratories for analysis. The microbiology laboratory is often part of the pathology department in a large hospital. This section examines words associated with microorganisms.

Microbiology is divided into the following specialities:

Bacteriology	study of bacteria
Mycology	study of fungi
Virology	study of viruses
Protozoology	the study of protozoa

Naming microorganisms

Species of microorganisms are given Latin names according to the binomial (two name) system . The first name denotes the group or **genus** to which the organism belongs and always begins with a capital letter. The second name is the **species or** specific name and this begins with a lower case letter for example:

Salmonella typhi	Salmonella is the genus, typhi the species
Clostridium tetani	Clostridium is the genus, tetani the species

Often the name of the genus is abbreviated if it is widely used, as in *E. coli* for *Escherichia coli* and *Staph. aureus* for *Staphylococcus aureus*.

The species name of microorganisms is sometimes formed from words that indicate:

their colour	e.g. *Staphylococcus aureus* (from aurum, meaning gold)
the place where they are found	e.g. *Staphylococcus epidermidis* (the epidermis of the skin)
the disease they cause	e.g. *Bacillus anthracis* (causes anthrax)
the scientist who studied or named them	e.g. *Escherichia coli* (after Dr Escherich)

Bacteriology

Bacteria are small single-celled organisms that can only be seen with an optical microscope. There are thousands of different types classified according to their shape, group arrangement, colony characteristics, structure and chemical characteristics. The combining form **bacteri/o** is used to mean bacteria (from Greek *bakterion* meaning staff).

CLASSIFICATION OF BACTERIA USING THE GRAM STAINING REACTION

For more than a century bacteria have been classified using the **Gram** staining reaction named after Christian Gram who devised it in 1884. His method is based upon the ability of bacteria to retain the purple crystal violet-iodine complex when stained and treated with organic solvents:

Gram-positive bacteria (Gram +ve)
retain the stain and appear purple.

Gram-negative bacteria (Gram −ve)
cannot retain the purple dye complex and need to be stained with a red dye before they can be seen with an optical microscope.

CLASSIFICATION BY SHAPE AND GROUPING

Individual bacteria have one of three basic shapes: they are either spherical, cylindrical or spiral. Spherical cells are called **cocci** (singular **coccus**), cylindrical cells **bacilli** (singular **bacillus**) and helical or spiral cells **spirilla** (singular **spirillum**).

The coccus (plural – cocci)

The word coccus comes from a Greek word *kokkos* meaning berry. They are usually round but can be ovoid or flattened on one side when adhering to another cell. Cocci can grow in several different arrangements or groups depending on the plane of cell division and whether the new cells remain together. Each arrangement is typical of a species and contributes to an organism's classification. When a coccus divides in one plane and the two new cells remain together the arrangement is called a **diplococcus**.

When cocci divide repeatedly in one plane and remain together to form a twisted row of cells they are called **streptococci** (*strepto-* from a Greek word meaning twisted, singular streptococcus). Others divide in three planes and remain together in irregular, grape-like patterns; these are called **staphylococci** (*staphylo-* from a Greek word meaning grapes, singular staphylococcus). See Figure 105 for examples:

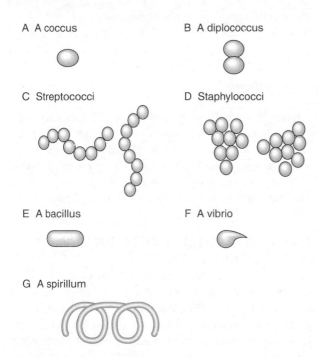

A   A coccus

B   A diplococcus

C   Streptococci

D   Staphylococci

E   A bacillus

F   A vibrio

G   A spirillum

Figure 105   *Shapes and group arrangements of bacteria*

Some cocci are of great medical importance, for example:

Gram +ve
  Streptococcus pneumoniae causes pneumonia and meningitis.

  Staphylococcus aureus causes serious infection in hospitals (MRSA – methicillin resistant *Staphylococcus aureus*).

Gram −ve
  Neisseria gonorrhoeae causes gonorrhoea.

  Neisseria meningitidis causes meningitis.

  (*Neisseria* are sometimes seen in pairs and are grouped as diplococci.)

The bacillus (plural – bacilli)

These are rod-shaped bacteria (*bacillus* is a Latin word meaning a stick or rod); they are also classified using the Gram staining procedure (see Fig. 105E). There are large differences in the length and width of bacilli and their ends can be square, rounded or tapered.

Some bacilli are of medical importance, for example:

Gram +ve
  Bacillus anthracis causes anthrax. It produces highly resistant spores that are difficult to destroy except at high temperatures.

  Clostridium tetani found in soil, causes tetanus.

Gram −ve
  Escherichia coli found in the human gut, certain strains are pathogenic.

  Salmonella typhi causes typhoid.

Gram-negative bacilli that appear curved in shape (like a comma) are called vibrios (see Fig. 105F), for example:

  Vibrio cholerae causes cholera, a water-borne infection.

The spirillum (plural – spirilla)

The spirilla are spiral or helical-shaped bacteria that look like tiny corkscrews (see Fig. 105G). Those that belong to the genus *Spirillum* consist of Gram −ve, non-flexous (non-flexible) spiral-shaped filaments. Another group distinguished by their flexibility belong to the genus *Spirochaeta*. (Note: the use of this group is becoming obsolete and most of the bacteria assigned to this group have been transferred to other genera). Examples are:

  Spirillum minus causes rat-bite fever in man.

  Treponema pallidum a spirochaete (Am. spirochete) that belongs to the order Spirochaetales and causes syphilis.

It should be noted that the cells of a given species are rarely arranged in exactly the same pattern. It is the predominant arrangement that is important when studying bacteria.

Some terms denoting shape, for example bacillus, may be used as generic names as in *Bacillus anthracis*.

CULTURE AND SENSITIVITY TESTING

Infected swabs, fluids and tissues are sent to microbiology laboratories for **culture and sensitivity testing**. To culture an organism, it is placed at an optimum temperature in a special culture medium (broth or agar jelly) that contains all the nutrients required for growth. In ideal conditions the microorganism multiplies rapidly producing a huge clone of identical cells. Samples from the culture are then exposed to a range of different antibiotics. If an organism is sensitive to a particular antibiotic, it will be destroyed or its growth inhibited. Antibiotics that are found to destroy the cultured organisms are administered to the patient to try and rid them of the infection.

WORD EXERCISE 15

Match a description in Column A with a bacterium in Column C by inserting a number in Column B.

Column A	Column B	Column C
(a) A bacterium that appears rod-shaped and purple following staining with the Gram staining procedure		1. diplococci
(b) A rod that appears comma-shaped and pink following staining with the Gram staining procedure		2. *Staphylococcus aureus*
(c) Cocci arranged into a twisted chain that infects the lungs		3. Gram −ve *Vibrio cholerae*
(d) Gold coloured cocci arranged into irregular grape-like groups that cause serious suppurative infections sometimes resistant to common antibiotics		4. Gram −ve *E. coli*
(e) Cocci belonging to the genus Neisseria that arrange themselves into pairs		5. Gram +ve *Bacillus anthracis*
(f) A helical bacterium that causes syphilis		6. *Streptococcus pneumoniae*
(g) A bacterium that appears rod-shaped and pink following staining with the Gram staining procedure		7. *Treponema pallidum* (a spirochaete)

WORD EXERCISE 16

Using your Exercise Guide write the meaning of:

(a) **bacterio**/logist

(b) **streptococc**/al

(c) **bacteri**/uria

(d) **bacteri**/cid/al

(e) **bacterio**/static

(f) **bacterio**/lytic

(g) **bacill**/aemia
(Am. **bacill**/emia)

(h) **bacillo**/genic

(i) **streptococci**/cide

(j) **strepto**/septic/aemia
(Am. **strepto**/septic/emia)

(k) **spirill**/osis

Mycology

Fungi are non-green plants that act as decomposers in the environment, breaking down the dead bodies of plants and animals. The group includes the familiar mushrooms and toadstools and microscopic moulds and yeasts.

Certain types of moulds and yeasts are pathogenic and infect the body causing disease. When they infect the skin they are called **dermatophytes** (*dermat/o* meaning skin, *-phyte* meaning plant). A common condition is Athlete's foot caused by several species of fungi (e.g. *Trichophyton rubrum*) that infect skin between the toes. In warm, moist conditions the fungi grow and digest the skin causing it to itch and split. The fungal spores that generate the infection are usually picked up on changing room floors so the condition is common among sports enthusiasts. Athlete's foot is easily treated and harmless, unlike some fungal infections found in tropical climates.

When round, red patches of skin infected with fungi begin to heal they often take on a ring-like appearance and because of this the infection became inaccurately known as 'ringworm'. The medical name for Athlete's foot is **Tinea pedis** or ringworm of the foot (*Tinea* is a Latin word meaning gnawing worm, and *-pedis* means the foot). Other superficial fungal infections of the skin are named in a similar way: **Tinea capitis** (ringworm of the head), **Tinea corporis** (ringworm of the body).

Fungal infections are life-threatening in patients whose immune system is compromised; for example, *Candida albicans* can cause serious infections of the mouth, digestive system and reproductive systems in AIDS patients. This type of infection is known as Candidiasis (*-iasis* meaning abnormal condition).

Fungi are named according to the binomial system with a generic and specific name as in *Candida albicans*.

Root	Myc
	*(From a Greek word **mykes**, meaning fungus.)*
Combining forms	**Myc/o**

WORD EXERCISE 17

Without using your Exercise Guide, write the meaning of:

(a) **myc**/osis   _____

(b) **myco**/tic   _____

(c) **myco**/tox/in   _____

(d) **myco**/toxic/osis   _____

Root	Fung
	(From a Greek word **fungus**, *meaning mushroom. Here it is used to mean fungus or fungal infection.)*
Combining forms	**Fung/i/o**

WORD EXERCISE 18

Without using your Exercise Guide, write the meaning of:

(a) **fungi**/form   _____

(b) **fungi**/toxic   _____

(c) **fungi**/cide   _____

(d) **fungi**/static   _____

Using your Exercise Guide, find the meaning of:

(e) **fung**/oid   _____

(f) **fungos**/ity   _____

Virology

A virus (virion) is an extremely small infectious particle that does not show the usual characteristics of life; for example, it does not move, respire, feed or respond to stimuli.

Viruses do reproduce but only within a specific host cell. (Note: a host is an organism that harbours a parasite.) When a virus comes into contact with a host cell, it inserts its genes. Once inside the viral genes alter the metabolism of the host cell and instruct it to make new viruses. The host cell fills with copies of the original virus and may burst, releasing the new infectious particles into the surrounding environment.

Viruses have characteristic shapes, different chemical structures and different methods of replication. They can only be seen in an electron microscope that produces a large magnification and has the ability to resolve their fine detail. Characteristics of viruses and the conditions they cause are incorporated into their names. In the examples given below the words have been split to show their meaning.

Onco/rna/virus
 type of virus that causes cancer (onc/o) and contains ribonucleic acid (-rna-).

Papo/va/virus
 type of virus that causes vacuoles (va) inside host cells and the formation of papillomas/tumours (papo – papilloma).

Pico/rna/virus
 type of virus that is very small (pico-) and contains ribonucleic acid (-rna-).

Retro/virus
 type of virus that carries the enzyme reverse transcriptase (retro – back).

Rhino/virus
 type of virus that infects the nose (rhin/o – nose).

Entero / virus
 type of virus that infects the intestines.

Bacterio/phage
 type of virus that uses a bacterium as a host.

Viruses may also be referred to by their genus and species name, for example *Herpes simplex*, a virus that causes cold sores around the mouth.

Root	Vir
	(From a Greek word **virus**, *meaning poison. Here it is used to mean virus, a minute infectious particle that replicates only within a living host cell. Each particle consists of viral genes enclosed in a protein coat.)*
Combining forms	**Vir/o/u**

WORD EXERCISE 19

Without using your Exercise Guide, write the meaning of:

(a) **viru**/cide   _____

(b) **viro**/logist _____

(c) anti/retro/**vir**/al _____

(d) **vir**/uria _____

Using your Exercise Guide, find the meaning of:

(e) **vir**/aemia _____
   (Am. **vir**/emia)

(f) **viro**/lact/ia _____

Protozoology

This is a branch of medicine concerned with single-celled animals called protozoa. Some of these organisms are pathogenic and responsible for serious disease. Infection with protozoa is generally referred to as a **pro-tozo**iasis (-*iasis* meaning abnormal condition/state of). Examples are given below:

Plasmodium falciparum
   (a type of sporozoan)   causes malaria

Trypanosoma gambiense
   (a type of flagellate)   causes African sleeping sickness

Entamoeba histolytica
   (a type of amoeba) causes amoebic (Am. amebic) dysentery

CASE HISTORY 21

The object of this exercise is to understand words associated with a patient's medical history. To complete the exercise:

• read through the passage on HIV infection; unfamiliar words are underlined and you can find their meaning using the Word Help

• write the meaning of the medical terms shown in bold print.

HIV infection

Mr U, a 38-year-old homosexual man, presented to the Accident and Emergency Department with a fever, non-productive cough and dyspnoea. During the previous 7 days he had become increasingly short of breath and complained of an inability to sleep because he was hot and sweating profusely. He was a non-smoker and had no haemoptysis (Am. hemoptysis). Mr U informed the medical staff that he had been diagnosed HIV positive 3 years earlier but had declined **antiretro-viral** therapy.

On examination he appeared pale, and thin and he indicated that he had lost a considerable amount of weight over the past 2 months. He was pyrexial (Temp. 39.1°C), tachycardic (121 beats/min), and tachypnoeic (Am. tachypneic) (28 breaths/min).

Examination of his mouth revealed white patches with surrounding inflammation indicative of a severe **candidiasis**; swabs were taken and sent for analysis. He was short of breath with poor lung expansion and a chest X-ray showed diffuse bilateral shading. His serum biochemistry and liver function were normal.

Mr U was admitted to the ward with a clinical diagnosis of PCP or other atypical pneumonia and started on the **antibacterial** co-trimoxazole in two daily doses and the **antibiotic** erythromycin given as an infusion over 1 hour. He was also given an intravenous steroid methylprednisolone to reduce inflammation in his alveoli and improve gaseous exchange.

The next day a bronchoscopy was performed, and the washings sent to the **microbiology** laboratory for culture and sensitivity testing. The results confirmed the diagnosis of *Pneumocystis carinii* infection and haematology reported a CD4 count of less than 50 cells mm^{-3}, indicating Mr U had developed AIDS. His mouth infection was confirmed as *Candida albicans* and he was prescribed the **antifungal** itraconazole.

Following administration of his high dose of co-trimoxazole Mr U developed severe nausea and was given the **anti-emetic** metoclopramide parenterally before his infusions.

Two weeks later he was clinically much improved, and a **pharmaceutical plan** was devised prior to his discharge. He was advised that he required antiretroviral therapy and counselled on the possibility of side-effects. He was given a discharge medication of sufficient oral co-trimoxazole to complete his initial course of treatment and instructed on a prophylactic dose regimen.

WORD HELP

AIDS acquired immune deficiency syndrome

atypical not conforming to the usual type/in microbiology applied to strains of unusual type

bilateral pertaining to both sides

bronchoscopy technique of viewing/examining the bronchial tree

Candida albicans a yeast-like fungus belonging to the genus *Candida* that infects the digestive and reproductive systems

CD4 cluster designation/cluster of differentiation. Refers to clusters of chemicals (cell surface markers)

WORD HELP (Contd.)

found on the surface of leucocytes (Am. leukocytes). CD4 molecules are found on T-cells (lymphocytes) and they act as the receptor molecules for HIV. The depletion of CD4 lymphocytes by HIV leads to the development of AIDS

culture and sensitivity testing growing microorganisms in the laboratory and testing them for sensitivity to antibiotics

dyspnoea difficult/laboured breathing

haemoptysis (Am. hemoptysis) spitting / coughing up of blood

infusion slow introduction of a therapeutic agent into a vein

non-productive not producing (sputum)

HIV positive presence of antibodies to the human immunodeficiency virus in the blood, it indicates the virus has infected the body

parenterally the word means pertaining to beyond the intestine but in practice it means administered by injection into the skin or muscle

PCP *Pneumocystis carinii* pneumonia

Pneumocystis carinii a protozoa-like organism that causes pneumonia, an opportunistic infection commonly seen in AIDS patients

prophylactic pertaining to preventative treatment

pyrexial having a fever/elevation of body temperature above normal

regimen regulated scheme (e.g. of taking drugs/medication)

tachycardic pertaining to fast heart beat

tachypnoeic pertaining to fast breathing

washing solution that has contacted a surface and is to be used for analysis

Now write the meaning of the following words from the case study without using your dictionary lists:

(a) antiretroviral _____

(b) candidiasis _____

(c) antibacterial _____

(d) antibiotic _____

(e) microbiology _____

(f) antifungal _____

(g) anti-emetic _____

(h) pharmaceutical plan _____

(Answers to the case history exercise are given in the Answers to Word Exercises beginning on page 275.)

Quick Reference

Combining forms relating to the pharmacology and microbiology:

cocc/o	coccus (berry-shaped bacterium)
bacill/o	bacillus (rod-like bacterium)
bacteri/o	bacterium/bacteria
fung/i	fungus
helmint/h/o	worm
myc/o	fungus
pharmac/o	drug
spirill/o	spiral-shaped bacteria of genus *Spirillum*
staphylococc/o	staphylococcus/a bunch of cocci
streptococc/o	streptococcus/a chain of cocci
toxic/o	poison
vibri/o	comma-shaped bacterium of genus *Vibrio*
vir/o	virus/virion

Abbreviations

You should learn common abbreviations related to microbiology. Note, however, some are not standard and their meaning may vary from one health care setting to another. There is a more extensive list for reference on page 307.

ABX	antibiotics
AFB	acid-fast bacilli
BCG	bacille (bacillus) Calmette–Guérin (causes tuberculosis)
C+S	culture and sensitivity test
EBV	Epstein–Barr virus
HBV	Hepatitis B virus
HSV	*Herpes simplex* virus
Hib	*Haemophilus influenzae* type b
HIV	human immunodeficiency virus
MRSA	multiple-resistant or methicillin resistant *Staphylococcus aureus*
NGU	non-gonococcal urethritis
PCN	penicillin

 NOW TRY THE WORD CHECK

WORD CHECK

This self-check exercise lists all the word components used in this unit. First write down the meaning of as many word components as you can. Then check your answers using the Exercise Guide and Quick Reference box or the Glossary of Word Components (pp. 319–341).

Prefixes

a- _____

an- _____

anti- _____

auto- _____

dia- _____

neo- _____

oxy- _____

retro- _____

Roots/Combining forms

acid/o _____

aesthet/o
(Am. esthet/o) _____

anxi/o _____

alges/i/o _____

bacill/o _____

bacteri/o _____

bi/o _____

bronch/i/o _____

cocc/o _____

cycl/o _____

cyt/o _____

dynam/o _____

epilept/o _____

fibrin/o _____

fung/i _____

gonad/o _____

haem/o
(Am. hem/o) _____

helmint/h/o _____

hypn/o _____

immun/o _____

kerat/o _____

kinet/o _____

lact/i/o _____

muc/o _____

oestr/o
(Am. estr/o) _____

pharmac/o _____

plas/m/o _____

prurit/o _____

psych/o _____

(r)rhythm/o _____

septic/o _____

spasm/o/d _____

spirill/o _____

staphylococc/o _____

streptococc/o _____

thyroid/o _____

toc/o _____

tox/ic/o _____

troph/o _____

tuss/i _____

ur/o _____

vir/o _____

Suffixes

-aemia
(Am. emia) _____

-al _____

-ase _____

-cid(e) _____

-form _____

-gen _____

-gnosy _____

-ia _____

-ic _____

-ite _____

-ive _____

-logist _____

-logy _____

-lytic _____

-oid _____

-ose _____

-osis _____

-plegia _____

-rrhoea
(Am. -rrhea) _____

-tic _____

-uria _____

-y _____

> **NOW TRY THE SELF-ASSESSMENT** <

SELF-ASSESSMENT

Test 21A
Prefixes and Suffixes

Match each prefix or suffix in Column A with a meaning in Column C by inserting the appropriate number in Column B.

Column A	Column B	Column C
(a) an-	_____	1. quick
(b) anti-	_____	2. knowledge/ process of judgment
(c) -ase	_____	3. chemical derived from ammonia
(d) -gen	_____	4. abnormal condition/ disease
(e) -gnosy	_____	5. condition of rhythm
(f) -ose	_____	6. process /condition
(g) -ine	_____	7. study of
(h) -in	_____	8. drug that breaks down .../ pertaining to breakdown
(i) -ic	_____	9. without
(j) -ite	_____	10. end-product
(k) -ive	_____	11. excessive discharge/flow
(l) -logy	_____	12. enzyme
(m)-logist	_____	13. against
(n) -lytic	_____	14. non-specific suffix indicating a chemical
(o) -osis	_____	15. type of drug/ pertaining to (i)

Column A	Column B	Column C
(p) oxy	_____	16. type of drug/ pertaining to (ii)
(q) -rrhoea (Am. rrhea)	_____	17. type of drug/ pertaining to (iii)
(r) -rrhythmia	_____	18. specialist who studies
(s) -tic	_____	19. precursor/agent that produces
(t) -y	_____	20. sugar

Score

20

Column A	Column B	Column C
(n) pharmac/o	_____	14. force/power of movement
(o) prurit/o	_____	15. virus/virion
(p) psych/o	_____	16. pain
(q) toxic/o	_____	17. acid
(r) troph/o	_____	18. motion/ movement
(s) tuss/i	_____	19. sleep
(t) vir/o	_____	20. mucus

Score

20

Test 21B

Combining forms of word roots

Match each combining form of a word root from Column A with a meaning from Column C by inserting the appropriate number in Column B.

Column A	Column B	Column C
(a) acid/o	_____	1. poison
(b) aesthet/o	_____	2. worms
(c) alges/i/o	_____	3. itching
(d) anxi/o	_____	4. fungus (i)
(e) bacteri/o	_____	5. fungus (ii)
(f) bi/o	_____	6. bacteria
(g) dynam/o	_____	7. drug
(h) fungi	_____	8. life
(i) helmint/h/o	_____	9. sensation
(j) hypn/o	_____	10. mind
(k) kinet/o	_____	11. nourish/stimulate
(l) muc/o	_____	12. cough
(m) myc/o	_____	13. anxiety

Test 21C

Write the meaning of:

(a) toxicology _____

(b) mycotoxicosis _____

(c) pharmacist _____

(d) chemotherapeutic agent _____

(e) microbiologist _____

Score

5

Test 21D

Build words that mean:

(a) specialist who studies bacteria _____

(b) drug that acts against living things _____

(c) the study of protozoa _____

(d) agent that stops the growth of bacteria _____

(e) pertaining to killing viruses _____

Score

5

Test 21E

Match each drug action from Column A with a drug classification from Column C by inserting the appropriate number in Column B.

Column A	Column B	Column C
(a) acts against worms	_____	1. immuno-suppressant
(b) acts to reduce pain	_____	2. cytotoxic
(c) reduces sensation	_____	3. miotic
(d) acts to reduce coughing	_____	4. antipsychotic
(e) neutralises stomach acid	_____	5. anxiolytic
(f) acts to break up mucus	_____	6. antipruritic
(g) acts to promote the excretion of urine	_____	7. anthelmintic
(h) acts to dilate bronchi	_____	8. antihistamine
(i) used to treat schizophrenia	_____	9. antitussive
(j) used to induce labour	_____	10. antibiotic
(k) acts to lower blood sugar of non-insulin dependent diabetics	_____	11. gonadotrophin

Column A	Column B	Column C
(l) acts to kill cancer cells	_____	12. analgesic
(m) reduces the immune response	_____	13. hypnotic
(n) used to treat glaucoma	_____	14. antihypertensive
(o) dilates the pupil for examination	_____	15. contraceptive
(p) promotes evacuation of the bowels	_____	16. anticoagulant
(q) prevents the effects of histamine	_____	17. bronchodilator
(r) used to induce sleep	_____	18. diuretic
(s) used to reduce high blood pressure	_____	19. anaesthetic (Am. anesthetic)
(t) used to reduce anxiety	_____	20. antacid
(u) used to prevent itching	_____	21. mucolytic
(v) used to prevent conception/ pregnancy	_____	22. mydriatic
(w) stimulates/ nourishes the reproductive organs	_____	23. antidiabetic
(x) prevents blood clotting	_____	24. laxative
(y) destroys bacteria and fungi	_____	25. oxytocic

Score

25

Test 21F

Match each description from Column A with the name of an organism from Column C by inserting the appropriate number in Column B.

Column A	Column B	Column C
(a) a round, berry-like bacterium	_____	1. staphylococci
(b) a rod-like bacterium	_____	2. spirillum
(c) a comma-shaped bacterium	_____	3. rhinovirus
(d) a spiral-shaped bacterium	_____	4. bacillus
(e) a cancer forming virus that contains RNA	_____	5. streptococci
(f) a plant (fungus) that infects the skin	_____	6. diplococci
(g) round berry-like bacteria that occur in chains	_____	7. a bacteriophage
(h) round berry-like bacteria that occur in bunches	_____	8. coccus
(i) virus that infects the nose	_____	9. vibrio
(j) berry-like bacteria that group in pairs	_____	10. dermatophyte
(k) single-celled animal that causes malaria	_____	11. a protozoan *Plasmodium*
(l) a virus that infects bacteria	_____	12. oncornavirus

Score

12

Check answers to Self-Assessment Tests on page 299.

Answers to word exercises

Introduction

Word Exercise 1
(a) Gastropathy
(b) Gastroscopy
(c) Hepatitis
(d) Hepatomegaly
(e) Hepatoma

Word Exercise 2
(a) Duodenojejunostomy
(b) Tracheobronchitis
(c) Gastroenterostomy
(d) Laryngopharyngectomy
(e) Osteoarthropathy

Word Exercise 3
(a) Endodontic
(b) Prosthodontist
(c) Pararectal
(d) Monocular
(e) Perisplenitis

Unit 1 Levels of organization

Word Exercise 1
(a) Cyt – word root meaning cell, o – combining vowel, pathy – suffix meaning disease
(b) Disease of cells
(c) Study of disease
(d) Study of disease of cells
(e) Breakdown/disintegration of cells
(f) Pertaining to poisonous to cells
(g) Specialist who studies cells

Word Exercise 2
(a) Erythr – word root meaning red, o – combining vowel, cyte – word root meaning cell
(b) Red cell

Word Exercise 3
(a) Melanocyte
(b) Fibrocyte
(c) Lympho/lymphocyte (lymph cell)
    Spermato/spermatocyte (sperm cell)
    Oo/oocyte (egg cell)
    Granulo/granulocyte (granular cell)
    Chondro/chondrocyte (cartilage cell)

Word Exercise 4
(a) Bone forming cell/immature bone cell
(b) Fibre forming cell/immature fibre cell
(c) Immature blood cell/cell that forms blood cells

Word Exercise 5
(a) The chemistry of tissues (refers to study of)
(b) Study of diseased tissues
(c) Person who specializes in study of tissues
(d) Breakdown/disintegration of tissues

Word Exercise 6
(a) Small
(b) Instrument to view small objects
(c) Technique of viewing very small objects with a microscope
(d) Person who specializes in microscopy
(e) Study of small life/microorganisms

Word Exercise 7
(a) The formation of organs
(b) Pertaining to formation/genesis of organs
(c) Pertaining to nourishing/stimulating organs

Case History 1
(a) The study of tissues/department that studies tissues
(b) Specialist who studies disease/diseased organs
(c) Pertaining to the study of cells
(d) Technique of viewing small things (here cells)
(e) White (blood) cell
(f) Lymph cell
(g) Study of small forms of life i.e. bacteria, fungi and protozoa etc.
(h) Pertaining to causing disease

Unit 2 The digestive system

Word Exercise 1
(a) Instrument to view the oesophagus
(b) Removal of oesophagus
(c) Incision into the oesophagus
(d) Inflammation of the oesophagus

Word Exercise 2
(a) Instrument to view the stomach
(b) Removal of part or all of stomach
(c) Incision into stomach

(d)   Inflammation of the stomach, especially the lining
(e)   Gastropathy
(f)   Gastrology
(g)   Epigastric

Word Exercise 3

(a)   Inflammation of the intestines
(b)   Disease of the intestines
(c)   Incision into the intestine
(d)   Opening into the intestine (often to connect to stomach, ileum, jejunum or abdominal wall)
(e)   Intestinal stone (compacted material in intestine)
(f)   Enterology
(g)   Enterologist
(h)   Study of intestines and stomach (+associated structures, e.g. liver and pancreas)
(i)   Disease of intestines and stomach
(j)   Inflammation of the intestines and stomach (often due to infection)
(k)   Technique of viewing the intestines and stomach

Word Exercise 4

(a)   Removal of stomach and pylorus
(b)   Technique of viewing pylorus (with an endoscope)

Word Exercise 5

(a)   Formation of an opening (anastomosis) between the intestine and duodenum
(b)   Formation of an opening (anastomosis) between one part of the jejunum and another part of the jejunum
(c)   Pertaining to the jejunum and duodenum
(d)   Ileostomy
(e)   Ileitis

Word Exercise 6

(a)   Large colon
(b)   Inflammation of the appendix
(c)   Removal of the colon
(d)   Opening into the colon (usually a connection between the colon and the abdominal wall; it acts as an artificial anus)
(e)   Caecostomy (Am. cecostomy)
(f)   Appendicectomy (Am. appendectomy)
(g)   Gastrocolostomy

Word Exercise 7

(a)   Technique of viewing the sigmoid colon
(b)   Pertaining to beside the rectum
(c)   Inflammation around anus/rectum
(d)   Administration of fluid into anus/rectum (enema)
(e)   Condition of pain in the anus/rectum
(f)   Proctoscope
(g)   Proctocaecostomy (Am. proctocecostomy)
(h)   Caecosigmoidostomy (Am. cecosigmoidostomy)

Word Exercise 8

(a)   Inflammation of the peritoneum
(b)   Infusion/injection into peritoneum

Word Exercise 9

(a)   Breaking down of the pancreas
(b)   Enlargement of the liver
(c)   Liver tumour
(d)   Pertaining to poisonous to the liver
(e)   Formation of an opening between the stomach and hepatic duct
(f)   Pertaining to the duodenum and pancreatic duct

Word Exercise 10

(a)   Condition of absence of bile
(b)   Bile stone
(c)   Abnormal condition of stones in bile duct (or gall bladder)
(d)   Condition of bile in blood
(e)   Condition of bile in urine
(f)   Incision into gall bladder
(g)   Removal of gall bladder
(h)   Abnormal condition of stones in gall bladder
(i)   X-ray film demonstrating bile ducts (vessels)
(j)   Technique or process of making a cholangiogram
(k)   Abnormal condition of stones in common bile duct
(l)   Incision into common bile duct to remove stones

Word Exercise 11

(a)   Visual examination of the abdomen (i.e. abdominal cavity) with a laparoscope
(b)   Incision into the abdomen

Word Exercise 12

(a)   Enteroscope (4)
(b)   Endoscope (6)
(c)   Enteroscopy (7)
(d)   Endoscopy (9)
(e)   Endoscopist (8)
(f)   Colonoscopy (3)
(g)   Proctoscope (1)
(h)   Sigmoidoscopy (10)
(i)   Panendoscopy (5)
(j)   Photoendoscopy (2)

Case History 2

(a)   Abnormal condition of stones in the bile (in gall bladder or bile duct)
(b)   Pertaining to the region upon/above the stomach (epigastrium)
(c)   Pertaining/relating to bile
(d)   Study of the intestines and stomach
(e)   Pertaining to using a laparoscope (instrument to view the abdomen)

(f)   Removal of the gall bladder
(g)   Inflammation of the gall bladder
(h)   Pertaining to the stomach and nose (here a tube passed through the nose into the stomach)

Unit 3 The breathing system

Word Exercise 1

(a)   Technique of viewing the nose
(b)   Disease of the nose
(c)   Condition of pain in the nose
(d)   Inflammation of the nose
(e)   Excessive flow/discharge from the nose
(f)   Surgical repair of the nose

Word Exercise 2

(a)   A tube that passes from nose to stomach (for suction or feeding)
(b)   A tube that passes from nose to oesophagus (for suction or feeding)

Word Exercise 3

(a)   Condition of pain in pharynx
(b)   Excessive flow/discharge from the pharynx
(c)   Pharyngoplasty
(d)   Pharyngorhinitis

Word Exercise 4

(a)   Study of the larynx
(b)   Removal of the pharynx and larynx
(c)   Laryngoscopy
(d)   Laryngorhinology

Word Exercise 5

(a)   Incision into the trachea
(b)   Formation of an opening into the trachea (to establish a safe airway) or the opening itself

Word Exercise 6

(a)   Bronchorrhoea (Am. bronchorrhea)
(b)   Bronchogram
(c)   Bronchography
(d)   Bronchoscope
(e)   The windpipe itself – bronchus
(f)   Condition of paralysis of the bronchi
(g)   Suturing of the bronchi
(h)   Dilatation of the bronchi
(i)   Abnormal condition of fungi in bronchi
(j)   Originating in the bronchi/pertaining to formation of bronchi
(k)   Involuntary contraction of bronchi (smooth muscle)
(l)   Pertaining to the bronchi and trachea
(m)   Inflammation of bronchi, trachea and larynx
(n)   Formation of an opening between the oesophagus and bronchus

Word Exercise 7

(a)   Incision into the lung
(b)   Suturing of the lung
(c)   Disease/abnormal condition of lung
(d)   Pneumonectomy
(e)   Pneumonopathy
(f)   Puncture of the lung (by surgery)
(g)   Fixation of a lung by surgery (to thoracic wall)

Word Exercise 8

(a)   Blood and air in thorax (pleural cavity)
(b)   Technique of making an X-ray after injection of air
(c)   Without breathing (temporary, due to low levels of carbon dioxide in blood)
(d)   Difficult/painful breathing
(e)   Above normal breathing (higher rate and depth)
(f)   Below normal breathing (low rate and depth)
(g)   Fast breathing

Word Exercise 9

(a)   Lobotomy
(b)   Lobectomy

Word Exercise 10

(a)   Pertaining to the lungs
(b)   Pertaining to the lungs

Word Exercise 11

(a)   Inflammation of the pleura
(b)   Puncture of the pleura
(c)   Pleurography
(d)   Condition of pain in the pleura
(e)   Adhesion/fixation of pleura

Word Exercise 12

(a)   Pertaining to the stomach and diaphragm
(b)   Pertaining to the liver and diaphragm
(c)   Condition of paralysis of the diaphragm

Word Exercise 13

(a)   Thoracopathy
(b)   Thoracotomy
(c)   Puncture of the thorax (by surgery)
(d)   Instrument to view the thorax
(e)   Abnormal condition of narrowing of the thorax

Word Exercise 14

(a)   Pertaining to between the ribs
(b)   Pertaining to originating in the ribs/pertaining to forming ribs
(c)   Inflammation of cartilage of the ribs

Word Exercise 15

(a)   Bronchoscope (3)
(b)   Laryngoscopy (4)
(c)   Rhinoscope (8)
(d)   Pharyngoscope (6)

(e) Bronchoscopy (7)
(f) Rhinologist (1)
(g) Tracheostomy tube (5)
(h) Laryngoscope (2)

Word Exercise 16

(a) Thoracoscope (5)
(b) Stethoscope (7)
(c) Spirometer (6)
(d) Spirography (3)
(e) Nasal speculum (1)
(f) Nasogastric tube (8)
(g) Pleurography (2)
(h) Spirometry (4)

Case History 3

(a) Pertaining to the lungs
(b) Removal of a lobe (here of the lung)
(c) Difficult/painful breathing
(d) Abnormal condition of blue (appearance of skin and mucous membranes)
(e) Spasmodic (involuntary) contractions of the bronchi/bronchial tubes
(f) Condition of below normal supply of oxygen (to tissues)
(g) Condition of above normal carbon dioxide (in the blood)
(h) Condition of the lung (in which there is inflammation of the spongy tissue of the lung due to infection)

Unit 4 The cardiovascular system

Word Exercise 1

(a) Pertaining to the heart
(b) Condition of pain in the heart
(c) Instrument to view the heart
(d) Instrument that records the heart (beat – force and form of)
(e) Tracing/recording made by a cardiograph
(f) Condition of fast heart rate
(g) Cardiomegaly
(h) Cardioplasty
(i) Cardiopathy
(j) Cardiology
(k) The heart muscle
(l) Disease of heart muscle
(m) Stitching/suturing of heart
(n) Instrument that records electrical activity of heart
(o) Inflammation inside heart (lining)
(p) Inflammation of all of heart
(q) Condition of slow heart beat
(r) Condition of right heart (heart displaced to right)
(s) Technique of recording heart sounds
(t) Technique of recording (ultrasound) echoes of heart
(u) Tracing of electrical activity of heart

Word Exercise 2

(a) Pericarditis
(b) Fixation of the pericardium to the heart
(c) Puncture of the pericardium (by surgery)
(d) Removal of the pericardium

Word Exercise 3

(a) Valvoplasty
(b) Valvectomy
(c) Instrument for cutting a heart valve
(d) Pertaining to a valve
(e) Incision into a valve

Word Exercise 4

(a) Sudden contraction of a blood vessel
(b) Pertaining to without blood vessels
(c) Vasculitis
(d) Vasculopathy

Word Exercise 5

(a) X-ray picture of blood vessels (usually arteries)
(b) X-ray picture of heart and major vessels
(c) Technique of making angiocardiogram
(d) Angiology
(e) Angioplasty
(f) Tumour formed from blood vessels (non-malignant)
(g) Dilatation of blood vessels
(h) Formation of blood vessels
(i) Abnormal condition of hardening of blood vessels

Word Exercise 6

(a) Aortopathy
(b) Aortography

Word Exercise 7

(a) Arteriorrhaphy
(b) Arteriosclerosis
(c) Removal of lining of artery
(d) Abnormal condition of decay of arteries
(e) Abnormal condition of narrowing of arteries

Word Exercise 8

(a) X-ray picture of a vena cava
(b) Technique of making an X-ray/tracing of the venae cavae

Word Exercise 9

(a) Dilatation of a vein (varicosity or varicose vein)
(b) Injection or infusion into a vein (of nutrients or medicines)
(c) Pertaining to veins/of the nature of veins
(d) Venogram
(e) Venography

Word Exercise 10

(a) General dilatation of arteries and veins
(b) Injection/infusion into a vein
(c) Incision into vein
(d) Cessation of movement of blood in a vein
(e) Instrument to measure pressure within a vein
(f) Concretion or stone within a vein

Word Exercise 11

(a) Formation of a clot
(b) Inflammation of a vein associated with a thrombus
(c) Removal of the lining of an artery and a thrombus
(d) Thrombosis
(e) Thrombectomy
(f) Formation of clots
(g) Disintegration/breakdown of clots

Word Exercise 12

(a) Formation of atheroma
(b) Blockage caused by atheroma and embolus

Word Exercise 13

(a) Surgical repair of an aneurysm
(b) Suturing/stitching of an aneurysm

Word Exercise 14

(a) Instrument that measures the force of the pulse (pressure and volume)
(b) Instrument that measures pressure of the pulse (arterial blood pressure)
(c) Technique of measuring the pulse
(d) Instrument that records the pulse
(e) Tracing/picture/recording of the pulse
(f) Instrument that records the heart beat and pulse

Word Exercise 15

(a) Cardioscope (6)
(b) Cardiograph (4)
(c) Electrocardiograph (5)
(d) Cardiovalvotome (2)
(e) Angiocardiography (3)
(f) Sphygmomanometer (1)

Word Exercise 16

(a) Echocardiography (6)
(b) Sphygmocardiograph (5)
(c) Stethoscope (2)
(d) Phonocardiogram (1)
(e) Electrocardiogram (3)
(f) Phlebomanometer (4)

Case History 4

(a) Study of the heart
(b) Pertaining to veins/of the nature of veins
(c) Condition of fast heart beat

(d) Instrument that records the electrical activity of the heart
(e) Enlargement of the heart
(f) Pertaining to two ventricles (right and left)
(g) Pertaining to the heart
(h) Drug that induces dilatation of blood vessels

Unit 5 The blood

Word Exercise 1

(a) The study of blood
(b) Study of diseases of the blood
(c) Pertaining to the force and movement of the blood (study of)
(d) Formation of the blood
(e) Cessation of blood flow/stopping of bleeding by clotting
(f) Blood in the pericardial sac (around heart)
(g) Spitting up of blood
(h) Haematoma (Am. hematoma)
(i) Haemolysis (Am. hemolysis)
(j) Haematuria (Am. hematuria)
(k) Haemorrhage (Am. hemorrhage)
(l) Too many blood cells (refers to conditions in which there is an increase in the number of circulating red blood cells)
(m) Without blood (refers to condition of reduced number of red cells and/or quantity of haemoglobin)
(n) Condition of decay of blood (due to infection)
(o) Instrument that measures haemoglobin
(p) Blood protein
(q) Condition of haemoglobin in the urine
(r) Condition of abnormal decrease of haemoglobin (colour)
(s) Condition of abnormal increase of haemoglobin (colour)
(t) Pertaining to normal concentration of haemoglobin (colour)

Word Exercise 2

(a) Condition of reduction in number of red blood cells
(b) Formation of red blood cells
(c) Immature germ cell that gives rise to red blood cells
(d) Formation of red blood cells
(e) Breakdown of red blood cells
(f) Condition of erythrocyte blood, i.e. too many red blood cells
(g) Abnormal condition of too many small cells (small erythrocytes)
(h) Abnormal condition of too many large cells (large erythrocytes)
(i) Abnormal condition of too many elliptical cells (elliptical erythrocytes)
(j) Abnormal condition of too many unequal cells (unequal sized erythrocytes)

(k) Abnormal condition of too many irregular/
varied cells (variable shaped erythrocytes)
(l) Pertaining to normal cells (red blood cells of
normal size)

Word Exercise 3

(a) Reticuloblast
(b) Reticulocytosis
(c) Reticulopenia

Word Exercise 4

(a) Leucopenia (Am. leukopenia)
(b) Leucopoiesis (Am. leukopoiesis)
(c) Formation of white blood cells
(d) Condition of white blood (synonymous with
leukocythaemia, a malignant cancer of white
blood cells)
(e) Abnormal condition of white cells (an increase in
white blood cells, usually transient in response to
infection)
(f) Tumour of leucocytes (Am. leukocytes)
(g) Immature germ cell that gives rise to leucocytes
(Am. leukocytes)
(h) Abnormal condition of too many white germ
cells (results in proliferation of leucocytes (Am.
leukocytes))
(i) Pertaining to poisonous to white cells

Word Exercise 5

(a) Marrow cell
(b) Condition of fibres in marrow
(c) Myeloblast
(d) Myeloma

Word Exercise 6

(a) Condition of reduction in the number of
platelets
(b) Formation of platelets
(c) Breakdown of platelets
(d) Disease of platelets
(e) Instrument that measures volume of
thrombocytes in a sample, or the actual value
of the measured volume of thrombocytes in a
sample of blood
(f) Withdrawal of blood, removal of red cells and
retransfusion of remainder
(g) Withdrawal of blood, removal of thrombocytes
and retransfusion of remainder
(h) Withdrawal of blood, removal of leucocytes and
retransfusion of remainder

Word Exercise 7

(a) Plasmapheresis (4)
(b) Differential count (3)
(c) Haematocrit (2)
(d) Haemoglobinometer (5)
(e) Blood count (1)

Case History 5

(a) Spitting/coughing up of blood
(b) Condition of reduction of all cells (i.e. all types of
cells in the blood)
(c) Pertaining to leukaemia/white blood (cancer of
the white blood cells)
(d) Pertaining to normal colour (here meaning
haemoglobin)
(e) Pertaining to normal cells (here normocyte refers
to an erythrocyte of a typical shape and size)
(f) Condition of a reduction in granulocytes (types of
white blood cells)
(g) Condition of reduction in thrombocytes/platelets
(h) Condition of without blood (actually a reduction
in erythrocytes and haemoglobin (Am.
hemoglobin))

Unit 6 The lymphatic system and immunology

Word Exercise 1

(a) Abnormal condition of lymph cells (too many
cells)
(b) Condition of bursting forth of lymph (from
lymph vessels)
(c) Technique of making an X-ray/tracing of
lymphatic vessels
(d) X-ray picture/tracing of a lymph vessel
(e) Dilatation of lymph vessels
(f) Tumour of a lymph node
(g) Removal of a lymph node
(h) Disease of a lymph node
(i) Inflammation of a lymph node

Word Exercise 2

(a) Enlargement of the spleen
(b) Enlargement of the liver and spleen
(c) Surgical fixation of the spleen
(d) Hernia/protrusion of the spleen
(e) Condition of softening of spleen
(f) Breakdown/disintegration of spleen
(g) X-ray picture of the spleen
(h) X-ray picture of portal vein and spleen

Word Exercise 3

(a) Tonsillitis
(b) Tonsillectomy
(c) Pertaining to the pharynx and tonsils
(d) Instrument to cut the tonsils

Word Exercise 4

(a) Thymocyte
(b) Thymopathy
(c) Thymocele
(d) Abnormal condition of ulceration of thymus
(e) Pertaining to lymphatics and thymus

Word Exercise 5

(a) Immunology
(b) Immunopathology
(c) Formation of immunity
(d) Self immunity (immune system acts against self, producing an autoimmune disease)
(e) Protein of immune system (antibody)

Word Exercise 6

(a) Serology

Word Exercise 7

(a) Condition of pus in blood (infection in blood)
(b) Pertaining to generating pus
(c) Flow of pus (usually referring to pus flowing from teeth sockets)
(d) Formation of pus

Word Exercise 8

(a) Tonsillotome (3)
(b) Lymphangiography (4)
(c) Lymphadenography (6)
(d) Lymphogram (2)
(e) Splenoportogram (1)
(f) Lymphography (5)

Case History 6

(a) Inflammation of the tonsils
(b) Enlargement of the spleen
(c) Disease of the lymph glands i.e. lymph nodes
(d) Pertaining to a lymph node
(e) Study of disease of tissues (here refers to a section of the pathology laboratory)
(f) Tumour of the lymph (tissue)
(g) Lymph cell
(h) Type of lymphocyte that secretes antibodies (named after the Bursa of Fabricus in birds)

Unit 7 The urinary system

Word Exercise 1

(a) Pertaining to the stomach and kidney
(b) X-ray/tracing of the kidney
(c) Technique of making an X-ray/tracing of kidney

Word Exercise 2

(a) Falling kidney (downward displacement)
(b) Abnormal condition of water in kidney (swelling)
(c) Swelling/hernia of a kidney
(d) Condition of pain in a kidney
(e) Nephropexy
(f) Nephroplasty
(g) Nephrotomy
(h) Nephrolithiasis

(i) Nephrectomy
(j) Inflammation of glomeruli (producing pus)
(k) Disease of glomeruli
(l) Abnormal condition of hardening of glomeruli

Word Exercise 3

(a) Inflammation of kidney and renal pelvis
(b) Incision to remove stone from renal pelvis
(c) Disease/abnormal condition of the kidney and renal pelvis
(d) Pyeloplasty
(e) Pyelogram

Word Exercise 4

(a) Hernia/protrusion of the ureter
(b) Removal of a ureterocele
(c) Condition of excessive flow of blood from the ureter
(d) Suturing of the ureter
(e) Dilatation of a ureter
(f) Visual examination of the kidney and ureters
(g) Formation of an opening into the ureter
(h) Ureteroenterostomy
(i) Ureterocolostomy

Word Exercise 5

(a) Inflammation of the bladder
(b) Removal of stones from bladder
(c) Inflammation of renal pelvis and bladder
(d) Falling/displacement of bladder
(e) Instrument to view the bladder
(f) Formation of an opening between rectum/anus and bladder
(g) Cystometer
(h) Cystometry
(i) Cystometrogram

Word Exercise 6

(a) Vesicostomy
(b) Vesicotomy
(c) Infusion/injection into the bladder
(d) Pertaining to the bladder
(e) Opening between sigmoid colon and bladder (to drain urine)
(f) Pertaining to the ureter and bladder

Word Exercise 7

(a) Process of measuring the urethra
(b) Inflammation of trigone and urethra
(c) Fixation (by surgery) of the urethra
(d) Urethralgia
(e) Urethrorrhagia
(f) Urethroscopy
(g) Tumour/boil in urethra
(h) Instrument for cutting urethra
(i) Abnormal condition of narrowing of urethra
(j) Condition of pain in the urethra

Word Exercise 8

(a) Of the nature of/pertaining to carrying urine
(b) Urine splitting/separating for analysis
(c) Instrument to measure urine

Word Exercise 9

(a) Technique of recording the urinary tract (X-ray)
(b) Person specializing in the study of the urinary tract
(c) Formation of urine
(d) Condition of little urine (diminished secretion of)
(e) Condition of albumin in urine
(f) Condition of urea (too much) in urine
(g) Condition of much urine
(h) Condition of painful difficult (flow) of urine
(i) Condition of blood in urine
(j) Condition of pus in urine
(k) Condition of too much calcium in urine

Word Exercise 10

(a) Inflammation of kidney due to stones
(b) Condition of calculus or stones in urine
(c) Formation of stones
(d) Instrument to crush stones
(e) Washing of stones from bladder following crushing
(f) Instrument that uses shock waves to destroy stones
(g) The procedure of breaking stones using shock waves/lithotriptor
(h) Excretion of stones in the urine

Word Exercise 11

(a) Diathermy (8)
(b) Cystoscope (10)
(c) Lithotriptor (7)
(d) Urinometer (9)
(e) Haemodialyser (2)
(f) Ureteroscopy (4)
(g) Urethrotome (3)
(h) Cystometer (5)
(i) Urethroscope (6)
(j) Lithotrite (1)

Case History 7

(a) Abnormal condition of stones in the urinary tract
(b) Pertaining to the urethra
(c) Condition of painful/difficult urine (urination)
(d) Condition of blood in urine
(e) Disease of the urinary tract
(f) Technique of making a tracing/X-ray of the renal pelvis
(g) Technique of breaking up stones using a lithotriptor
(h) Condition of above normal calcium in the urine

Unit 8 The nervous system

Word Exercise 1

(a) Study of nerves/nervous system
(b) Disease of the nervous system
(c) Condition of pain in nerves
(d) Nerve fibre tumour (arises from connective tissue around nerves)
(e) Inflammation of many nerves
(f) Pertaining to formation of nerves/originating in nerves
(g) Neurosclerosis
(h) Neuromalacia
(i) Neurologist
(j) Wasting/decay of nerves
(k) Pertaining to affinity for/stimulating nervous tissue
(l) Injury to nerve
(m) Nerve glue cell
(n) Tumour of gliocytes/gliacytes (nerve glue cells)

Word Exercise 2

(a) Disease of a plexus
(b) Pertaining to the formation of a plexus/originating in a plexus

Word Exercise 3

(a) Hernia/protrusion from head
(b) Pertaining to without a head
(c) Pertaining to tumour of blood within the head (actually a collection of blood in sub-periosteal tissue, the result of an injury)
(d) Thing (baby) with water in head
(e) Microcephalic
(f) Cephalogram
(g) Cephalometry
(h) Thing (baby) with large head
(i) Pertaining to turning motion of head

Word Exercise 4

(a) Tumour of brain
(b) Abnormal condition of pus (infection) of brain
(c) Pertaining to without a brain
(d) Instrument that records electrical activity of the brain
(e) Encephalography
(f) Pneumoencephalography
(g) Electroencephalography
(h) Encephalopathy
(i) Encephalocele
(j) Tracing/picture of brain made using reflected ultrasound (echoes)
(k) Middle brain
(l) Inflammation of grey matter of brain

Word Exercise 5

(a) Cerebrosclerosis
(b) Cerebromalacia
(c) Cerebrosis

Word Exercise 6

(a) Ventriculoscopy
(b) Ventriculotomy
(c) Technique of making X-ray of brain ventricles
(d) Opening between the cistern (subarachnoid space) and ventricles

Word Exercise 7

(a) Craniotomy
(b) Craniometry
(c) Intracranial

Word Exercise 8

(a) Ganglioma
(b) Pertaining to before a ganglion
(c) Pertaining to after a ganglion
(d) Removal of a ganglion

Word Exercise 9

(a) Meningitis
(b) Meningocele
(c) Meningorrhagia
(d) Hernia/protrusion of brain through meninges
(e) Inflammation of brain and meninges
(f) Disease of brain and meninges
(g) Tumour of the meninges
(h) Pertaining to above/upon the dura
(i) Swelling/tumour of blood beneath the dura

Word Exercise 10

(a) Inflammation of the ganglia and spinal roots
(b) Inflammation of nerves and spinal nerve roots
(c) Incision into a spinal root

Word Exercise 11

(a) Inflammation of the meninges and spinal cord
(b) Hernia/protrusion of the spinal cord through the meninges
(c) Inflammation of spinal nerve roots and spinal cord
(d) Inflammation of brain and spinal cord
(e) Wasting of the spinal cord
(f) Inflammation of grey matter of spinal cord
(g) Myelosclerosis
(h) Myelomalacia
(i) Myelography
(j) Condition of abnormal/difficult development/ growth (of cells) of the spinal cord
(k) Without nourishment of the spinal cord (wasting away/poor growth)
(l) Abnormal condition of a tube (cavity) in spinal cord

Word Exercise 12

(a) Instrument to measure spine (curvature)
(b) Puncture of spine
(c) Splitting of spine

Word Exercise 13

(a) Condition of paralysis of all four limbs
(b) Condition of paralysis of half body, right or left side
(c) Condition of near/beside paralysis (lower limbs)
(d) Condition of two parts paralyzed (similar parts on either side of body)
(e) Condition of paralysis of four limbs (synonymous with quadriplegia)

Word Exercise 14

(a) Condition of without sensation/state of being anaesthetized
(b) Pertaining to a drug that reduces sensation
(c) Study of anaesthesia
(d) Person who administers anaesthesia/specialist in anaesthesia
(e) Condition of anaesthesia of half the body (one side)
(f) Condition of decreased sensation
(g) Condition of increased sensation
(h) Post-anaesthesic/anaesthetic/anaesthesia
(i) Pre-anaesthesic/anaesthetic/anaesthesia

Word Exercise 15

(a) Abnormal condition of stupor/deep sleep (drug induced)
(b) Treatment with narcotics

Word Exercise 16

(a) Condition of sensing pain
(b) Condition of without sensation of pain
(c) Condition of excessive/above normal sensation of pain
(d) Pertaining to a loss of pain/drug that reduces pain

Word Exercise 17

(a) Study of the mind (behaviour)
(b) Pertaining to the mind
(c) Disease of the mind
(d) Abnormal condition/disease of the mind
(e) Drug that acts on/has an affinity for the mind
(f) Pertaining to body and mind (actually body symptoms of mental origin)
(g) Study/treatment of mind/mental illness/treatment of the mind by a doctor

Word Exercise 18

(a) Condition of fear of heights (peaks, extremities)
(b) Condition of fear of open spaces
(c) Condition of fear of water
(d) Condition of fear of cancer
(e) Condition of fear of death/dead bodies

Word Exercise 19

(a) Pertaining to forming/causing epileptic fit
(b) Pertaining to following/after an epileptic fit
(c) Having form of epilepsy

Word Exercise 20
(a)   Encephalography (5)
(b)   Pneumoencephalography (4)
(c)   Ventriculoscopy (6)
(d)   Tendon hammer (1)
(e)   Tomograph (2)
(f)   Craniometry (3)

Word Exercise 21
(a)   MRI (3)
(b)   Lumbar puncture (6)
(c)   Myelography (5)
(d)   CAT (1)
(e)   Electroencephalography (2)
(f)   Ventriculography (4)

Case History 8
(a)   Pertaining to the (blood) vessels of the cerebrum/brain
(b)   Condition of half paralysis (one side of the body)
(c)   Condition of beyond sensation (numbness) of half (one side) of the body/abnormal sensations
(d)   Loss of sensation of half (one side) of the body
(e)   Pertaining to the cerebrum/cerebral hemispheres
(f)   Pertaining to within the cranium/skull
(g)   Study of nerves/nervous system, here refers to a department that studies and treats disorders of the nervous system
(h)   Pertaining to above normal/exaggerated reflexes

Unit 9 The eye

Word Exercise 1
(a)   Ophthalmoscope
(b)   Ophthalmologist
(c)   Ophthalmoplegia
(d)   Ophthalmitis
(e)   Ophthalmomycosis
(f)   Pertaining to pain in the eye
(g)   Pertaining to circular movement of eye
(h)   Inflammation of optic nerve
(i)   Inflammation of all eye
(j)   Instrument to measure tension (pressure) within the eye
(k)   Condition of inflammation of eye with mucus discharge
(l)   Condition of inflammation due to dryness of eye
(m)   In eye (displacement of eyes into sockets)
(n)   Out eye (bulging eyes)

Word Exercise 2
(a)   Pertaining to one eye
(b)   Pertaining to one eye
(c)   Pertaining to two eyes
(d)   Nerve that stimulates eye movement/action

(e)   Pertaining to nose and eye
(f)   Picture/tracing of electrical activity of eye
(g)   Pertaining to circular movement of eye

Word Exercise 3
(a)   Instrument that measures sight
(b)   Technique of measuring sight
(c)   Person who measures sight (specializes in optometry)
(d)   Instrument for measuring the muscles of sight (power of ocular muscles)
(e)   Condition of sensation of sight (ability to perceive visual stimuli)

Word Exercise 4
(a)   Condition of double vision
(b)   Condition of old man's vision
(c)   Condition of dim vision
(d)   Condition of half colour vision (faulty colour vision in half field of view)
(e)   Condition of painful/difficult/bad vision
(f)   Condition of without half vision (blindness in one half of visual field in one or both eyes)

Word Exercise 5
(a)   Blepharoplegia
(b)   Blepharospasm
(c)   Blepharoptosis
(d)   Blepharorrhaphy
(e)   Flow of pus from eyelid
(f)   Inflammation of eyelid glands (meibomian glands)
(g)   Condition of sticking together of eyelids
(h)   Slack, loose eyelids (causes drooping)

Word Exercise 6
(a)   Incision into sclera
(b)   Dilatation of sclera
(c)   Instrument to cut sclera

Word Exercise 7
(a)   Inflammation of cornea and sclera
(b)   Measurement of cornea (actually curvature of cornea)
(c)   Instrument to cut cornea
(d)   Surgical repair of cornea (corneal graft)
(e)   Puncture of the cornea
(f)   Abnormal condition of ulceration of cornea
(g)   Puncture of the cornea
(h)   To carve the cornea
(i)   Cone-like protrusion of the cornea

Word Exercise 8
(a)   Iridoptosis
(b)   Iridokeratitis
(c)   Motion/movement of iris (contraction and expansion)
(d)   Separation of iris

(e)   Hernia/protrusion of iris (through cornea)
(f)   Separation of iris and sclera
(g)   Incision into iris and sclera
(h)   Inflammation of iris and cornea

Word Exercise 9

(a)   Inflammation of ciliary body and iris
(b)   Condition of paralysis of ciliary body
(c)   Heating through the ciliary body (to destroy tissue)

Word Exercise 10

(a)   Goniometer
(b)   Gonioscope
(c)   Goniotomy

Word Exercise 11

(a)   Condition of paralysis of pupil
(b)   Measurement of pupil (diameter)

Word Exercise 12

(a)   Condition of equal pupils
(b)   Condition of unequal pupils
(c)   Surgical fixation of pupil into new position
(d)   Surgical repair of pupil

Word Exercise 13

(a)   Inflammation of ciliary body and choroid
(b)   Inflammation of choroid and sclera

Word Exercise 14

(a)   Tumour of germ cells of retina
(b)   Condition of softening of retina
(c)   Splitting (separation of retina)
(d)   Disease of the retina
(e)   Technique of viewing the retina
(f)   Electroretinogram
(g)   Retinochoroiditis
(h)   Choroidoretinitis

Word Exercise 15

(a)   Swelling of the optic disc
(b)   Retinopapillitis

Word Exercise 16

(a)   Phacomalacia
(b)   Phacoscope
(c)   Phacosclerosis
(d)   Aphakia
(e)   Removal of lens bladder (capsule)
(f)   Sucking out of lens

Word Exercise 17

(a)   Instrument to measure scotomas
(b)   Technique of measuring scotomas
(c)   Instrument to record scotomas

Word Exercise 18

(a)   Lacrimotomy
(b)   Nasolacrimal

Word Exercise 19

(a)   Tear bladder (lacrimal sac)
(b)   Technique of making an X-ray of the lacrimal sac
(c)   Formation of an opening between the nose and lacrimal sac
(d)   Tear stone
(e)   Abnormal condition of narrowing lacrimal duct (apparatus)
(f)   Pertaining to stimulation of tears
(g)   Flow of mucus from lacrimal sac
(h)   Condition of pus in lacrimal sac

Word Exercise 20

(a)   Ophthalmoscope (4)
(b)   Dacryocystogram (1)
(c)   Keratome (5)
(d)   Pupillometry (8)
(e)   Optometry (7)
(f)   Scotometry (2)
(g)   Ophthalmotonometer (3)
(h)   Optomyometer (6)

Word Exercise 21

(a)   Sclerotome (5)
(b)   Optometer (4)
(c)   Keratometry (6)
(d)   Pupillometer (8)
(e)   Phacoscope (7)
(f)   Retinoscopy (1)
(g)   Tonography (2)
(h)   Dacryocystography (3)

Case History 9

(a)   Specialist who measures site (optician)
(b)   Condition of double vision
(c)   Condition of pain in the eye
(d)   Inflammation of the optic nerve
(e)   Inflammation of the optic disc
(f)   Dark area/region of reduced vision within a visual field
(g)   Pertaining to the eye
(h)   Condition of paralysis of the eye

Unit 10 The ear

Word Exercise 1

(a)   Otology
(b)   Otoscope
(c)   Otosclerosis
(d)   Otopyosis
(e)   Technique of viewing the ear (with an otoscope)
(f)   Study of the larynx, nose and ear
(g)   Abnormal condition of fungi in the ear

(h)   Excessive flow of pus from the ear
(i)   Condition of small ears
(j)   Condition of large ears

Word Exercise 2

(a)   Auriscope
(b)   Pertaining to two ears
(c)   Pertaining to within the ear
(d)   Pertaining to having two ear flaps (pinnae)

Word Exercise 3

(a)   Myringotomy
(b)   Myringotome
(c)   Myringomycosis

Word Exercise 4

(a)   Tympanoplasty
(b)   Tympanocentesis
(c)   Tympanostomy
(d)   Inflammation of the middle ear/ear drum
(e)   Incision into the middle ear/ear drum

Word Exercise 5

(a)   Blocking up of Eustachian tube
(b)   Pertaining to pharynx and Eustachian tube

Word Exercise 6

(a)   Stapedectomy
(b)   Cutting of tendon of stapes

Word Exercise 7

(a)   Incision into the malleus

Word Exercise 8

(a)   Pertaining to malleus and incus
(b)   Pertaining to stapes and incus
(c)   Pertaining to the incus and malleus

Word Exercise 9

(a)   Cochleostomy
(b)   Electrocochleography

Word Exercise 10

(a)   Labyrinthitis
(b)   Labyrinthectomy

Word Exercise 11

(a)   Incision into the vestibule
(b)   Pertaining to originating in the vestibule

Word Exercise 12

(a)   Mastoidalgia
(b)   Mastoidotomy
(c)   Mastoidectomy
(d)   Tympanomastoiditis

Word Exercise 13

(a)   Audiology
(b)   Instrument that measures hearing
(c)   Tracing/recording made by an audiometer
(d)   Technique of measuring hearing/using an audiometer

Word Exercise 14

(a)   Audiometer (6)
(b)   Audiometry (1)
(c)   Aural speculum (7)
(d)   Auriscope (2)
(e)   Otoscopy (3)
(f)   Aural syringe (4)
(g)   Grommet (5)

Case History 10

(a)   Condition of pain in the ear
(b)   Technique of viewing/examining the ear
(c)   Technician who measures hearing
(d)   Tracing/recording of hearing (ability)
(e)   Study of the ear and its disorders
(f)   Technique of measuring the tympanic membrane (actually the measurement of the mobility and impedance of the membrane)
(g)   Incision into the tympanic membrane/ear drum
(h)   Opening into the tympanum/tympanic membrane

Unit 11 The skin

Word Exercise 1

(a)   Abnormal condition of the skin
(b)   Above/upon skin/the outer layer of the skin
(c)   Skin plant (fungus that infects skin)
(d)   Thick skin
(e)   Yellow skin
(f)   Self surgical repair of skin (using one's own skin for a graft)
(g)   Condition of dry skin
(h)   Specialist who studies skin and diseases of the skin
(i)   Dermatomycosis
(j)   Dermatome
(k)   Hypodermic/subdermal
(l)   Intradermal

Word Exercise 2

(a)   Abnormal condition of the epidermis caused by excessive exposure to sun
(b)   Abnormal condition of the epidermis (above normal thickening)
(c)   Tumour of the epidermis
(d)   Breakdown/disintegration of the epidermis

Word Exercise 3

(a)   Nerve that performs an action to move hair (erects hair)

Word Exercise 4

(a) Abnormal condition of hair plants (fungal infection)
(b) Abnormal condition of hair
(c) Condition of sensitive hairs
(d) Condition of split hairs
(e) Broken/ruptured hairs

Word Exercise 5

(a) Excessive flow of sebum
(b) Sebaceous stone (actually hardened sebum)
(c) Pertaining to stimulating the sebaceous glands

Word Exercise 6

(a) Abnormal condition of sweating (excess)
(b) Condition of increased/above normal sweating
(c) Formation of sweat
(d) Abnormal condition of without sweating
(e) Inflammation of sweat glands

Word Exercise 7

(a) Abnormal condition of hidden nail (ingrowing)
(b) Condition of increased growth of nails
(c) Difficult/poor growth of nails (malformation)
(d) Without nourishment/wasting away of nails
(e) Condition beside a nail (inflammation)
(f) Splitting/parting of nails
(g) Condition of nail eating (actually biting)
(h) Onycholysis
(i) Onychomycosis
(j) Onychitis
(k) Rupture/breaking of nails
(l) Condition of without nails
(m) Condition of thickened nails

Word Exercise 8

(a) Melanocyte
(b) Melanosis
(c) Tumour of melanin (melanocytes), highly malignant

Word Exercise 9

(a) Excision biopsy (4)
(b) Dermatome (5)
(c) Medical laser (2)
(d) PUVA (6)
(e) Epilation (1)
(f) Electrolysis (3)

Case History 11

(a) Study of the skin
(b) Specialist who studies the skin and its disorders
(c) Pertaining to above normal epidermis i.e. a thickening of the epidermis
(d) Pertaining to the skin/of the nature of skin
(e) Disintegration/break-down of the nails
(f) Pertaining to the epidermis/keratin

(g) Tumour formed from an epithelium/epithelial cell
(h) Tumour of melanin/melanocytes

Unit 12 The nose and mouth

Word Exercise 1

(a) Study of mouth
(b) Condition of excessive flow (of blood) from mouth
(c) Disease of mouth
(d) Stomatodynia/stomatalgia
(e) Stomatomycosis

Word Exercise 2

(a) Pertaining to the mouth
(b) Pertaining to inside the mouth
(c) Pertaining to the pharynx and mouth
(d) Pertaining to the nose and mouth

Word Exercise 3

(a) Glossology
(b) Glossodynia/glossalgia
(c) Glossopharyngeal (e.g. glossopharyngeal nerve IX)
(d) Condition of paralysis of the tongue
(e) Condition of hairy tongue
(f) Protrusion/swelling of tongue
(g) Condition of large tongue
(h) Surgical repair of the tongue

Word Exercise 4

(a) Removal of a salivary gland
(b) Technique of making X-ray/tracing of salivary vessels/ducts
(c) Condition of much saliva (excess secretion)
(d) X-ray of salivary glands and ducts
(e) Sialolith
(f) A drug that stimulates saliva (production)
(g) Condition of eating air and saliva (excessive swallowing)

Word Exercise 5

(a) Pertaining to formation of saliva/originating in saliva
(b) Excessive flow of saliva
(c) Stone in the saliva

Word Exercise 6

(a) Gnathalgia/gnathodynia
(b) Gnathoplasty
(c) Gnathology
(d) Stomatognathic
(e) Instrument that measures force of jaw (closing force)
(f) Split or cleft jaw
(g) Inflammation of the jaw

Word Exercise 7

(a) Surgical repair of mouth and lip
(b) Split/cleft lip
(c) Suturing of lips
(d) Cheilitis

Word Exercise 8

(a) Pertaining to larynx, tongue and lips
(b) Labioglossopharyngeal

Word Exercise 9

(a) Gingivitis
(b) Gingivectomy
(c) Pertaining to gums and lips
(d) Pertaining to (the part) behind the palate

Word Exercise 10

(a) Palatoplegia
(b) Palatognathic
(c) Palatoschisis
(d) Pertaining to after the palate

Word Exercise 11

(a) Uvulectomy
(b) Uvulotomy

Word Exercise 12

(a) Condition of without speech/loss of voice
(b) Condition of difficult speech

Word Exercise 13

(a) Odontology
(b) Odontopathy
(c) Odontalgia
(d) Pertaining to around the teeth (study of tissues that support the teeth)
(e) Study of inside of teeth (pulp, dentine, etc.)
(f) Pertaining to straight teeth (branch of dentistry dealing with the straightening of teeth and associated facial abnormalities)
(g) Person who specializes in orthodontics
(h) Pertaining to adding teeth (branch of dentistry dealing with the construction of artificial teeth and other oral components)

Word Exercise 14

(a) Condition of nasal voice (speech through nose)
(b) Technique of measuring pressure (air flow) in nose
(c) Tumour/swelling/boil of nose
(d) Technique of viewing the nose (internally)
(e) Study of the larynx, nose and ear
(f) Condition of excessive flow of blood (from nose)

Word Exercise 15

(a) Hollow/cavity in bone/anatomical part
(b) Inflammation of bronchi and sinuses

(c) Inflammation of a sinus
(d) X-ray/tracing of sinus

Word Exercise 16

(a) Antroscope
(b) Antrotympanitis
(c) Incision into the antrum
(d) Pertaining to the nose and antrum
(e) Swelling/protrusion of antrum
(f) Pertaining to the cheek and antrum
(g) Formation of an opening into the antrum

Word Exercise 17

(a) Pertaining to the face
(b) Condition of paralysis of the face
(c) Surgical repair of the face

Word Exercise 18

(a) Antroscope (3)
(b) Sialangiography (5)
(c) Gnathodynamometer (1)
(d) Rhinomanometer (6)
(e) Prosthesis (4)
(f) Glossography (2)

Case History 12

(a) Inflammation of the nose
(b) Technique of viewing/examining the nose
(c) Inflammation of a sinus
(d) Study of the larynx, nose and ears (here referring to the department that studies disorders of these areas)
(e) Pertaining to towards the back of the nose
(f) Pertaining to the antrum (here the maxillary sinus or antrum of Highmore)
(g) Pertaining to within the nose
(h) Formation of an opening into the antrum (maxillary sinus or antrum of Highmore)

Unit 13 The muscular system

Word Exercise 1

(a) Pertaining to nerve and muscle
(b) Disease of heart muscle
(c) Poor nourishment (growth) of muscle
(d) Inflammation of a muscle
(e) Abnormal condition of fibres in muscle
(f) Myosclerosis
(g) Myoma
(h) Myoglobin
(i) Myospasm
(j) Condition of involuntary twitching of muscle
(k) Condition of muscle tone (abnormal increased tone)
(l) Slight paralysis of muscle
(m) Rupture of a muscle
(n) Condition of softening of a muscle

(o) Myography
(p) Electromyography
(q) Myogram

Word Exercise 2

(a) Tumour of striated muscle
(b) Breakdown of striated muscle

Word Exercise 3

(a) Pertaining to affinity for/stimulating muscle
(b) Pertaining to the diaphragm muscles
(c) Poor nourishment (growth) of muscle. An inherited disease

Word Exercise 4

(a) Condition of sensation of movement
(b) Instrument that measures muscular movement
(c) Pertaining to forming movements
(d) Condition of above normal movement
(e) Dyskinesia

Word Exercise 5

(a) Condition of pain in a tendon
(b) Instrument to cut tendons
(c) Inflammation of tendons
(d) Study of tendons
(e) Tenomyoplasty
(f) Tenomyotomy
(g) Suturing of an aponeurosis
(h) Inflammation of an aponeurosis

Word Exercise 6

(a) Pertaining to straight child, a branch of surgery that deals with the restoration of function in the musculoskeletal system

Word Exercise 7

(a) Myography (5)
(b) Electromyography (4)
(c) Myogram (2)
(d) Myokinesiometer (6)
(e) Orthosis (1)
(f) Electromyogram (3)

Case History 13

(a) Difficult/poor nourishment (of a tissue)
(b) False above normal nourishment (here the muscles look large and over nourished but the enlargement is due to disease processes within the muscle)
(c) Pertaining to dystrophy
(d) Technique of recording the electrical activity of muscle
(e) Pertaining to disease of muscle
(f) Recording/tracing of the electrical activity of muscle
(g) Without nourishment (wasting away)
(h) Pertaining to heart muscle

Unit 14 The skeletal system

Word Exercise 1

(a) Bone plant (plant-like growth of bone)
(b) Abnormal condition of passages (pores) in bone
(c) Abnormal condition of stone-like bones
(d) Breaking down of bone
(e) Cell that breaks down bone
(f) Bad nourishment of bone (poor growth)
(g) Osteoblast
(h) Osteolytic
(i) Osteotome
(j) Osteologist

Word Exercise 2

(a) Instrument to view within a joint
(b) Abnormal condition of pus in joint
(c) Technique of making an X-ray of joints
(d) Inflammation of many joints
(e) Fixation of a joint by surgery
(f) Breaking of a joint (actually breaking adhesions within a joint to improve mobility)
(g) Arthroscopy
(h) Arthrocentesis
(i) Arthrogram
(j) Arthropathy
(k) Arthrolith
(l) Arthroplasty

Word Exercise 3

(a) Inflammation of a synovial joint
(b) Removal of the synovial membranes/synovia
(c) Tumour/swelling of a synovial membrane

Word Exercise 4

(a) Plant-like growth of cartilage
(b) Pertaining to/of the nature of bone and cartilage
(c) Abnormal condition of passages (pores) in cartilage
(d) Bad nourishment of cartilage (poor growth)
(e) Pertaining to rib cartilage
(f) Pertaining to within cartilage
(g) Chondralgia
(h) Chondromalacia
(i) Chondrogenesis
(j) Chondrolysis
(k) Abnormal condition of calcified cartilage/ abnormal increase in calcium in cartilage

Word Exercise 5

(a) Condition of pain in the vertebrae
(b) Abnormal condition of pus in vertebrae
(c) Spondylolysis
(d) Spondylopathy
(e) Slipping/dislocation of vertebrae

Word Exercise 6

(a) Resembling a disc
(b) Pertaining to forming a disc/originating in a disc

(c) Discography
(d) Discectomy

Word Exercise 7

(a) Inflammation of bone marrow
(b) Abnormal condition of fibres in marrow

Word Exercise 8

(a) Osteotome (4)
(b) Arthrodesis (3)
(c) Replacement arthroplasty (5)
(d) Arthrocentesis (1)
(e) Arthrography (2)

Word Exercise 9

(a) Claviculoplasty
(b) Craniomalacia
(c) Intercostal
(d) Phalangectomy
(e) Pelvic
(f) Olecranarthritis
(g) Tibiofemoral
(h) Scapulodesis
(i) Metatarsalgia
(j) Acetabuloplasty

Word Exercise 10

(a) Pertaining to between finger/toe bones
(b) Condition of pain in a metatarsus
(c) Pertaining to a tarsus and metatarsus
(d) Pertaining to a metacarpus

Case History 14

(a) Specialist who studies rheumatism
(b) Condition of pain in the joints
(c) Inflammation of a bursa
(d) Inflammation of many joints
(e) Pertaining to the phalanges and metacarpals
(f) Pertaining to between the phalanges
(g) Pertaining to the phalanges and the metatarsal bones
(h) Disease of joints

Unit 15 The male reproductive system

Word Exercise 1

(a) Disease of the testes
(b) Hernia/protrusion/swelling of testes (through scrotum)
(c) Process of hidden testes, i.e. undescended
(d) Surgical fixation of the testes, i.e. into their normal position
(e) Orchiotomy/orchidotomy
(f) Orchioplasty/orchidoplasty
(g) Orchidectomy/orchiectomy

(h) Orchialgia/orchidalgia
(i) Surgical fixation of hidden testes, i.e. into their normal position

Word Exercise 2

(a) Scrotectomy
(b) Scrotoplasty
(c) Scrotocele
(d) Pertaining to through/across the scrotum

Word Exercise 3

(a) Phallitis
(b) Phallic
(c) Phallectomy

Word Exercise 4

(a) Balanitis
(b) Condition of bursting forth (of blood) from the glans penis
(c) Inflammation of the prepuce and glans penis

Word Exercise 5

(a) Epididymitis
(b) Epididymectomy
(c) Inflammation of the testes and epididymis

Word Exercise 6

(a) Removal of the vas deferens (a section of it to prevent transfer of sperm)
(b) Formation of an opening between the epididymis and the vas deferens
(c) Technique of making an X-ray of the epididymis and vas deferens
(d) Cutting/excision of the vas deferens
(e) Suturing of the vas deferens
(f) Formation of an opening between the testes and the vas deferens
(g) Formation of an opening between the vas deferens and another part of the vas deferens
(h) Incision into the vas deferens

Word Exercise 7

(a) Vesiculography
(b) Vesiculotomy
(c) Removal of the seminal vesicles and vas deferens

Word Exercise 8

(a) Incision into the bladder and prostate gland
(b) Enlargement of the prostate gland
(c) Removal of the prostate gland
(d) Removal of the seminal vesicles and prostate gland

Word Exercise 9

(a) Pertaining to/of the nature of carrying semen
(b) Condition of semen in the urine
(c) Tumour of semen (actually the germ cells of the testis)

Word Exercise 10

(a) Condition of being without sperm
(b) Condition of few sperm (low sperm count)
(c) Killing of sperms (actually an agent used as a contraceptive for killing sperm)
(d) Spermatopathia
(e) Spermatogenesis
(f) Spermatolysis
(g) Spermatorrhoea (Am. spermatorrhea)

Word Exercise 11

(a) Sperm count (5)
(b) Transurethral resection (4)
(c) Vasectomy (6)
(d) Orchidometer (3)
(e) In vitro fertilization (1)
(f) Vasoligature (2)

Case History 15

(a) Process of hidden testicles (i.e. undescended testicles)
(b) Fixation of testicles by surgery (operation to fix undescended testicles in their correct position)
(c) Inflammation of the testes/testicles
(d) Pertaining to within a testicle
(e) Removal of a testicle
(f) Pertaining to sperm
(g) Pertaining to through the scrotum
(h) Tumour of the semen (arising from undifferentiated germ cells in the testis)

Unit 16 The female reproductive system

Word Exercise 1

(a) Germ cell that produces eggs
(b) Egg cell (ovum)
(c) Formation of eggs

Word Exercise 2

(a) Oophorectomy
(b) Oophoropexy
(c) Oophorotomy
(d) Removal of bladder (cyst) of ovary (an ovarian cyst)
(e) Opening into an ovary/formation of an opening into an ovary

Word Exercise 3

(a) Ovariectomy
(b) Ovariotomy
(c) Rupture/breaking of ovary
(d) Pertaining to the oviduct and ovary
(e) Puncture of an ovary

Word Exercise 4

(a) Removal of an ovary and oviduct
(b) Removal of an oviduct and ovary
(c) Fixation of a Fallopian tube (by surgery)
(d) Hernia/protrusion/swelling of oviduct
(e) Inflammation of ovary and oviduct
(f) Salpingography
(g) Salpingolithiasis
(h) Salpingoplasty

Word Exercise 5

(a) Uteralgia/uterodynia
(b) Uterosclerosis
(c) Pertaining to the tubes (Fallopian) and uterus
(d) Technique of making an X-ray of the oviduct and uterus
(e) Pertaining to the bladder and uterus
(f) Pertaining to the rectum and uterus
(g) Pertaining to the placenta and uterus

Word Exercise 6

(a) Hysteroscope
(b) Hysteroptosis
(c) Hysterogram
(d) Technique of making an X-ray of the oviduct and uterus
(e) Formation of an opening between the oviduct and uterus
(f) Removal of ovary, oviduct and uterus
(g) Suturing of the neck of the womb
(h) Incision into the neck of the womb

Word Exercise 7

(a) Excessive dripping/bleeding from womb
(b) Condition of disease of womb with excessive loss of blood
(c) Inflammation of the peritoneum around the womb
(d) Inflammation of veins of womb
(e) Abnormal condition of cysts in the womb
(f) Abnormal condition of falling/prolapsed womb
(g) Metrostenosis
(h) Metromalacia
(i) Inflammation within the lining of the womb (endometrium)
(j) Tumour of the endometrium
(k) Abnormal condition of the endometrium

Word Exercise 8

(a) Excessive dripping of menses/prolonged menstruation
(b) Beginning of menstruation
(c) Stopping of menstruation (occurs in women aged 45–50 years approximately)
(d) Without menstrual flow (menstruation), e.g. as in pregnancy
(e) Difficult/painful/bad menstruation

(f)   Reduced flow of menses/infrequent menstruation

(g)   Before menstruation

Word Exercise 9

(a)   Cervicitis

(b)   Cervicectomy

Word Exercise 10

(a)   Visual examination of the vagina

(b)   Microscope used to view the lining of the vagina in situ

(c)   Picture (in this case a differential list) of vaginal cells

(d)   Suturing of the perineum and vagina

(e)   Removal of the uterus through vagina

(f)   Hernia/protrusion/swelling of the uterus into vagina

(g)   Inflammation of the vagina and cervix

(h)   Colpoperineoplasty

(i)   Colpopexy

Word Exercise 11

(a)   Incision into the perineum and vagina

(b)   Suturing of the perineum and vagina

(c)   Pertaining to the bladder and vagina

(d)   Vaginomycosis

(e)   Vaginopathy

Word Exercise 12

(a)   Inflammation of the vagina and vulva

(b)   Surgical repair of the vagina and vulva

Word Exercise 13

(a)   Instrument to view the rectouterine pouch

(b)   Technique of viewing the rectouterine pouch

(c)   Puncture of the rectouterine pouch

Word Exercise 14

(a)   Study of women (particularly diseases of the female reproductive tract)

(b)   Pertaining to woman-forming (feminizing)

Word Exercise 15

(a)   A woman's first pregnancy

(b)   A woman's second pregnancy

(c)   A woman who is pregnant and has been pregnant more than twice before

(d)   Before pregnancy

Word Exercise 16

(a)   A woman who has had one pregnancy that resulted in a viable child

(b)   A woman who has had two pregnancies that resulted in viable offspring

(c)   A woman who has had more than two pregnancies that resulted in viable offspring

(d)   A woman who has never borne a viable child

Word Exercise 17

(a)   Study of the fetus

(b)   Instrument to view the fetus

(c)   Pertaining to the placenta and fetus

(d)   Fetotoxic

(e)   Fetometry

Word Exercise 18

(a)   Instrument to cut the amnion

(b)   Pertaining to the amnion and fetus

(c)   Amniotomy

(d)   Amnioscope

(e)   Technique of making an X-ray of the amnion

(f)   An X-ray picture of the amnion

(g)   Puncture of the amnion to remove amniotic fluid

(h)   Pertaining to the amnion and chorion (fetal membranes)

(i)   Inflammation of the amnion and chorion

Word Exercise 19

(a)   Placentography

(b)   Placentopathy

Word Exercise 20

(a)   Condition of difficult/painful/bad birth

(b)   Study of labour/birth

(c)   Condition of good (normal) birth

Word Exercise 21

(a)   Pertaining to new birth

(b)   Pertaining to before birth

(c)   Pertaining to around/near birth

(d)   Pertaining to before birth

(e)   Study of neonates (new births)

Word Exercise 22

(a)   Technique of making a breast X-ray

(b)   Surgical reconstruction/repair of the breast

(c)   Pertaining to affinity for/affecting the breast

Word Exercise 23

(a)   Mastography

(b)   Mastoplasty

(c)   Mastectomy

(d)   Condition of women's breasts (abnormal condition seen in males)

Word Exercise 24

(a)   Agent stimulating/promoting milk production

(b)   Pertaining to carrying milk

(c)   Instrument to measure milk (specific gravity)

(d)   Hormone that nourishes (develops/stimulates) milk

(e)   Hormone that acts before milk, i.e. on breast to stimulate lactation

(f)   Agent that stops milk

(g)   Pertaining to forming milk/originating in milk

Word Exercise 25

(a) Agent that stimulates milk production
(b) Excessive flow of milk
(c) Condition of holding back/stopping milk
(d) Formation of milk

Word Exercise 26

(a) Vaginal speculum (9)
(b) Colposcope (5)
(c) Pap test (7)
(d) Culdoscopy (3)
(e) Fetoscope (10)
(f) Hysteroscope (2)
(g) Amniotome (4)
(h) Lactometer (6)
(i) Obstetrical forceps (8)
(j) Tocography (1)

Case History 16

(a) Woman pregnant for the first time
(b) Without menstruation/menstrual flow
(c) Technique of recording labour (uterine contractions) and the heart rate (of the fetus) during delivery
(d) Pertaining to before birth
(e) Pertaining to around birth
(f) Doctor who specializes in probems associated with childbirth/midwifery
(g) Period following birth when reproductive organs return to their normal condition (approx. 6 weeks)
(h) Pertaining to the amnion

Unit 17 The endocrine system

Word Exercise 1

(a) Process of secreting below normal level of pituitary secretion
(b) Process of secreting above normal level of pituitary secretion
(c) Condition of small extremities, i.e. hands and feet (due to deficiency of growth hormone)
(d) Large extremities, i.e. hands and feet (due to excess production of growth hormone in adults)

Word Exercise 2

(a) Pertaining to the tongue and thyroid gland
(b) Inflammation of the thyroid gland
(c) Thyroid protein
(d) Incision into thyroid cartilage
(e) Condition of poisoning by thyroid (due to overstimulation of thyroid gland)
(f) Near/beside the thyroid/the parathyroid gland
(g) Removal of the parathyroid gland
(h) Process of secreting above normal levels of parathyroid hormones

(i) Enlargement of the thyroid gland
(j) Hyperthyroidism
(k) Hypothyroidism
(l) Thyroptosis
(m) Thyrotropic
(n) Thyrogenic

Word Exercise 3

(a) Pertaining to affinity for/acting on pancreas
(b) Formation of insulin (from Islets of Langerhans)
(c) Tumour of Islets of Langerhans
(d) Inflammation of Islets of Langerhans
(e) Process of secreting above normal level of insulin
(f) Condition of below normal levels of sugar in blood
(g) Condition of above normal levels of sugar in blood
(h) Condition of sugar in urine
(i) Pertaining to a constant glucose level (controlled level)

Word Exercise 4

(a) Adrenomegaly
(b) Adrenotoxic
(c) Adrenotropic
(d) Condition of above normal levels of sodium in blood
(e) Condition of below normal levels of potassium in blood
(f) Secretion of excess sodium in urine
(g) Pertaining to nourishing the adrenal cortex
(h) Condition of above normal growth of cells of adrenal cortex

Word Exercise 5

(a) Pertaining to male and female
(b) Tumour of germ cells of male, i.e. testis

Word Exercise 6

(a) Adrenal function test (4)
(b) Glucose tolerance test (3)
(c) PBI test (2)
(d) Glucose oxidase paper strip test (5)
(e) Thyroid scan (1)

Case History 17

(a) Condition of too much urine
(b) Condition of sugar in the urine
(c) Condition of above normal concentration of sugar in the blood
(d) Condition of ketones in the blood
(e) Abnormal acidity caused by ketones
(f) Pertaining to the pancreas
(g) Condition of below normal levels of sugar in the blood
(h) Pertaining to sugar

Unit 18 Radiology and nuclear medicine

Word Exercise 1

(a) Specialist who studies radiology (medically qualified)
(b) An X-ray picture
(c) Technique of making an X-ray
(d) One who makes an X-ray (technician, not medically qualified)
(e) Specialist who treats disease using radiation (medically qualified)

Word Exercise 2

(a) Technique of making an X-ray/roentgenogram
(b) Specialist who studies roentgenology/X-rays (medically qualified)
(c) An X-ray picture
(d) X-ray picture of the heart
(e) Fluoroscope
(f) Fluorography

Word Exercise 3

(a) Moving X-ray picture
(b) Technique of making a moving X-ray
(c) Technique of making a moving X-ray of the heart and vessels
(d) Moving X-ray picture of the oesophagus

Word Exercise 4

(a) X-ray picture of a slice/section through body
(b) Technique of making an X-ray of a slice/section through the body

Word Exercise 5

(a) Picture of sparks, i.e. distribution of radioactivity within body (synonymous with scintiscan) image/tracing produced by a scintiscanner
(b) Technique of making a scintigram

Word Exercise 6

(a) Treatment by radiation
(b) Specialist who treats disease with radiation (medically qualified)

Word Exercise 7

(a) Picture/tracing produced using ultrasound
(b) Technique of making a picture/tracing using ultrasound
(c) An instrument that uses ultrasound to make a picture/tracing

Word Exercise 8

(a) Picture/tracing of the brain made using ultrasound echoes
(b) Echogenic
(c) Echogram
(d) Echoencephalograph

(e) Echocardiogram
(f) Echography

Word Exercise 9

(a) Picture/tracing of infrared heat within body
(b) Technique of making a thermogram of infrared heat from the scrotum (used to detect testicular cancer)

Word Exercise 10

(a) Radiography (4)
(b) Fluoroscopy (7)
(c) Thermography (8)
(d) Ultrasonograph (5)
(e) Computerized tomograph (6)
(f) Radiotherapy (9)
(g) Cineradiography (10)
(h) Gamma camera (1)
(i) Echocardiography (2)
(j) Contrast medium (3)

Case History 18

(a) Recording/picture produced using X-rays
(b) Technique of recording/producing an image of a 'slice'/cross-section through the body
(c) Specialist who treats disease using radiation (medically qualified)
(d) Treatment using radiation/X-rays etc.
(e) X-ray picture of a slice/section through body
(f) Pertaining to the killing of a tumour
(g) Device that produces high energy beams of electrons/X-rays for radiotherapy
(h) Technique of making a recording using high frequency sound waves

Unit 19 Oncology

Word Exercise 1

(a) Abnormal condition of tumours
(b) Formation of tumours
(c) Pertaining to affinity for a tumour
(d) Oncogenic
(e) Oncolysis
(f) Oncologist

Word Exercise 2

(a) Pertaining to the formation of a carcinoma (malignant tumour of an epithelium)
(b) Destruction/disintegration of a carcinoma
(c) Pertaining to stopping growth of a carcinoma

Word Exercise 3

(a) Malignant tumour of cartilage
(b) Malignant tumour of smooth muscle
(c) Malignant tumour of striated muscle
(d) Malignant tumour of meninges
(e) Malignant tumour of blood vessels
(f) Abnormal condition of sarcomas

Case History 19

(a) New growth (of cancer cells)
(b) Parts of a tumour that have spread from one site to another
(c) Tumour of the meninges
(d) Lump of matter (here meaning a tumour)
(e) Tumour of glial cells (neurogliacytes) in the brain
(f) Specialist who studies tumours/cancers
(g) Specialist who treats disease using radiation/ X-rays etc. (medically qualified)
(h) Treatment using chemicals (cytotoxic drugs that kill cancer cells)

Unit 20 Anatomical position

Word Exercise 1

(a) Superior
(b) Inferior
(c) Lateral
(d) Medial
(e) Anterior
(f) Dorsal
(g) Distal
(h) Proximal
(i) Superficial

Word Exercise 2

(a) Inferior
(b) Superior
(c) Medial
(d) Proximal
(e) Anterior
(f) Dorsal

Word Exercise 3

(a) Region pertaining to below cartilage (of rib cage)
(b) Region pertaining to upon/above the stomach
(c) Region pertaining to the flank/hip

Word Exercise 4

(a) 6
(b) 1
(c) 7
(d) 2
(e) 5
(f) 8
(g) 3
(h) 4

Word Exercise 5

Leg regions
(a) femoral region
(b) patella region
(c) crural region
(d) tarsal region
(e) digital/phalangeal region
(f) hallux region
(g) pedal region

Arm regions
(a) brachial region
(b) antebrachial region
(c) pollex region
(d) axillary region
(e) carpal region
(f) palmar/volar region
(g) digital/phalangeal region

Word Exercise 6

(a) 3
(b) 1
(c) 4
(d) 2

Word Exercise 7

(a) Paranasal
(b) Intervertebral
(c) Epigastric
(d) Post-ganglionic
(e) Dextrocardia
(f) Infra-orbital/sub-orbital

Word Exercise 8

(a) Pertaining to around the heart
(b) Pertaining to within a vein
(c) Pertaining to between the ribs
(d) Uterus turned backwards
(e) Pertaining to above the liver
(f) Pertaining to below the sternum
(g) Pertaining to before/in front of a ganglion
(h) Pertaining to outside the placenta
(i) Under the epidermis

Case History 20

(a) Pertaining to near the point of attachment/ origin
(b) Pertaining to near the surface of the body or structure
(c) Towards the front
(d) Pertaining to the median line along the centre of the body
(e) Flexing/bending back
(f) Pertaining to the side
(g) Pertaining to further away from the point of attachment/origin
(h) From the front to the back

Unit 21 Pharmacology and microbiology

Word Exercise 1

(a) (Scientific) study of drugs
(b) Specialist who studies drugs
(c) Drug psychosis/abnormal condition of psychosis due to drugs/abnormal condition of drugged mind

Word Exercise 2

(a) 3
(b) 1
(c) 5
(d) 2
(e) 4

Word Exercise 3

(a) Drug that acts against bacteria
(b) Drug that acts against life (actually against living cells bacteria and fungi)
(c) Drug that acts against fungi
(d) Drug that acts against viruses/virions
(e) Drug that acts against itching
(f) Drug that acts against acid (neutralizes acid)
(g) Drug that acts against worms, e.g. thread worms/tapeworms

Word Exercise 4

(a) The word means without pain, therefore a drug that reduces pain
(b) The word means without sensation, therefore a drug that reduces sensation

Word Exercise 5

(a) Drug that acts against (reduces symptoms of) diarrhoea/against excessive discharge through (the body)
(b) Drug that acts against (prevents) spasm (these reduce the motility of the intestines)

Word Exercise 6

(a) Drug that breaks down mucus (reduces viscosity of mucus)
(b) Drug that acts against (prevents) coughing
(c) Drug that dilates the bronchi

Word Exercise 7

(a) Drug that breaks down fibrin of blood clots (used to remove clots/thrombi)
(b) Drug that prevents the breakdown of fibrin/clots (used to promote clotting in severe haemorrhage (Am. hemorrhage))
(c) The word means against without rhythm, therefore drug that acts against arrhythmias (an arrhythmia is an abnormal heart beat, i.e. one without rhythm)
(d) Drug that stops blood flow thereby stimulating the clotting of blood

Word Exercise 8

(a) The word means pertaining to sleep, therefore a drug that induces sleep
(b) The word means breaking down anxiety, therefore a drug that reduces anxiety
(c) Drug that acts against (prevents) epilepsy
(d) Drug that acts against (prevents) psychosis, e.g. schizophrenia

Word Exercise 9

(a) Drug that paralyzes the ciliary body of the eye (used for eye examination)

Word Exercise 10

(a) Drug that acts against (prevents) itching
(b) Drug that breaks down epidermis/keratin (used to remove warts – overgrowths of epidermis caused by a viral infection)

Word Exercise 11

(a) Drug that produces quick labour/birth (used to induce birth)
(b) Drug that nourishes/stimulates the gonads
(c) Drug that acts against oestrogen (Am. estrogen) (used for infertility treatment in women)

Word Exercise 12

(a) Drug that acts against the thyroid (especially the synthesis of thyroid hormones)

Word Exercise 13

(a) Drug that is poisonous to cells and kills them, used to destroy cancer cells
(b) Drug that acts against new growths (tumours/cancer cells) and kills them

Word Exercise 14

(a) Drug that suppresses the immune system/response
(b) Drug used to suppress the cell-mediated immune response by killing cells (used to prevent rejection of transplanted organs)

Word Exercise 15

(a) 5
(b) 3
(c) 6
(d) 2
(e) 1
(f) 7
(g) 4

Word Exercise 16

(a) Specialist who studies bacteria
(b) Pertaining to streptococci
(c) Condition of bacteria in the urine
(d) Pertaining to killing bacteria
(e) Pertaining to stopping bacteria (growing)
(f) Pertaining to breakdown/disintegration of bacteria
(g) Condition of bacilli in the blood
(h) Pertaining to the formation of bacilli
(i) Agent that kills streptococci
(j) Condition of blood poisoning (septicaemia (Am. septicemia)) caused by streptococci
(k) Abnormal condition/disease caused by spirilli

Word Exercise 17

(a) Abnormal condition/disease of fungi (fungal infection)
(b) Pertaining to fungi
(c) Toxin/poison produced by fungi
(d) Abnormal condition/disease due to fungal toxin/ poison

Word Exercise 18

(a) Having the form of a fungus
(b) Pertaining to toxic/poisonous to fungi
(c) Agent that kills fungi
(d) Pertaining to stopping fungi (growth)
(e) Resembling fungi
(f) State/condition of fungi

Word Exercise 19

(a) Agent that kills viruses
(b) Specialist who studies viruses

(c) Agent that acts against retroviruses (e.g. HIV)
(d) Condition of (excreting) viruses in urine
(e) Condition of viruses in the blood
(f) Condition of (excreting) viruses in milk

Case History 21

(a) Drug that acts against retroviruses (e.g. HIV)
(b) Abnormal condition resulting from *Candida* (a yeast-like fungal infection)
(c) Drug that acts against bacteria
(d) Drug that acts against life (antibiotics are derived or are derivatives of chemicals produced by living microorganisms and have the capacity to kill other organisms)
(e) The study of small organisms (bacteria, fungi, protozoa etc.)
(f) Drug that acts against fungi (e.g. *Candida albicans*)
(g) Drug that acts to prevent vomiting
(h) Pertaining to a treatment regimen involving drugs

Answers to self-assessment tests

Levels of organization

Test 1A

(a)	7	(h)	4	(o)	16
(b)	14	(i)	17	(p)	20
(c)	18	(j)	12	(q)	11
(d)	19	(k)	5	(r)	15
(e)	8	(l)	10	(s)	6
(f)	3	(m)	1	(t)	13
(g)	9	(n)	2		

Test 1B

(a) Breakdown of cartilage
(b) Breakdown of white cells
(c) Pertaining to poisonous to tissues
(d) Disease of bone
(e) Immature lymph cell/cell that forms lymphocytes

Test 1C

(a) Microcyte
(b) Pathologist
(c) Cytopathologist
(d) Chondrology
(e) Cytopathic

The digestive system

Test 2A

(a)	15	(f)	4	(k)	3
(b)	14	(g)	13/12	(l)	7
(c)	10/11	(h)	5	(m)	8
(d)	2	(i)	12	(n)	6
(e)	9	(j)	1	(o)	11

Test 2B

(a)	14	(h)	17	(o)	11
(b)	20	(i)	15	(p)	13
(c)	2	(j)	7	(q)	10
(d)	5	(k)	12	(r)	4
(e)	19	(l)	3	(s)	18
(f)	9	(m)	16	(t)	8
(g)	6	(n)	1		

Test 2C

(a)	6	(h)	7	(o)	18
(b)	20	(i)	5	(p)	3
(c)	17	(j)	12	(q)	10
(d)	14	(k)	19	(r)	1
(e)	16	(l)	4	(s)	9
(f)	8	(m)	15	(t)	2
(g)	11	(n)	13		

Test 2D

(a) Inflammation of colon, intestine and stomach
(b) Technique of making an X-ray/recording of liver
(c) Pertaining to the rectum and ileum
(d) Instrument to view the sigmoid colon and rectum
(e) Enlargement of the pancreas

Test 2E

(a) Duodenitis
(b) Gastralgia
(c) Hepatotomy
(d) Proctology
(e) Ileoproctostomy

The breathing system

Test 3A

(a)	3	(e)	4	(i)	9
(b)	10	(f)	7/6	(j)	1
(c)	5	(g)	2		
(d)	6/7	(h)	8		

Test 3B

(a)	14	(h)	18	(o)	15
(b)	16	(i)	4	(p)	20
(c)	7	(j)	1	(q)	9
(d)	12	(k)	19	(r)	3
(e)	8	(l)	5	(s)	10
(f)	2	(m)	6	(t)	17
(g)	11	(n)	13		

Test 3C

(a)	3	(h)	13	(o)	17
(b)	19	(i)	12	(p)	9
(c)	5	(j)	10/11	(q)	11/10
(d)	18	(k)	14	(r)	20
(e)	7	(l)	2	(s)	4
(f)	15	(m)	6	(t)	8
(g)	1	(n)	16		

Test 3D

(a) Originating in bronchi/pertaining to formation of bronchi
(b) Abnormal condition of narrowing of trachea

(c)   Specialist who studies lungs
(d)   Instrument that records diaphragm
      (movement)
(e)   Condition of paralysis of larynx

Test 3E

(a)   Bronchoplasty
(b)   Bronchoscopy
(c)   Tracheorrhaphy
(d)   Rhinology
(e)   Costophrenic

The cardiovascular system

Test 4A

(a)	6	(c)	4	(e)	2
(b)	1	(d)	5	(f)	3

Test 4B

(a)	8	(h)	20	(o)	3/2
(b)	5	(i)	2/3	(p)	14
(c)	15	(j)	1	(q)	13
(d)	4	(k)	19	(r)	6
(e)	10	(l)	18	(s)	17
(f)	7	(m)	11	(t)	16
(g)	12	(n)	9		

Test 4C

(a)	12	(h)	1	(o)	18
(b)	9/10	(i)	13	(p)	20
(c)	6	(j)	14	(q)	17
(d)	2	(k)	3	(r)	5
(e)	7	(l)	15/16	(s)	10/9
(f)	8	(m)	4	(t)	16/15
(g)	11	(n)	19		

Test 4D

(a)   Inflammation of heart valves
(b)   Suturing of the aorta
(c)   Instrument to view vessels
(d)   Abnormal condition of narrowing of veins
(e)   Inflammation of lining of artery due to a
      clot

Test 4E

(a)   Thromboarteritis
(b)   Cardiocentesis
(c)   Arteriopathy
(d)   Phlebectomy
(e)   Angiocardiology

The blood

Test 5A

(a)	5	(c)	3/1	(e)	4
(b)	1/3	(d)	2		

Test 5B

(a)	10	(i)	3	(q)	5
(b)	17	(j)	12	(r)	11
(c)	9	(k)	7	(s)	16
(d)	6	(l)	2	(t)	15
(e)	13	(m)	21	(u)	24
(f)	19	(n)	4	(v)	14
(g)	20	(o)	18	(w)	8
(h)	22	(p)	23	(x)	1

Test 5C

(a)   Condition of white blood cells/leucocytes
      (Am. leukocytes) in urine
(b)   Abnormal condition of marrow cells (too
      many)
(c)   Condition of erythrocytes in urine
(d)   Condition of blood with thrombocytes (too many
      platelets)
(e)   Breakdown of phagocytes

Test 5D

(a)   Haemopathy (Am. hemopathy)
(b)   Erythrocytopenia
(c)   Haematologist (Am. hematologist)
(d)   Haemotoxic/haematotoxic (Am. hemotoxic/
      hematotoxic)
(e)   Neutropenia

The lymphatic system and immunology

Test 6A

(a)	5	(c)	2	(e)	4
(b)	3	(d)	1		

Test 6B

(a)	14	(h)	10	(o)	15
(b)	5	(i)	3	(p)	11
(c)	8	(j)	13	(q)	9
(d)	4	(k)	18	(r)	20
(e)	2	(l)	17	(s)	7
(f)	1	(m)	19	(t)	12
(g)	16	(n)	6		

Test 6C

(a)   Excessive flow of lymph
(b)   Pertaining to the spleen
(c)   Dilatation of a lymph node
(d)   Breakdown of thymus
(e)   Specialist who studies sera

Test 6D

(a)   Lymphoma
(b)   Lymphography
(c)   Splenectomy

(d)   Splenorrhagia
(e)   Lymphangioma

The urinary system

Test 7A

(a)	4	(d)	3	(g)	5
(b)	2	(e)	7	(h)	8
(c)	1	(f)	6		

Test 7B

(a)	9	(h)	17	(o)	10
(b)	7	(i)	18	(p)	6
(c)	15	(j)	2	(q)	20
(d)	16	(k)	5	(r)	1
(e)	14	(l)	13	(s)	3
(f)	11	(m)	8	(t)	4
(g)	12	(n)	19		

Test 7C

(a)	17	(h)	18	(o)	16
(b)	8/9	(i)	12	(p)	7
(c)	11	(j)	5	(q)	13
(d)	15	(k)	3/2	(r)	14
(e)	1	(l)	4	(s)	10
(f)	19	(m)	20	(t)	9 or 8
(g)	2/3	(n)	6		

Test 7D

(a)   Incision to remove stones from the renal pelvis and kidney
(b)   Abnormal condition of narrowing of the ureter
(c)   Technique of recording/making an X-ray of urethra and bladder
(d)   Hernia/protrusion of the bladder
(e)   Dilatation of the pelvis

Test 7E

(a)   Ureterectasis
(b)   Sigmoidoureterostomy
(c)   Cystography
(d)   Urogram
(e)   Nephrosclerosis

The nervous system

Test 8A

(a)	3	(e)	6	(h)	8
(b)	1	(f)	4	(i)	7
(c)	9	(g)	2	(j)	5
(d)	10				

Test 8B

(a)	7/8	(h)	13	(o)	20
(b)	19	(i)	4/3	(p)	12
(c)	15	(j)	14	(q)	1
(d)	8/7	(k)	6	(r)	11
(e)	3/4	(l)	2	(s)	9/10
(f)	18	(m)	17	(t)	10/9
(g)	16	(n)	5		

Test 8C

(a)	20	(h)	7	(o)	3
(b)	10	(i)	18	(p)	2
(c)	13	(j)	6	(q)	1
(d)	8	(k)	17	(r)	14
(e)	11	(l)	16	(s)	5
(f)	19	(m)	4	(t)	9
(g)	12	(n)	15		

Test 8D

(a)	14	(h)	2	(o)	4
(b)	7	(i)	17	(p)	6
(c)	19	(j)	11	(q)	15
(d)	13	(k)	8	(r)	20
(e)	3	(l)	1	(s)	9
(f)	18	(m)	16	(t)	5
(g)	12	(n)	10		

Test 8E

(a)   Inflammation of the spinal cord and nerves
(b)   Incision into the spine
(c)   Condition of softening of the meninges
(d)   Disease of spinal cord and brain
(e)   Instrument to view ventricles

Test 8F

(a)   Meningopathy
(b)   Cephalometer
(c)   Radiculomyelitis
(d)   Encephalorrhagia
(e)   Neurocytology

The eye

Test 9A

(a)	3	(e)	1	(h)	9
(b)	4	(f)	7	(i)	6
(c)	2	(g)	8	(j)	10
(d)	5				

Test 9B

(a)	12	(h)	20	(o)	8
(b)	10	(i)	15	(p)	7
(c)	18	(j)	6	(q)	17
(d)	19	(k)	16	(r)	2
(e)	1	(l)	4/5	(s)	9
(f)	14	(m)	3	(t)	5/4
(g)	13	(n)	11		

Test 9C

(a)	17	(h)	10	(o)	3
(b)	14	(i)	4	(p)	11
(c)	9	(j)	2	(q)	5
(d)	18	(k)	20/19	(r)	8
(e)	1	(l)	16/15	(s)	13
(f)	12	(m)	15/16	(t)	7
(g)	19/20	(n)	6		

Test 9D

(a) Surgical repair/reconstruction of the eye
(b) Surgical fixation of the retina
(c) Excessive flow of pus from tear ducts
(d) Inflammation of the iris and sclera
(e) Nerve that stimulates movement/action of the eye

Test 9E

(a) Ophthalmoscopy
(b) Blepharitis
(c) Keratopathy
(d) Retinoscope
(e) Iridoplegia

The ear

Test 10A

(a)	8	(e)	3	(h)	1
(b)	5	(f)	4	(i)	6
(c)	7	(g)	10	(j)	2
(d)	9				

Test 10B

(a)	8/9/10	(h)	3	(o)	11
(b)	9/8/10	(i)	15	(p)	13
(c)	14	(j)	17	(q)	2
(d)	10/9/8	(k)	6	(r)	5
(e)	16	(l)	18	(s)	4
(f)	19	(m)	7	(t)	1
(g)	12	(n)	20		

Test 10C

(a)	12	(h)	17	(o)	3
(b)	5/6	(i)	11	(p)	4
(c)	7	(j)	13	(q)	1
(d)	15	(k)	18	(r)	14
(e)	20	(l)	6/5	(s)	8
(f)	2	(m)	16	(t)	9
(g)	10	(n)	19		

Test 10D

(a) Study of the larynx and ear
(b) Condition of hardening within middle ear (around ear ossicles)

(c) Pertaining to the vestibular apparatus and stapes
(d) Pertaining to the malleus and tympanic membrane
(e) Pertaining to the cochlea and vestibular apparatus

Test 10E

(a) Mastoidocentesis
(b) Myringectomy
(c) Otoplasty
(d) Otalgia
(e) Tympanogenic

The skin

Test 11A

(a)	5	(c)	1	(e)	2
(b)	4	(d)	6	(f)	3

Test 11B

(a)	18	(h)	4	(o)	20
(b)	19	(i)	3	(p)	1
(c)	17	(j)	14	(q)	7
(d)	8	(k)	6	(r)	12
(e)	13	(l)	5	(s)	15
(f)	2	(m)	10	(t)	9
(g)	16	(n)	11		

Test 11C

(a)	11	(e)	12	(i)	8
(b)	7	(f)	2	(j)	4/5
(c)	9	(g)	3	(k)	10
(d)	1	(h)	6	(l)	5/4

Test 11D

(a) Abnormal condition of skin plants (fungal infection)
(b) Epidermal cell
(c) Condition of without hair sensation
(d) Tumour of a sweat gland
(e) Abnormal condition of fungi in the epidermis

Test 11E

(a) Dermatitis
(b) Onychosis
(c) Melanonychia
(d) Dermatology
(e) Pachyonychia

The nose and mouth

Test 12A

(a)	4	(d)	5	(g)	3
(b)	8	(e)	2	(h)	1
(c)	6	(f)	7		

Test 12B

(a)	19	(h)	8	(o)	6
(b)	14	(i)	7	(p)	11
(c)	13	(j)	9	(q)	20
(d)	15	(k)	18	(r)	10
(e)	16	(l)	5	(s)	3
(f)	4	(m)	1	(t)	2
(g)	17	(n)	12		

Test 12C

(a)	9	(h)	12	(o)	8
(b)	13	(i)	16/15	(p)	20/19
(c)	15/16	(j)	5	(q)	3
(d)	17	(k)	4	(r)	11
(e)	18	(l)	2	(s)	10
(f)	1	(m)	14	(t)	6
(g)	7	(n)	19/20		

Test 12D

(a) Instrument to measure power/force of the tongue
(b) Measurement of saliva
(c) Inflammation of the tongue and mouth
(d) Splitting of the palate and jaw
(e) Pertaining to formation of/originating in teeth

Test 12E

(a) Sialadenotomy
(b) Palatorrhaphy
(c) Rhinomycosis
(d) Labial
(e) Palatoplasty

The muscular system

Test 13A

(a)	18	(h)	17/16	(o)	7
(b)	15	(i)	3	(p)	10
(c)	8	(j)	19	(q)	20
(d)	13	(k)	1	(r)	11
(e)	9	(l)	5	(s)	12
(f)	2	(m)	4	(t)	14
(g)	16/17	(n)	6		

Test 13B

(a) Instrument that measures electrical activity of muscle
(b) Study of movement
(c) Incision into a tendon and muscle
(d) Without nourishment of muscle (muscle wasting)
(e) Pertaining to an aponeurosis and muscle

Test 13C

(a) Myomalacia
(b) Myogenic

(c) Myopathy
(d) Tenorrhaphy
(e) Tenotomy

The skeletal system

Test 14A

(a)	4	(c)	2	(e)	6
(b)	3	(d)	1	(f)	5

Test 14B

(a)	14/15	(h)	13	(o)	3
(b)	4	(i)	15/14	(p)	2
(c)	18	(j)	20	(q)	6
(d)	12	(k)	11	(r)	16
(e)	7	(l)	8	(s)	5
(f)	19	(m)	9	(t)	10
(g)	17	(n)	1		

Test 14C

(a)	5	(h)	15	(o)	19
(b)	7	(i)	16	(p)	18
(c)	9	(j)	11	(q)	4
(d)	12	(k)	10	(r)	13
(e)	17	(l)	2	(s)	6
(f)	20	(m)	1	(t)	3
(g)	14	(n)	8		

Test 14D

(a) Inflammation of cartilage of a joint
(b) Stone in a bursa
(c) Binding together of vertebrae
(d) Cell that breaks down cartilage
(e) Pertaining to having a hump/hunch back

Test 14E

(a) Arthralgia
(b) Osteosynovitis
(c) Spondylomalacia
(d) Osteoarthropathy
(e) Synovioblast

The male reproductive system

Test 15A

(a)	3	(d)	6	(g)	4
(b)	7	(e)	2	(h)	8
(c)	5	(f)	1		

Test 15B

(a)	16	(h)	13	(o)	14
(b)	18	(i)	20	(p)	19
(c)	3	(j)	12/11	(q)	2
(d)	9	(k)	1	(r)	5
(e)	15	(l)	7	(s)	6

(f)	17	(m)	10	(t)	4
(g)	11/12	(n)	8		

Test 15C

(a)	4	(f)	15	(k)	13
(b)	14	(g)	2	(l)	7
(c)	8	(h)	3	(m)	9
(d)	1	(i)	6	(n)	10
(e)	12	(j)	5	(o)	11

Test 15D

(a) Removal of the epididymes and testes
(b) Flow from the penis (abnormal)
(c) Removal of the vas deferens and epididymes
(d) Tying off of the vas deferens
(e) Condition of sperm in the urine

Test 15E

(a) Orchidorrhaphy/orchiorrhaphy
(b) Prostatalgia
(c) Epididymovasostomy
(d) Scrotitis
(e) Prostatorrhoea (Am. prostatorrhea)

The female reproductive system

Test 16A

(a)	3	(d)	6	(g)	8
(b)	4	(e)	2	(h)	7
(c)	1	(f)	5		

Test 16B

(a)	5	(h)	17	(o)	18
(b)	10/11	(i)	7	(p)	8
(c)	12	(j)	15	(q)	16
(d)	19	(k)	3	(r)	1
(e)	20	(l)	13	(s)	14
(f)	2	(m)	6	(t)	9
(g)	4	(n)	11/10		

Test 16C

(a)	22	(j)	4	(r)	9
(b)	17/18	(k)	13/12/14	(s)	7
(c)	16	(l)	5	(t)	23
(d)	8	(m)	10	(u)	15
(e)	1	(n)	19	(v)	14/12/13
(f)	12/13/14	(o)	20/21	(w)	18/17
(g)	24	(p)	21/20	(x)	25
(h)	2/3	(q)	11	(y)	6
(i)	3/2				

Test 16D

(a) Instrument that measures labour (uterine contractions)
(b) Removal of the uterus and ovaries
(c) Surgical fixation of the breasts

(d) Rupture of the uterus
(e) Disease of the uterus

Test 16E

(a) Culdoplasty
(b) Salpingostomy
(c) Amniorrhexis
(d) Colpoptosis
(e) Colpocytology

The endocrine system

Test 17A

(a)	4	(d)	2	(g)	1
(b)	3	(e)	5	(h)	8
(c)	7	(f)	6		

Test 17B

(a)	16	(h)	10	(o)	9
(b)	11	(i)	15	(p)	4
(c)	20	(j)	2	(q)	5
(d)	1	(k)	7	(r)	12
(e)	19	(l)	3	(s)	14
(f)	8	(m)	17	(t)	13
(g)	18	(n)	6		

Test 17C

(a) Removal of the parathyroid and thyroid gland
(b) Pituitary cell
(c) Enlargement of the adrenal
(d) Pertaining to acting on/affinity for sugar
(e) Condition of above normal level of ketones in the blood

Test 17D

(a) Hyperinsulinism
(b) Hyponatraemia (Am. hyponatremia)
(c) Thyrotrophic
(d) Adrenotropic
(e) Hypoparathyroidism

Radiology and nuclear medicine

Test 18A

(a)	11	(h)	19	(o)	10
(b)	13	(i)	9	(p)	7
(c)	15	(j)	3	(q)	4
(d)	20	(k)	1	(r)	8
(e)	17	(l)	2	(s)	6
(f)	14	(m)	18	(t)	5
(g)	12	(n)	16		

Test 18B

(a) Treatment with X-rays
(b) Specialist who studies sound (ultrasound images)

(c)   Treatment with X-rays and heat
(d)   Instrument that produces a moving X-ray picture
(e)   Technique of making a recording/picture of a slice through the body using ultrasound

Test 18C

(a)   Ultrasonotherapy
(b)   Fluoroscopic
(c)   Scintiangiography
(d)   Thermograph
(e)   Echoencephalography

Oncology

Test 19A

(a)	9	(h)	16	(o)	11
(b)	20	(i)	17	(p)	6
(c)	10	(j)	18	(q)	5
(d)	14	(k)	4	(r)	15
(e)	12	(l)	2	(s)	7
(f)	3	(m)	19	(t)	8
(g)	1	(n)	13		

Test 19B

(a)   Malignant tumour of fibrous tissue
(b)   Malignant glandular tumour of stomach
(c)   Malignant tumour of liver cells
(d)   Malignant, disordered tumour of the thyroid (refers to appearance of backward growth, i.e. becoming disordered)
(e)   Malignant tumour originating in the bronchus

Test 19C

(a)   Lymphosarcoma
(b)   Chondroma
(c)   Osteosarcoma
(d)   Neoplasia
(e)   Oncotherapy

Anatomical position

Test 20A

(a)	13	(h)	8/9	(o)	10
(b)	18	(i)	12	(p)	9/8
(c)	17	(j)	3	(q)	11
(d)	20	(k)	19	(r)	4
(e)	1	(l)	5/6	(s)	15
(f)	14	(m)	7	(t)	6/5
(g)	2	(n)	16		

Test 20B

(a)	9	(h)	15	(o)	8/7
(b)	12	(i)	19	(p)	13
(c)	7/8	(j)	5	(q)	10
(d)	14	(k)	18	(r)	3
(e)	1/2	(l)	6	(s)	17
(f)	20	(m)	11	(t)	4
(g)	16	(n)	2/1		

Test 20C

(a)   Pertaining to between the phalanges (fingers and toes)
(b)   A turning to the right
(c)   Pertaining to behind/back of cheek
(d)   Pertaining to above the ribs
(e)   Pertaining to within the nose

Test 20D

(a)   Lateral
(b)   Laevoversion (Am. levoversion)
(c)   Post ganglionic
(d)   Infrahepatic
(e)   Transdermal

Pharmacology and microbiology

Test 21A

(a)	9	(h)	14	(o)	4
(b)	13	(i)	15/16/17	(p)	1
(c)	12	(j)	10	(q)	11
(d)	19	(k)	15/16/17	(r)	5
(e)	2	(l)	7	(s)	15/16/17
(f)	20	(m)	18	(t)	6
(g)	3	(n)	8		

Test 21B

(a)	17	(h)	4/5	(o)	3
(b)	9	(i)	2	(p)	10
(c)	16	(j)	19	(q)	1
(d)	13	(k)	18	(r)	11
(e)	6	(l)	20	(s)	12
(f)	8	(m)	5/4	(t)	15
(g)	14	(n)	7		

Test 21C

(a)   Study of poisons
(b)   Abnormal condition/disease caused by poisoning with fungi/fungal toxins
(c)   Drug specialist (a person who dispenses drugs)
(d)   Chemical/drug used for treatment of disease (used in treatment of cancer – chemotherapy)
(e)   Specialist who studies microorganisms

Test 21D

(a)   Bacteriologist
(b)   Antibiotic
(c)   Protozoology
(d)   Bacteriostatic
(e)   Virucidal

Test 21E

(a)	7	(h)	17	(o)	22	(v)	15
(b)	12	(i)	4	(p)	24	(w)	11
(c)	19	(j)	25	(q)	8	(x)	16
(d)	9	(k)	23	(r)	13	(y)	10
(e)	20	(l)	2	(s)	14		
(f)	21	(m)	1	(t)	5		
(g)	18	(n)	3	(u)	6		

Test 21F

(a)	8	(h)	1
(b)	4	(i)	3
(c)	9	(j)	6
(d)	2	(k)	11
(e)	12	(l)	7
(f)	10		
(g)	5		

Abbreviations

The abbreviations listed here have been extracted from recent health care publications and the medical records of patients. Students should be aware that whilst certain abbreviations are standard, others are not and their meaning may vary from one health care setting to another. Abbreviations with several meanings should be carefully interpreted to avoid confusion.

A	anaemia (Am. anemia)
AAA	abdominal aortic aneurysm/acute anxiety attack
AAAAA	aphasia, agnosia, agraphia, alexia and apraxia
AAFB	acid alcohol fast bacilli
AB1	one abortion
Ab, ab	abortion/antibody
ABC	airway, breathing, circulation
Abdo	abdomen
ABE	acute bacterial endocarditis
ABG	arterial blood gases
abor	abortion
ABX	antibiotics
AC	air conduction
ac	ante cibum (before meals/food)
ACBS	aortocoronary bypass surgery
Accom	accommodation of eye
ACE	angiotensin converting enzyme
ACh	acetyl choline
ACS	acute confused state
ACTH	adrenocorticotrophic hormone
ACU	acute care unit
AD or ad	Alzheimer's disease/auris dextra (right ear)
ADA	adenosine deaminase
ADC	AIDS dementia complex
ADD	attention deficit disorder
ADH	antidiuretic hormone
ADL	aids to daily living
ADR	adverse drug reaction
ADU	acute duodenal ulcer
A&E	accident and emergency
AED	anti-epileptic drug
AEM	ambulatory electrocardiogram monitoring
AF	amniotic fluid/atrial fibrillation
AFB	acid-fast bacilli
AFP	alphafeto protein
A/G	albumin/globulin ratio
Ag	antigen
AGA	appropriate for gestational age
AGL	acute granulocytic leukaemia (Am. leukemia)
AGN	acute glomerulonephritis
AI	aortic incompetence/aortic insufficiency/artificial insemination
AID	artificial insemination by donor
AIDS	acquired immunodeficiency syndrome
AIH	artificial insemination by husband
A/K	above knee (amputation)
ALD	alcoholic liver disease
ALG	anti-lymphocyte immunoglobulin
ALL	acute lymphocytic leukaemia (Am. leukemia)
ALS	amyotrophic lateral sclerosis
ALs	activities of living
ALT	alanine aminotransferase/alanine transaminase
amb	ambulant/ambulatory
AMI	acute myocardial infarction
AML	acute myeloid leukaemia (Am. leukemia)
ANC	absolute neutrophil count
ANF	antinuclear factor
ANS	autonomic nervous system
ANT or ant	anterior
antib	antibiotic
A&O	alert and orientated
AOB	alcohol on breath
AP	antepartum/anteroposterior/appendicectomy/auscultation and percussion
APB	atrial premature beat
APH	antepartum haemorrhage (Am. hemorrhage)
APPY	appendicectomy
APSAC	acylated plasminogen streptokinase activator complex (anistreplase)
APTT	activated partial thromboplastin time
A–R	apical–radial (pulse)
ARC	aids related complex
ARD	acute respiratory disease
ARDS	adult respiratory distress syndrome
ARF	acute renal failure
AS	alimentary system/aortic stenosis/auris sinistra (left ear)
A–S	Adams–Stokes attack
5-ASA	5-aminosalicylic acid
ASC	altered state of consciousness
ASCVD	arteriosclerotic cardiovascular disease
ASD	atrial septal defect
ASHD	arteriosclerotic heart disease
ASO	antistreptolysin O
ASOM	acute suppurative otitis media
AST	aspartate transaminase

Astigm	astigmatism of eye	BT	bedtime/bone tumour/brain tumour/breast tumour
ASX	asymptomatic		
ATG	anti-thymocyte immunoglobulin	BTS	blood transfusion service
ATN	acute tubular necrosis	BUN	blood urea nitrogen
ATP	adenosine triphosphate	BW	body weight
ATS	antitetanus serum	BX, Bx or bx.	biopsy
aud	audiology		
aur dextr	to the right ear	C	Celsius
AV	arteriovenous/atrioventricular bundle/atrioventricular node/aortic valve	c	with
		C 1–7	cervical vertebra
		CA, Ca or ca.	cancer/carcinoma/cardiac arrest/coronary artery
AVM	arteriovenous malformation		
AVP	vasopressin	CABG	coronary artery bypass grafting
AVR	aortic valve replacement	CACX	cancer of the cervix
A&W	alive and well	CAD	coronary artery disease
AXR	abdominal X-ray	CAG	closed angle glaucoma
AZT	azidothymidine	CAH	chronic active hepatitis/congenital adrenal hyperplasia
Ba	barium	CAL	computer assisted learning
BaE	barium enema	CAPD	continuous ambulatory peritoneal dialysis
BAL	blood alcohol level		
BBA	born before arrival	CAT	computer assisted tomography/computerized axial tomography
BBB	blood brain barrier/bundle branch block		
BBBB	bilateral bundle branch block	CAVH	continuous arteriovenous haemofiltration (Am. hemofiltration)
BBT	basal body temperature		
BBx	breast biopsy	CAVHD	continuous arteriovenous haemodialysis (Am. hemodialysis)
BC	birth control/bone conduction		
BCC	basal cell carcinoma	CBC	complete blood count
BCG	bacille Calmette–Guérin	CBE	clinical breast examination
BD or b.d.	bis diurnal (twice a day)	CBF	cerebral blood flow
BDA	British Diabetic Association	CCCC	closed-chest cardiac compression
BE	bacterial endocarditis/barium enema	CCF	chronic cardiac failure/congestive cardiac failure
BI	bone injury		
BID	brought in dead	CCIE	counter current immuno electrophoresis
bid	bis in die (twice daily)		
B/KA	below knee (amputation)	CCU	coronary care unit
BM	bowel movement	CD	Crohn's disease/cluster designation
BMI	body mass index	CDH	congenital dislocation of the hip joint
BMR	basal metabolic rate	CEA	carcino embryonic antigen
BM (T)	bone marrow (trephine)	CF	cancer free/cardiac failure/cystic fibrosis
BMT	bone marrow transplant		
BNF	British National Formulary	CFT	complement fixation test
BNO	bowels not open	CFTR	cystic fibrosis transmembrane regulator
BOR	bowels open regularly		
BP	blood pressure/British Pharmacopoeia/bypass	CGL	chronic granulocytic leukaemia
		CGN	chronic glomerulonephritis
BPD	bronchopulmonary dysplasia	CH	cholesterol
BPH	benign prostatic hypertrophy	CHD	coronary heart disease
BPM	beats per minute	CHF	congestive heart failure
BRO	bronchoscopy	CHI	creatinine height index
BS	blood sugar/bowel sounds/breath sounds	CHOP	cyclophosphamide, hydroxydaunorubicin, oncovin and prednisolone
BSA	body surface area		
BSE	bovine spongiform encephalopathy/breast self-examination	CHR	chronic
		CI	cardiac index/cerebral infarction
		CIBD	chronic inflammatory bowel disease/disorder
BSS	blood sugar series		

CIN	cervical intraepithelial neoplasia
CJD	Creutzfeldt–Jakob disease
CK	creatine kinase
CL	clubbing
CLD	chronic liver disease/chronic lung disease
CLL	chronic lymphocytic leukaemia (Am. leukemia)
CMF	cyclophosphamide, methotrexate, 5-fluorouracil
CML	chronic myeloid leukaemia (Am. leukemia)
CMV	cytomegalovirus
CN	cranial nerve
CNS	central nervous system
CO	carbon monoxide/cardiac output/complains of
COAD	chronic obstructive airways disease
COD	cause of death
COLD	chronic obstructive lung disease
COPD	chronic obstructive pulmonary disease
COP	colloid osmotic pressure
C&P	cystoscopy and pyelogram
CP	cor pulmonale/cerebral palsy
CPA	cardiopulmonary arrest
CPAP	continuous positive airways pressure
CPK	creatinine phosphokinase
CPN	community psychiatric nurse
CPPV	continuous positive pressure ventilation
CPR	cardiopulmonary resuscitation
CrCl	creatine clearance
CRD	chronic renal disease
CRF	chronic renal failure
CRH	corticotrophin-releasing hormone
C + S	culture and sensitivity (test)
C-sect, or c/sect	caesarean section (Am. cesarean)
CSF	cerebrospinal fluid
CSH	chronic subdural haematoma (Am. hematoma)
CSM	cerebrospinal meningitis
CSOM	chronic suppurative otitis media
CSR	Cheyne–Stokes respiration/correct sedimentation rate
CSU	catheter specimen of urine
CT	cerebral tumour/clotting time/computerized tomography/ continue treatment/coronary thrombosis
CUG	cystourethrogram
CV	cardiovascular/cerebrovascular
CVA	cerebrovascular accident (stroke)/costovertebral angle
CVD	cardiovascular disease
CVP	central venous pressure
CVS	cardiovascular system/chorionic villus sampling

CVVH	continuous venovenous haemofiltration (Am. hemofiltration)
CVVHD	continuous venovenous haemodialysis (Am. hemodialysis)
Cx	cervical/cervix
CXR	chest X-ray
Cy	cyanosis
cyclic AMP	cyclic adenosine monophosphate
Cysto	cystoscopy
D	diagnosis
db	decibel
DBP	diastolic blood pressure
D&C	dilatation and curettage
DC or d/c	decrease/direct current/discharge/discontinue
DCCT	diabetes control and complications trial
DD	differential diagnosis
DDA	Dangerous Drugs Act
DDAVP	desmopressin (synthetic vasopressin)
ddC/DDC	dideooxycytidine/zalcitabine
ddI/DDI	didanosine/dideoxyinosine
DDx	differential diagnosis
D&E	dilatation and evacuation
Derm, derm	dermatology
DES	diethylstilbestrol
DH	delayed hypersensitivity/drug history
DIC	disseminated intravascular coagulation
DIDMOAD	diabetes insipidus, diabetes mellitus, optic atrophy and deafness
Diff	differential blood count (of cell types)
DIMS	disorders of initiating and maintaining sleep
DIOS	distal intestinal obstruction syndrome
DIP	distal interphalangeal
DJK	degenerative joint disease
DKA	diabetics ketoacidosis
DLE	discoid lupus erythematosus/disseminated lupus erythematosus
DM	diabetes mellitus/diastolic murmur
DMD	Duchenne muscular dystrophy
dmft	decayed missing and filled teeth (deciduous)
DMFT	decayed missing and filled teeth (permanent)
D/N	day/night (frequency of urine)
DNA	deoxyribose nucleic acid/did not attend
DOA	dead on arrival
DOB	date of birth
DOD	date of death
DOE	dyspnoea on exertion (Am. dyspnea)
DOES	disorders of excessive somnolence
DS	Down's syndrome

D/S	dextrose and saline
DSA	digital subtraction angiography
DTP	diphtheria, tetanus and pertussis (vaccine)
DTR	deep tendon reflex
DTs	delerium tremens
DU	duodenal ulcer
DUB	dysfunctional uterine bleeding
D&V	diarrhoea and vomiting
DVT	deep venous thrombosis
Dx	diagnosis
DXT	deep X-ray therapy
DXRT	deep X-ray radiotherapy
EBM	expressed breast milk
EBV	Epstein–Barr virus
ECF	extracellular fluid
ECFV	extracellular fluid volume
ECG	electrocardiogram
ECHO	echocardiogram
ECSL	extra corporeal shockwave lithotripsy
ECT	electroconvulsive therapy
EDC	expected date of confinement
EDD	expected date of delivery
EDV	end-diastolic volume
EEG	electroencephalography/gram
EENT	eyes, ears, nose and throat
EFM	electronic fetal monitoring
ELBW	extremely low birth weight
ELISA	enzyme-linked immunosorbent assay
Em	emmetropia (good vision)
EMD	electromechanical dissociation
EMG	electromyogram/electromyography
EMI	elderly mentally infirm/**e**toposide-**m**ethotrexate-**i**fosfamide
EMU	early morning urine
EN	erythema nodosum
ENG	electronystagmogram
ENT	ear, nose and throat
EOG	electrooculogram
EOM	extraocular movement
EP	ectopic pregnancy
EPSP	excitatory postsynaptic potential
ERCP	endoscopic retrograde cholangiopancreatography
ERT	estrogen replacement therapy (Am.)
ERV	expiratory reserve volume
ESM	ejection systolic murmur
ESN	educationally subnormal
ESP	end-systolic pressure
ESR	erythrocyte sedimentation rate
ESRD	end-stage renal disease
ESRF	end-stage renal failure
ESV	end-systolic volume
ESWL	extracorporeal shock wave lithotripsy
ET	embryo transfer/endotracheal/endotracheal tube

ET CPAP	endotracheal continuous positive airways pressure
ETF	Eustachian tube function
ETT	endotracheal tube/exercise tolerance test
EUA	examination under anaesthesia (Am. anesthesia)
EX	examination
EXP	expansion
Ez	eczema
F	Fahrenheit
FA	folic acid
FAS	fetal alcohol syndrome
FB	fasting blood sugar/finger breadth/foreign body
FBC	full blood count
FBE	full blood examination
FBS	fasting blood sugar
FDIU	fetal death in utero
FET	forced expiratory technique
FEV	forced expiratory volume
FEV_1	forced expiratory volume in 1 sec
FFA	free fatty acids
FFP	fresh frozen plasma
FH	family history
FLP	fasting lipid profile
FMH	family medical history
FNAB	fine needle aspiration biopsy
FOB	faecal occult blood (Am. fecal)
FOBT	faecal occult blood testing (Am. fecal)
FP	false positive
FRC	functional reserve capacity/functional residual capacity
FROM	full range of movement
FSH	follicle stimulating hormone
FSHRH	follicle stimulating hormone releasing hormone
FT	full term
FT_4	free thyroxine
FTI	free thyroxine index
FTND	full term, normal delivery
FUO	fever of unknown origin
FVC	forced vital capacity
FX, Fx or fx.	fracture
g	gauge
GI and GII	gravida I and gravida II (first and second pregnancy)
GA	general anaesthesia (Am. anesthesia)/general appearance
GABA	gamma-aminobutyric acid
GB	gall bladder/Guillain–Barré (syndrome)
GC	gonococci
GCSF	granulocyte colony stimulating factor
GE	gastroenterology
GF	glomerular filtration/gluten-free

GFR	glomerular filtration rate
GGTP	gamma glutamyl transpeptidase
γGT	gamma glutamyl transferase
GH	growth hormone
GHIH	growth hormone inhibiting hormone
GHRH	growth hormone releasing hormone
GHRIH	growth hormone release-inhibiting hormone
GI	gastrointestinal
GIFT	gamete intrafallopian transfer
ging	gingiva (gum)
GIS	gastrointestinal system
GIT	gastrointestinal tract
GKI	glucose/potassium/insulin
GM	grand mal seizure
GN	glomerulonephritis
GNDC	Gram-negative diplococci
GnRH	gonadotrophin releasing hormone
GP	general practitioner
GR1	one pregnancy
grav	gravid (pregnant)
GS	general surgery/genital system
G&S/XM	group and save/cross match
GTN	glyceryl trinitrate
gtt	guttae (drops)
GTT	glucose tolerance test
GU	gastric ulcer/genitourinary/ gonococcal urethritis
GUS	genitourinary system
GVHD	graft versus host disease
Gyn	gynaecology (Am. gynecology)
H	hypodermic
HAV	hepatitis A virus
HB	heart block
Hb	haemoglobin (Am. hemoglobin)
HBAg	hepatitis B antigen
HBGM	home blood glucose monitoring
HBO	hyperbaric oxygenation
HBP	high blood pressure
HBsAg	hepatitis B surface antigen
HBV	hepatitis B virus
HC	head circumference
HCG(hCG)	human chorionic gonadotrophin
H/ct or /h.ct	haematocrit (Am. hematocrit)
HCV	hepatitis C virus
HCVD	hypertensive cardiovascular disease
HD	haemodialysis (Am. hemodialysis)/Hodgkin's disease/Huntington's disease
HDLs	high density lipoproteins
HDN	haemolytic disease of newborn (Am. hemolytic)
HDV	hepatitis delta virus
HEENT	head, eyes, ears, nose and throat
HF	heart failure
HGH or hGH	human growth hormone

HGP	human genome project
HHNK	hyperglycaemic (Am. hyperglycemic) hyperosmolar nonketonic
HHV	human herpes virus
Hib	*Haemophilus influenzae* type b
Hist.	histology (lab)
HIV	human immunodeficiency virus
HIVD	herniated intervertebral disc
H&L	heart and lungs
HLA	human leucocyte antigen (Am. leukocyte)
HMG(hMG)	human menopausal gonadotrophin
HOCM	hypertrophic obstructive cardiomyopathy
HO	house officer
H&P	history and physical
HPC	history of present condition
HPEN	home parenteral and enteral nutrition
hpf	high power field
HPI	history of present illness
HR	heart rate
HRM	human resource management
HRT	hormone replacement therapy
HSA	human serum albumin
HSV	*Herpes simplex* virus
5-HT	5-hydroxytryptamine
HT	hypertension
HTLV	human T-cell leukaemia-lymphoma virus (Am. leukemia)
HTN	hypertension
HTVD	hypertensive vascular disease
HUS	haemolytic uraemic syndrome (Am. hemolytic uremic syndrome)
HVD	hypertensive vascular disease
Hx	history
IABP	intra-aortic balloon pump
IBC	iron binding capacity
IBD	inflammatory bowel disease
IBS	irritable bowel syndrome
IC	intercostal/intracerebral/intracranial
ICA	islet cell antibody
ICF	intracellular fluid
ICH	intracerebral haemorrhage (Am. hemorrhage)
ICM	intracostal margin
ICP	intracranial pressure
ICS	intercostal space
ICSH	interstitial cell stimulating hormone
ICU	intensive care unit
ID or id	identity/intradermal
I&D	incision and drainage
IDDM	insulin dependent diabetes mellitus
IDL	intermediate-density lipoprotein
IFN	interferon
Ig	immunoglobulin (e.g. IgA, IgG)
IGT	impaired glucose tolerance
IHD	ischaemic heart disease (Am. ischemic)

IHR	intrinsic heart rate	IVU	intravenous urography
i.m.	intramuscular		
IM	infectious mononucleosis/intramuscular	J	jaundice
		JVD	jugular venous distension
IMHP	intramuscular high potency	JVP	jugular vein pressure/jugular venous pressure
IMI	inferior myocardial infarction		
IMP	impression		
IMV	intermittent mandatory ventilation	KA	ketoacidosis
IN	internist (Am.)	KCCT	kaolin-cephalin clotting time
inf	inferior	KCO	transfer factor for carbon monoxide
inf.MI	inferior myocardial infarction	KJ	knee jerk
INR	international normalized ratio	KLS	kidney, liver, spleen
int	between/inter	KO	keep open
I&O	intake and output	KS	Karposi's sarcoma
IOFB	intraocular foreign body	KUB	kidney, ureters and bladder
IOL	intraocular lens	KVO	keep vein open
IOP	intraocular pressure		
in utero	within uterus	L	lymphadenopathy
i.p.	intraperitoneal	(L)	left/lower
IPA	immunosuppressive acid protein	L 1–5	lumbar vertebrae
IPD	idiopathic Parkinson's disease	L&A	light and accommodation
IPF	idiopathic pulmonary fibrosis	LA	left arm/left atrium/local anaesthetic (Am. anesthetic)
IPPA	inspection, palpation, percussion, auscultation		
		La	labial (lips)
IPPB	intermittent positive pressure breathing	LAD	left axis deviation
		LaG	labia and gingiva (lips and gums)
IPPV	intermittent positive pressure ventilation	LAS	lymphadenopathy syndrome
		LAT or lat.	lateral
IQ	intelligence quotient	LBBB	left bundle branch block
IRDS	idiopathic respiratory distress syndrome	LBM	lean body mass
		LBW	low birth weight
IRV	inspiratory reserve volume	LCCS	low cervical caesarean section (Am. cesarean)
ISQ	idem status quo (i.e. unchanged)		
IT	intrathecal	LD	lethal dose/loading dose
ITCP	idiopathic thrombocytopenia purpura	LDH	lactic dehydrogenase
ITP	idiopathic thrombocytopenic purpura	LDL	low density lipoprotein
ITT	insulin tolerance test	LE	lupus erythematosus
ITU	intensive therapy unit	LFT	liver function test
IU	international units	LGA	large for gestational age
IUC	idiopathic ulcerative colitis	LH	luteinizing hormone
IUCD	intrauterine contraceptive device	LHRH	luteinizing hormone releasing hormone
IUD	intrauterine death/intrauterine device		
		LIF	left iliac fossa
IUFB	intrauterine foreign body	LIH	left inguinal hernia
IUGR	intrauterine growth retardation	LKKS	liver, kidney, kidney, spleen
IV or i.v.	intravenous	LL	left leg/left lower/lower lobe
IVC	inferior vena cava/intravenous cholecystogram	LLETZ	large loop excision of the transformation zone
IVD	intervertebral disc		
IVF	in vitro fertilization/in vivo fertilization	LLL	left lower lid (eye)/left lower lobe (lung)
IVH	intraventricular haemorrhage (Am. hemorrhage)	LLQ	left lower quadrant
		LMN	lower motor neuron
IVHP	intravenous high potency	LMP	last menstrual period
IVI	intravenous infusion	LN	lymph node
IVP	intravenous pyelogram/intravenous pyelography	LNMP	last normal menstrual period
		LOC	level of consciousness
IVSD	interventricular septal defect	LOM	limitation of movement
IVT	intravenous transfusion	LP	lumbar puncture

LPA	left pulmonary artery	MFT	muscle function test
LPN	licensed practical nurse (Am.)	MG	myasthenia gravis
LRI	lower respiratory infection	MGN	membranous glomerulonephritis
LS	left side/liver and spleen/lumbosacral/lymphosarcoma	MH	medical history/menstrual history
		MHC	major histocompatability complex
LSB	long stay bed (geriatric)	MHz	megahertz (megacycles per second)
LSCS	lower section caesarean section	MI	mitral incompetence/mitral
LSD	lysergic acid diethylamide		insufficiency/myocardial infarction
LSK	liver, spleen, kidneys	MIBG	meta-iodobenzyl guanidine
LSM	late systolic murmur	MIC	minimum inhibitory concentration
LTC	long term care	MID	multi-infarct dementia
LTOT	long term oxygen therapy	ML	middle lobe/midline
L&U	lower and upper	MLT	medical laboratory
LUL	left upper lobe		technician/technologist
LUQ	left upper quadrant	mm^3	cubic millimetre
LV	left ventricle	mmHg	millimetres of mercury
LVDP	left ventricular diastolic pressure	MMM	mitozantrone, methotrexate,
LVE	left ventricular enlargement		mitomycin C
LVEDP	left ventricular end-diastolic pressure	mmol	millimole
		MNJ	myoneural junction
LVEDV	left ventricular end-diastolic volume	MODY	maturity onset diabetes of the young
LVET	left ventricular ejection time	MOFS	multiple organ failure syndrome
LVF	left ventricular failure	MOPP	mustine, oncovin (vincristine),
LVH	left ventricular hypertrophy		procarbazine, prednisolone
LVP	left ventricular pressure	MPJ	metacarpophalangeal joint
L&W	living and well	MPQ	McGill Pain Questionnaire
Lymphos	lymphocytes	MR	mitral regurgitation
		MRDM	malnutrition-related diabetes mellitus
M	male/married/murmur	MRI	magnetic resonance imaging
MAb	monoclonal antibody	mRNA	messenger ribonucleic acid
MABP	mean arterial blood pressure	MRSA	methicillin resistant *Staphylococcus*
MAC	mid-arm circumference/ *Mycobacterium avium* complex		*aureus*
		MS	mitral stenosis/multiple
MAMC	mid-arm muscle circumference		sclerosis/muscle shortening/muscle
mane	in the morning		strength/musculoskeletal/musculo-
MAOI	mono-amine oxidase inhibitor		skeletal system
MAP	mean arterial pressure/muscle action potential	MSAFP	maternal serum alphafetoprotein
		MSE	mental state examination
MCH	mean corpuscular (red cell) haemoglobin (Am. hemoglobin)	MSH	melanocyte-stimulating hormone
		MSL	midsternal line
MCHC	mean corpuscular haemoglobin concentration (Am. hemoglobin)	MSOF	multisystem organ failure
		MSSU	midstream specimen of urine
MCL	mid clavicular line	MSU	midstream urine
MCP	metacarpophalangeal	MTA	mid-thigh amputation
MCV	mean corpuscular (cell) volume	MTP	metatarsophalangeal
MD	maintenance dose/mitral disease/muscular dystrophy	MV	mitral valve
		MVP	mitral valve prolapse
MDI	metered dose inhaler	MVR	minute volume of respiration/mitral
MDM	mid diastolic murmur		valve replacement
MDRTB	multidrug resistant tuberculosis	My, my	myopia
ME	myalgic encephalopathy		
med	medial	N	normal
MEN	multiple endocrine neoplasia	NAD	nothing abnormal discovered/no
meQ	milliequivalent		acute distress/normal axis deviation
mEq/l	milliequivalent per litre	NAG	narrow angle glaucoma
Metas	metastasis	NANB	non A, non B viruses
MF	mycoses fungoides/myocardial fibrosis	NAP	neutrophil alkaline phosphatase
		NAS, nas	nasal/no added salt

NBM	nil (nothing) by mouth	OPA	outpatient appointment
NCVs	nerve conduction velocities	OPD	outpatient department
NEC	necrotizing enterocolitis	Ophth	ophthalmology
NFTD	normal full term delivery	OPT	orthopantomogram
NG	nasogastric	OR	operating room
NGU	non-gonococcal urethritis	ORT	operating room technician
NHL	non-Hodgkin's lymphoma	Ortho	orthopaedics (Am. orthopedics)
NHS	national health service	Orthop	orthopnoea (Am. orthopnea)
NIDDM	non-insulin-dependent diabetes mellitus	OS	oculus sinister (left eye), oculo sinistro (in left eye)
NK	natural killer (cells)	Os	mouth
NMR	nuclear magnetic resonance	osteo	osteomyelitis
NO	nitric oxide	OT	occupational therapy/old tuberculin/oxytocin
#NOF	fractured neck of femur		
NP	nasopharynx	OTC	over the counter (remedies)
NPN	non-protein nitrogen	oto	otology
NPO, npo	non per os/nothing by mouth	OU	oculus unitas (both eyes together)/oculus uterque (for each eye)/oculus utro (in each eye)
NREM	non-rapid eye movement (sleep)		
NRS	numerical rating scale		
NS	nephrotic syndrome/nervous system/no specimen	P	pressure
NSAIDs	non-steroidal anti-inflammatory drugs	PA	pernicious anaemia (Am. anemia)/posteroanterior/ pulmonary artery
NSFTD	normal spontaneous full-term delivery	P&A	percussion and auscultation
NSR	normal sinus rhythm	PABA	para-aminobenzoic acid
NST	non-shivering thermogenesis	PACG	primary angle closure glaucoma
NSU	nonspecific urethritis	PADP	pulmonary artery diastolic pressure
NT	nasotracheal/nasotracheal tube	PAH	pulmonary artery hypertension
N&T	nose and throat	PAP	primary atypical pneumonia
NTP	normal temperature and pressure	Pap.	Papanicolaou smear test
N&V	nausea and vomiting	PAS	p-aminosalicylic acid
NVD	nausea, vomiting and diarrhoea	PAT	paroxysmal atrial tachycardia
		PAWP	pulmonary artery wedge pressure
O	oedema (Am. edema)	PBC	primary biliary cirrhosis
O&A	observation and assessment	PBI	protein bound iodine
OA	on admission/osteoarthritis	pc	post cibum (after meals/food)
OAD	obstructive airway disease	PCA	patient controlled analgesia
OAG	open angle glaucoma	PCAS	patient controlled analgesia system
OB	occult blood	PCN	penicillin
Ob-Gyn	obstetrics and gynaecology (Am. gynecology)	PCNL	percutaneous nephrolithotomy
Obst-Gyn	obstetrics and gynaecology (Am. gynecology)	PCO_2	partial pressure carbon dioxide
OC	oral cholecystogram/oral contraceptive	PCP	*Pneumocystis carinii* pneumonia
		PCT	prothrombin clotting time
OCP	oral contraceptive pill	PCV	packed cell volume
OD	oculus dexter (right eye), oculo dextro (in the right eye)/overdose	PCWP	pulmonary capillary wedge pressure
		PD	Parkinson's disease/peritoneal dialysis
od	every day		
Odont	odontology	PDA	patent ductus arteriosus
ODQ	on direct questioning	PE	physical examination/pleural effusion/pulmonary embolism
OE	on examination/otitis externa		
OGD	oesophago-gastro-duodenoscopy	PEC	pneumoencephalogram
OGTT	oral glucose tolerance test	PED	paediatrics (Am. pediatrics)
OH	occupational history	PEEP	positive end expiratory pressure
OHS	open heart surgery	PEF	peak expiratory flow
OM	olim mane (once daily in the morning)/otitis media	PEFR	peak expiratory flow rate
		PEG	percutaneous endoscopic gastrostomy/pneumoencephalogram
OOB	out of bed		

PEJ	percutaneous endoscopic jejunostomy	p.r. or PR	per rectum/plantar reflex
PEM	protein-energy malnutrition	PRH	prolactin releasing hormone
PERLAC	pupils equal, react to light, accommodation consensual	PRL	prolactin
		PRN or p.r.n.	pro re nata (as required)
PERRLA	pupils equal, round, react to light, accommodation consensual	PROG	progesterone
		PROM	premature rupture of membranes
PET	positron emission tomography/pre-eclamptic toxaemia (Am. toxemia)	PRV	polycythaemia rubra vera (Am. polycythemia)
PF	peak flow	pros	prostate
PFT	peak flow rate	prox	proximal
PFTs	pulmonary function tests	PS	pulmonary stenosis/pyloric stenosis
PG	prostaglandin	PSA	prostate specific antigen
PGL	persistent generalized lymphadenopathy	PSCT	pain and symptom control team
		PSD	personal and social development
PH	past history/patient history/prostatic hypertrophy/pulmonary hypertension	PSG	presystolic gallop
		PSVT	paroxysmal supraventricular tachycardia
pH	hydrogen-ion concentration		
PID	pelvic inflammatory disease/prolapsed intervertebral disc	pt or PT	patient/physical therapy/prothrombin time/physical therapist (Am.)
PIH	prolactin inhibiting hormone		
PIP	proximal interphalangeal	PTA	prior to admission
PIVD	protruded intervertebral disc	PTC	percutaneous transhepatic cholangiogram/graphy
PKU	phenylketonuria		
PM	post mortem	PTCA	percutaneous transluminal coronary angioplasty
PMB	post menopausal bleeding		
PMH	past medical history	PTD	permanent and total disability
PMI	past medical history/point of maximum impulse	PTH	parathormone/parathyroid hormone
		PTR	prothrombin ratio
PML	progressive multifocal leucoencephalopathy (Am. leukoencephalopathy)	PTT	partial thromboplastin time
		PTX	pneumothorax
		PU	peptic ulcer/per urethra
PMN	polymorphonuclear leucocytes (Am. leukocyte)	PUO	pyrexia of unknown origin
		PUVA	psoralen + ultraviolet light A
PMS	premenstrual syndrome	PV	per vagina
PMT	premenstrual tension	P&V	pyloroplasty and vagotomy
PMV	prolapsed mitral valve	PVC	premature ventricular contraction
PN	percussion note/peripheral nerve/peripheral neuropathy	PVD	peripheral vascular disease
		PVP	pulmonary venous pressure
PND	paroxysmal nocturnal dyspnoea (Am. dyspnea)/post nasal drip	PVT	paroxysmal ventricular tachycardia
		PX	physical examination
PNS	peripheral nervous system	Px	past history/prognosis
PO or po	per os/by mouth		
PO_2	partial pressure oxygen	QDS or qds	quater diurnale summensum (four times a day)
POAG	primary open angle glaucoma		
POLY	polymorphonuclear leucocytes (Am. leukocytes)	qid	quater in die (four times a day)
POP	plaster of Paris	(R)	right
pos	position	RA	rheumatoid arthritis/right auricle/atrium
post	posterior		
PPAM	pneumatic post-amputation mobility	Ra	radium
PPD	packs per day/purified protein derivative (of tuberculin)	RAD	radiation absorbed dose/right axis deviation
PPE	personal protective equipment	rad	radical
PPH	postpartum haemorrhage (Am. hemorrhage)	RAS	reticular activating system
		RAST	radio-allergosorbent test
PPS	plasma protein solution	RBBB	right bundle branch block
PPT	partial prothrombin time	RBC	red blood cell/red blood (cell) count
PPV	positive-pressure ventilation	RBS	random blood sugar

RCC	red cell concentrate/red cell count
RDA	recommended dietary allowance
rDNA	recombinant deoxyribose nucleic acid
RDS	respiratory distress syndrome
RE	rectal examination
REM	rapid eye movement (in sleep)
RES	reticulo endothelial system
RF	renal failure/rheumatoid factor/rheumatic fever
RFLA	rheumatoid factor-like activity
RFT	respiratory function tests
Rh	Rhesus
RHD	rheumatic heart disease
RHL	right hepatic lobe
RIA	radioimmunoassay
RIF	right iliac fossa
RK	radial keratotomy/right kidney
RL	right leg/right lung
RLC	residual lung capacity
RLD	related living donor
RLE	right lower extremity
RLL	right lower lobe
RLQ	right lower quadrant
RM	radical mastectomy
RN	registered nurse
RNA	ribose nucleic acid
R/O	rule out
ROM	range of movement (exercises)
ROS	review of symptoms
RP	radial pulse
RPE	retinal pigment epithelial (cells, layer)
RQ	respiratory quotient
RR	recovery room/respiratory rate
RR&E	round regular and equal
RRR	regular rate and rhythm
RS	respiratory system/Reye's syndrome
RSI	repetitive strain injury
RSV	respiratory syncytial virus
RT	radiologic technologist (Am.)/radiotherapy
RTA	renal tubular acidosis/road traffic accident
RUL	right upper lobe
RUQ	right upper quadrant
RV	residual volume/right ventricle
RVF	right ventricular failure
RVH	right ventricular hypertrophy
s	without
S1	first heart sound
S2	second heart sound
SA	sarcoma/sinoatrial (node)/sinus arrhythmia/Stokes-Adams (attacks)
SACD	subacute combined degeneration
SAD	seasonal affective disorder
SAH	subarachnoid haemorrhage (Am. hemorrhage)
SB	seen by

SBE	subacute bacterial endocarditis
SBO	small bowel obstruction
SBP	systolic blood pressure
s.c.	subclavian/subcutaneous
SCA	sickle-cell anaemia
SCC	squamous cell carcinoma
SCD	sequential pneumatic compression device/sudden cardiac death
SCID	severe combined immunodeficiency syndrome
SDH	subdural haematoma (Am. hematoma)
SDS	same day surgery
SED	skin erythema dose
SEM	systolic ejection murmur
SG	skin graft/specific gravity
SGA	small for gestational age
SGOT	serum glutamic oxaloacetic transaminase now serum aspartate transferase
SGPT	serum glutamic pyruvic transaminase
SF	synovial fluid
SH	social history
SIADH	syndrome of inappropriate antidiuretic hormone
SIDS	sudden infant death syndrome
SIG	sigmoidoscope/sigmoidoscopy
SIMV	synchronized intermittent mandatory ventilation
s.l.	sublingual
SLE	systemic lupus erythematosus
SLS	social and life skills
SMD	senile macular degeneration
SNS	somatic nervous system
SOA	swelling of ankles
SOB	short of breath/stools for occult blood
SOBOE	short of breath on exertion
SOS	swelling of sacrum
SP	systolic pressure
SPF	sun protection factor
SPP	suprapubic prostatectomy
SR	sedimentation rate/sinus rhythm
SS S/S	saline solution/signs and symptoms
ST	sinus tachycardia/skin test
STD	sexually transmitted disease/skin test dose
STS	serological tests for syphilis
STU	skin test unit
Subcu	subcutaneous
subling	sublingual/under the tongue
sup	superior
SV	stroke volume
SVC	superior vena cava
SVI	stroke volume index
SVR	systemic venous resistance
SVT	supraventricular tachycardia
SWS	slow wave sleep
Sx	symptoms
syph.	syphilis

T	temperature/tumour	TUIP	transurethral incision of the prostate
t	terminal	TUR	transurethral resection (of prostate)
T 1–12	thoracic vertebrae	TURB	transurethral resection of bladder
T_3, T_4	triiodothyronine, tetraiodothyronine (thyroid hormones)	TURP	transurethral resection of the prostate
T&A	tonsils and adenoids or tonsillectomy/adenoidectomy	TURT	transurethral resection of tumour
		TV	tidal volume
T.A.	toxin-antitoxin	Tx	therapy/transfusion/treatment
TAH	total abdominal hysterectomy	T&X	type and crossmatch
Tb or TB	tuberculosis (tubercle bacillus)		
TBA	to be arranged	U	unit
TBG	thyroid binding globulin	UA	uric acid/urinalysis
TBI	total body irradiation	UAC	umbilical artery catheter
TBW	total body water/total body weight	UC	ulcerative colitis
T&C	type and crossmatch	UDO	undetermined origin
TCP	thrombocytopenia	U&E	urea and electrolytes
TD	thymus dependent cells	UG	urogenital
TDM	therapeutic drug monitoring	UGH	uveitis + glaucoma + hyphaema syndrome (Am. hyphema)
TDS	ter diurnale summensum (three times a day)	UGI	upper gastrointestinal
TED	thromboembolic deterrent (stockings)	UIBC	unsaturated iron-binding capacity
TENS	transcutaneous electrical nerve stimulation	ung	ointment (unguentum)
		URI	upper respiratory (tract) infection
TH	thyroid hormone (thyroxine)	URT	upper respiratory tract
THR	total hip replacement	URTI	upper respiratory tract infection
TI	thymus independent cells	US	ultrasonography/ultrasound/urinary system
TIA	transient ischaemic attack (Am. ischemic)	USS	ultrasound scan
TIBC	total iron-binding capacity	UTI	urinary tract infection
t.i.d.	ter in die (three times daily)	UVA	ultra violet light A
TIP	terminal interphalangeal	UVB	ultra violet light B
TIPS	transjugular intrahepatic portosystemic shunting	UVC	ultra violet light C
TJ	triceps jerk	VA	visual acuity
TKVO	to keep vein open	VAC	vincristine, adriamycin, cyclophosphamide
TLC	tender loving care/total lung capacity	VAS	visual analogue scale
TLD	thoracic lymph duct	VC	vital capacity/vulvovaginal candidiasis
TM	tympanic membrane		
TMJ	temporomandibular joint	VD	venereal disease
TMR	transmyocardial revascularization	VDRL	venereal disease research laboratory (test)
TNF	tumour necrosis factor		
TNM	tumour, node, metastases	VE	vaginal examination
TOP	termination of pregnancy	VF	ventricular fibrillation/visual field
tPA	recombinant tissue-type plasminogen activator	VHD	valvular heart disease
		VLBW	very low birth weight
TPHI	*Treponema pallidum* haemagglutination inhibition (Am. hemagglutination)	VLDL	very low density lipoprotein
		VMA	vanillyl-mandelic acid
TPI	*Treponema pallidum* immobilization	VP	venous pressure
TPN	total parenteral nutrition	VPC	ventricular premature contraction
TPR	temperature, pulse, respiration	VRS	verbal rating scale
TRH	thyrotrophin-releasing hormone	VS	vital signs
TSA	tumour specific antigen	VSD	ventricular septal defect
TSF	triceps skinfold thickness	VT	ventricular tachycardia
TSH	thyroid stimulating hormone	VUR	vesicouretic reflux
TSS	toxic shock syndrome	VWF	von Willebrand factor
TT	tetanus toxoid/thrombin clotting time	VV	varicose veins/vulva and vagina
TTA	transtracheal aspiration		
TTO	to take out (to home)		

WBC	white blood (cell) count/white blood cell
WCC	white cell count
WNL	within normal limits
WPW	Wolff-Parkinson-White (syndrome)
WR	Wasserman reaction (test for syphilis)
X-match	cross-match
XR	X-ray
XRT	X-ray therapy
ZE	Zollinger-Ellison (syndrome)
ZN	Ziel-Nielsen Stain

Symbols

♂	male
♀	female
*	birth
α	alpha
β	beta
γ	gamma
Δ	delta/diagnosis
ΔΔ	differential diagnosis
#	fracture
†	dead

Glossary

The glossary contains a list of prefixes, suffixes and combining forms used in common medical terms. The meaning of each word component is given with an example of its use in a medical term. Use the list to decipher the meaning of unfamiliar words. Note, a dash is added to indicate whether the component usually precedes or follows the other elements of a compound word; for example, ante- precedes a word root as in **ante**natal whilst -stomy follows the root as in colo**stomy**. Some terms are composed of one or more roots with a prefix or suffix; for example **-algia** contains the root **alg** meaning pain and the suffix **-ia** meaning condition of. The vowels of combining forms are used or dropped by the application of 'rules' described in the introduction of this book. Some roots are listed with more than one combining vowel, for example, **ren**/i/o. Both vowels may be used as in **ren**ipelvic and **ren**ography.

	Meaning	Medical Term
a-	without, not (n is added before words beginning with a vowel)	**a**phasia
-a	noun ending/a name	burs**a**
ab-	away from	**ab**duct
abdomin/o	abdomen	**abdomino**pelvic
-able	capable of/having ability to	palp**able**
ac-	pertaining to/to/toward/near	**ac**cretion
acanth/o	spiny	**acanth**osis
acarin/o	mites of the order Acarina	**acarin**osis
acar/i/o	mites of the order Acarina	**acari**cide
acetabul/o	acetabulum	**acetabulo**plasty
acet/o	vinegar	*Aceto*bacter
aceton-	ketones/acetone	**aceton**aemia (Am. **aceton**emia)
achill/o	Achilles tendon	**achillo**tomy
acid/o	acid	**acido**phil
acin/i	sac-like dilatation	**acin**us
acne/o	acne/point/peak	**acne**genic
acou-	hear/hearing	**acou**metric
-acousia	condition of hearing	dys**acousia**
acoust/o	hear/hearing/sound	**acoust**ic
acro-	extremities, point	**acro**megaly
acromi/o	acromion (point of the shoulder)	**acromio**clavicular
act-	do, drive, act	**act**ion
actin/o	rays e.g. of sun/ultraviolet radiation	**actino**therapy
acu-	hear/hearing/severe/sudden	**acu**te
-acusia	condition/sense of hearing	dys**acusia**
ad-	to/toward/in the direction of the midline	**ad**duct
adamant/o	dental enamel	**adamant**ine
aden/o	gland	**aden**oid
adenoid-	adenoids	**adenoid**ectomy
adip/o	adipose tissue/fat	**adip**osity
adnex/o	bound to/conjoined	**adnex**a
adrenal/o	adrenal gland	**adrenal**ectomy
adren/o	adrenal gland	**adreno**genital
adrenocortic/o	adrenal cortex	**adrenocortic**al
-aem-	blood (Am. -em-)	an**aem**ia
-aemia	condition of blood (Am. -emia)	leuk**aemia**
aer/o	air/gas	**aero**phagia
aesthe/s/i/o	sensation/sensitivity (Am. esthe/s/i/o)	an**aesthesio**logy
aeti/o	cause (Am. eti/o)	**aeti**ology
af-	to/towards/near	**af**ferent
ag-	to/towards/near	**ag**glutinate

agglutin/o	sticking/clumping together	**agglutin**ation
-ago	abnormal condition/disease	lumb**ago**
-agogic	pertaining to inducing/stimulating	dacry**agogic**
-agogue	inducing/promoting	lact**agogue**
agora-	market place open space	**agora**phobia
-agra	seizure/sudden pain	pod**agra**
-aise	comfort/ease	mal**aise**
-al¹	pertaining to	bronchi**al**
-al²	used in pharmacology to mean a drug or drug action	antifung**al**
albin/o	white	**albin**ism
alb/i/o	white	**alb**us
album-	white	**album**in
albumin/o	albumin/albumen	**albumin**uria
-algesia	condition of pain	an**algesia**
alges/i/o	sense of pain	**algesio**meter
-algia	pain	neur**algia**
alg/e/i/o	pain	**alg**aesthesia
aliment/o	to nourish	**aliment**ary
all/o	other/different from normal	**allo**genic
alve/o	trough/channel/cavity	**alve**us
alveol/o	alveoli (of lungs)	**alveol**itis
ambi-	on both sides	**ambi**lateral
ambly/o	dull/dim	**ambly**opia
ameb/o (Am.)	ameba, a type of protozoan	**ameb**iasis
amel/o	dental enamel	**amelo**blast
-amine	nitrogen containing compound	catechol**amine**
amni/o	amnion/fetal membrane	**amnio**centesis
amnion/o	amnion/fetal membrane	**amnion**ic
amoeb/o	amoeba a type of protozoan (Am. ameb/o)	**amoeb**iasis
amph/i	both/doubly/both sides	**amphi**gonadism
amyl/o	starch	**amyl**oid
an-	without/not	**an**encephalic
-an	pertaining to/characteristic of	ovari**an**
ana-	backward/apart/up/again	**ana**plastic
ancyl/o	crooked/stiffening/fusing/bent	**ancylo**stomiasis
andr/o	male	**andro**logy
aneurysm/o	aneurysm	**aneurysmo**plasty
angi/o	vessel	**angio**plasty
aniso-	unequal/dissimilar	**aniso**coria
ankyl/o	crooked/stiffening/fusing/bent	**ankyl**osis
an/o	anus	**ano**rectal
-ant	having the characteristic of	stimul**ant**
ante-	before in time or place/in front	**ante**natal
anter/o	front/in front of/anterior to	**antero**lateral
anthrac/o	coal dust	**anthrac**osis
anthrop/o	man/human	**anthropo**metry
anti-	against	**anti**fungal
antr/o	antrum/maxillary sinus	**antro**tomy
anxi/o	anxiety	**anxio**lytic
aort/o	aorta	**aorto**rrhaphy
ap-	to/toward/near	**ap**position
-aph-	touch	hyper**aph**ia
-apheresis	removal	leuk**apheresis**
aphth/o	ulcer	**aphth**ous
apic/o	apex	**apic**al
ap/o	away from/detached/derived from	**apo**physis
aponeur/o	aponeurosis (flat tendon)	**aponeuro**rrhaphy
append/ic/o	appendix	**appendic**ectomy
aqu/a/e/o	water	**aqu**eous

-ar	pertaining to	lob**ar**
arachn/o	spider	**arachno**phobia
arc/o	arch/bow-shaped	**arc**us
-arch/e-	beginning	men**arch**
arrhen/o	male/masculine	**arrheno**blastoma
arter/i/o	artery	**arterio**sclerosis
arteriol/o	arteriole	**arteriolo**necrosis
arthr/o	joint	**arthro**desis
articul/o	joint	**articul**ate
-ary	pertaining to/connected with	pulmon**ary**
as-	to/towards/near	**as**sociation
-ase	an enzyme	amyl**ase**
-asia	state or condition	euthan**asia**
-asis	state or condition	elephanti**asis**
-asthenia	condition of weakness	my**asthenia**
asthen/o	weakness	**astheno**coria
astr/o	star-shaped/star	**astro**cyte
at-	to/towards/near	**at**traction
-ate	use/subject to	stimul**ate**
atel/o	imperfect/incomplete	**atelo**cardia
ather/o	porridge-like plaque lining blood vessel	**athero**sclerosis
-ation	action/condition	ejacul**ation**
-atresia	condition of occlusion/closure/absence of opening	anal **atresia**
atret/o	closure of a normal opening/imperforation	**atreto**metria
atri/o	atrium	**atrio**ventricular
audi/o	hearing/sense of hearing	**audio**metry
audit/o	hearing/sense of hearing	**audit**ory
-aural	pertaining to the ear	mon**aural**
auricul/o	ear/pinna	**auriculo**plasty
aur/i/o	ear/hearing	**aur**iscope
auto-	self	**auto**lysis
aux/i	increase	**aux**ilytic
-auxis	increase	onych**auxis**
aux/o	increase	**auxo**cardia
-ax	noun ending/a name	thor**ax**
axill/o	armpit	**axill**ary
ax/i/o	axis	**axi**petal
axon/o	axis/axon of neurone	**axon**al
azot/o	urea/nitrogen	**azot**aemia (Am. **azot**emia)
ba-	go/walk/stand	hypno**batia**
bacill/o	bacillus/a rod-shaped bacterium	**bacill**uria
bacter/i/o	baterium/bacteria	**bacterio**phage
balan/o	glans penis	**balan**itis
ball-	throw/movement	**ball**istocardiograph
bar/o	weight/pressure	**baro**trauma
bartholin/o	Bartholin's glands of vagina	**bartholin**itis
basi-	base/basic/alkaline	**basi**chromatin
baso-	base/basic/alkaline	**baso**phil
bathy-	deep	**bathy**pnoea
bi-	two/twice/life	**bi**pedal
bili-	bile	**bili**ary
bin-	two each/double	**bin**ocular
bio-	life/living	**bio**logy
-blast	germ cell/embryonic/immature growing thing	osteo**blast**
blast/o	early/growth/germ/development	retino**blast**oma
blenn/o	mucus	**blenn**oid
blephar/o	eyelid	**blephar**optosis
bol-	ball	**bol**us

brachi/o	arm	**brachi**al
brachy-	short	**brachy**gnathia
brady-	slow	**brady**cardia
brev/i	short	**brevi**flexor
bromidr/o	stench/smell of sweat	**bromidr**osis
bronch/i/o	bronchus/bronchial tube/windpipe	**broncho**scopy
bronchiol/o	bronchiole	**bronchiol**itis
bront/o	thunder	**bronto**phobia
bucca-	cheek	**bucca**l
bucc/o	cheek	**bucco**pharyngeal
burs/o	bursa (fluid filled sac)	**burs**itis
byssin/o	cotton dust	**byssin**osis
cac/o	bad/ill/abnormal	**caco**cholia
caec/o	caecum (Am. cecum)	**caeco**cele
calcane/o	calcaneus/heel bone	**calcaneo**plantar
calc/i/o	calcium/lime/heel	**calci**penia
calcin/o	calcium	**calcin**osis
calcul/o	stone/little stone	**calcul**us
cali/o	calyx/cup-shaped organ or cavity (Am. calix)	**cali**orrhaphy
calor/i	heat	**calor**imetry
cancer/o	cancer (general term)	**cancero**phobia
canth/o	canthus	**cantho**plasty
capill/o	hair/blood capillary	**capill**ary
capit-	head	**capit**ate
-capnia	condition of carbon dioxide	hyper**capnia**
caps-	container	**caps**itis
capsul/o	capsule	**capsul**ar
carb/o	carbon/bicarbonate	**carbo**hydrate
carcin/o	cancerous/malignant	**carcin**oma
-cardia	condition of heart	tachy**cardia**
cardi/o	heart	**cardio**logist
cari/o	rot/decay (of teeth)	**cario**genesis
carp/o	carpal/wrist bones	**carpo**ptosis
cary/o	nucleus	eu**caryo**tic
cat/a	down/negative	**cata**bolic
caud/o	tail/towards the tail/lower part of body	**caud**al
caus-	burn/corrosive	**caus**tic
caut-	burn	**caut**ery
cav-	hollow	**cav**ity
cec/o (Am.)	cecum	**ceco**cele
-cele	swelling/protrusion/hernia	vesico**cele**
celi/o	hollow/abdomen	**celio**scope
cell-	cell	**cell**ular
cel/o (Am.)	hollow/abdomen/celom	**celo**schisis
cen/o	new/empty/common	**ceno**genesis
-centesis	surgical puncture to remove fluid	amnio**centesis**
centi-	hundred/one hundredth	**centi**grade
centr/i/o	centre/central location	**centri**lobular
cephal/o	head	hydro**cephal**ic
cerat/o	horny/epidermis/cornea (syn: kerat/o)	**cerato**cricoid
cerebell/o	cerebellum	**cerebell**ar
cerebr/i/o	cerebrum/brain	**cerebr**oma
cer/o	wax	**cer**oma
cerumin/o	cerumen/ear wax	**cerumin**ous
cervic/o	cervix	**cervic**al
-chalasis	slackening/loosening	blepharo**chalasis**
chancr-	chancre, a destructive sore	**chancr**oid
cheil/o	lip	**cheilo**plasty

cheir/o	hand	**cheiro**megaly
chem/i/c/o	chemical	**chemo**receptor
chil/o	lip	**chilo**plasty
chir/o	hand	**chiro**pody
chlor/o	green/chlorine	**chlor**oma
cholangi/o	bile vessel/bile duct	**cholangio**gram
cholecyst/o	gall bladder	**cholecysto**lithiasis
choledoch/o	common bile duct	**choledocho**lithiasis
chol/e/o	bile	**chol**uria
cholester/o	cholesterol	**cholester**osis
chondr/i/o	cartilage	**chondro**sarcoma
chord/o	string/cord	**chordo**tomy
chore/o	dance/jerky movement	**chore**a
chori/o	chorion/outer fetal membrane	**chorio**allantois
choroid/o	choroid layer of eye	**choroid**itis
chromat/o	colour	**chromat**opsia
-chromia	condition of haemoglobin/colour (Am. hemoglobin)	hypo**chromia**
chrom/o	colour	**chromo**cystoscopy
chron/o	time	**chron**ic
chrys/o	gold	**chryso**derma
chyl/e/o	chyle-lymphatic fluid formed by lacteals in intestine/product of digestion	**chylo**thorax
chym/o	chyme, creamy material produced by digestion of food/to pour	**chymo**poiesis
-cidal	pertaining to killing	bacterio**cidal**
-cide	agent that kills/killing	acari**cide**
cili/o	cilia/ciliary body of eye/eyelash	**cili**ectomy
cinemat/o	movement/motion (picture)	**cinemato**graphy
cine/o	movement/motion	**cine**angiography
circum-	around	**circum**cision
cirrh/o	yellow	**cirrh**osis
cirs/o	varicose vein/varix	**cirs**ectomy
cis-	on the near side/this side	**cis** position
-cis-	cut/kill	ex**cis**ion
cistern/o	cistern/enclosed space (sub arachnoid space)	**cisterno**graphy
-clasia	condition of breaking	osteo**clasia**
-clasis	breaking	osteo**clasis**
-clast	a cell which breaks	osteo**clast**
claustr/o	barrier/enclosed	**claustro**phobia
clavic/o	clavicle	**clavico**tomy
clavicul/o	clavicle	**clavicul**ar
-cle	small	vesi**cle**
cleid/o	clavicle	**cleido**tomy
clin/o	bend/incline	**clino**dactyly
clitor/i/o	clitoris	**clitor**ism
-clonus	violent action	myo**clonus**
-clysis	infusion/injection/irrigation	veno**clysis**
co-	with/together	**co**factor
coccid/i	type of parasitic protozoa of order coccidia	**coccid**iosis
cocc/i/o	berry-shaped bacterium	**cocco**genous
-coccus	berry-shaped bacterium	strepto**coccus**
coccyg/o	coccyx	**coccyg**eal
cochle/o	cochlea	**cochleo**vestibular
-coel(e)	hollow/abdomen	blasto**coel(e)**
coel/o	hollow/abdomen/ceolom (Am. celom)	**coel**om
col-	with/together	**col**lateral
col/o	colon	**colo**stomy
colon/o	colon	**colon**ic
colp/o	vagina	**colpo**hysterectomy

com-	with/together	**com**mensal
con-	with/together	**con**centric
coni/o	dust	**coni**osis
conjunctiv/o	conjunctiva	**conjunctiv**itis
contra-	against/opposite	**contra**ception
-conus	cone-like protrusion	kerato**conus**
copr/o	faeces (Am. feces)	**copr**olith
cor-	with/together	**cor**rosive
cord/o	a cord	**cord**otomy
cor/e/o	pupil	**coreo**morphosis
-coria	condition of the pupils	aniso**coria**
corne/o	cornea/horny (consisting of keratin)	**corne**oblepharon
coron/o-	crown-like projection/encircling/coronary vessels of heart	**coron**ary
corpor/o	body	**corpor**al
-cortex-	outer part/bark	adrenal **cortex**
cortic/o	cortex/outer region	**cortic**otrophic
cost/o	rib	inter**cost**al
cox/o	hip/hip joint	**cox**ofemoral
crani/o	skull	**crani**otomy
cren/o	crenated	**creno**cytosis
-crescent	grow/crescent	epithelial **crescent**
-crine	secrete	exo**crine**
crin/o	secrete	endo**crin**ology
-crit	separate/device for measuring cells	haemato**crit** (Am. hemato**crit**)
crur/o	leg	**crur**al
cry/o	relating to cold	**cryo**stat
crypt/o	hidden	**crypt**orchism
cubit/o	elbow	**cubit**us
culd/o	cul-de sac/rectouterine pouch	**culdo**scope
-cule	small	animal**cule**
cult-	cultivate	**cult**ure
cune/i	wedge (shape)	**cunei**form
cutane/o	skin	**cutane**ous
cut/i	skin	**cut**icle
cyan/o	blue	**cyan**osis
cycl/o	ciliary body/circle	**cyclo**tomy
cyes/i/o	pregnancy	**cyesi**ology
-cyesis	pregnancy	pseudo**cyesis**
cyst/i/o	bladder	**cyst**ostomy
-cyte	cell	melano**cyte**
cyt/o	cell	**cyto**logy
-cytosis	abnormal increase/condition of cells	thrombo**cytosis**
dacry/o	tear/lacrimal apparatus	**dacry**olith
dacryocyst/o	lacrimal sac	**dacryocysto**tomy
dactyl/o	digits/fingers or toes	**dactylo**megaly
de-	down/away from/loss of/reversing	**de**calcification
deca-	ten	**deca**gram
deci-	one tenth	**deci**litre
demi-	half	**demi**facet
dendr/i/o	tree/tree-like (dendrite of neurone)	**dendri**tic
dentin/o	dentine of tooth (Am. dentin)	**dentino**genesis
dent/i/o	tooth	**dent**ist
derm/a/o	skin	**derm**abrasion
dermat/o	skin	**dermat**ology
descemet/o	Descemet's membrane (of cornea)	**descemeto**cele
-desis	fixation/to bind together by surgery/sticking together	arthro**desis**
desm/o	band/ligament	**desmo**pathy

dextro-	right	**dextro**cardia
di-	two/double	**di**coria
dia-	through/apart/across/between	**dia**physis
-dialysis	separate	haemo**dialysis**
		(Am. hemo**dialysis**)
diaphor/o	sweating (excessive)	**diaphor**esis
diaphragmat/o	diaphragm	**diaphragmat**algia
didym-	twin	epi**didym**is
digit/o	finger/toe	**digito**plantar
dipl/o-	double	**dipl**opia
dips/o	thirst	poly**dips**ia
dis-	reversal/separation/duplication	**dis**location
disc/o	intervertebral disc	**disc**ography
disk/o (Am.)	intervertebral disc	**disk**ectomy
dist/o	far from point of origin	**dist**al
diverticul/o	diverticulum	**diverticul**itis
doch/o	duct/to receive	chole**doch**itis
dolich/o	long	**dolicho**cranial
dolor/i/o	pain (dol – unit of pain)	**doloro**genic
-dorsal	pertaining to back (of body)	ventro**dorsal**
dors/i/o	back (of body)	**dorso**ventral
-drome	a course/conduction/flowing	syn**drome**
drom/o	a course/conduction/flowing	**dromo**tropic
-duct-	lead (to or away from)	ovi**duct**
duoden/o	duodenum	**duodeno**stomy
dur/o	dura mater/hard	epi**dur**al
dynam/o	force/power (of movement)	**dynam**ic
-dynia	condition of pain	pleuro**dynia**
dys-	difficult/disordered/painful/bad	**dys**phasia
e-	out from/outside/without	**e**masculation
-e	noun ending/a name	trigon**e**
-eal	pertaining to	oesophag**eal**
ec-	out/outside/away from	**ec**cyesis
ech/o	reflected sound/echo	**echo**lalia
ect-	out/outside/outer part	**ect**ethmoid
ecto-	out/outside/outer part	**ecto**derm
ectopia-	condition of displacement	**ectopia** lentis
ectop/o	displaced away from normal position	**ectop**ic
-ectasis	dilatation, stretching	bronchi**ectasis**
-ectomy	removal, excision	appendic**ectomy**
ectro-	congenital absence/miscarriage	**ectro**dactylia
edema- (Am.)	swelling due to fluid	**edema**tous
ef-	out/away from	**ef**ferent
eikon/o	icon	**eikono**meter
elae/o	oil	**elaeo**pathia
electro-	electrical	**electro**cardiograph
ellipto-	shaped like an ellipse	**ellipto**cytosis
em-	in	**em**pathy
-ema (Am.)	swelling/distension	myxed**ema**
embol/o	embolus/plug/blockage	**embol**ism
embry/o	embryo	**embryo**genesis
-emesis	vomiting	haemat**emesis**
		(Am. hemat**emesis**)
emet/o	vomiting	**emet**ic
-emia (Am.)	condition of blood	an**emia**
emmetr/o	in due measure/normally proportioned	**emmetr**opia
-emphraxis	blocking/stopping up	salping**emphraxis**
en-	within/in	**en**sheathed

encephal/o	brain	**encephal**itis
endo-	within, inside	**endo**scope
endocrin/o	endocrine (gland)	**endocrino**logist
endometri/o	endometrium of uterus (lining)	**endometri**osis
enter/o	intestine	**enter**itis
-ent	person/agent	dilu**ent**
ento-	within, inside	**ento**cranial
eosin/o	red/dawn coloured/like eosin, a red acid dye	**eosino**phil
ep-	above/upon/on	**ep**arterial
epi-	above/upon/on	**epi**dermis
epididym/o	epididymis	**epididymo**vasectomy
epiglott/o	epiglottis	**epiglott**itis
epilept/i/o	epilepsy	**epilepti**form
episi/o	vulva	**episio**tomy
epitheli/o	epithelium	**epitheli**al
-er	one who/person/agent	radiograph**er**
erg/o/n/o	work	**ergono**meter
-erysis	drag/draw/suck out	phaco**erysis**
erythr/o	red	**erythro**cyte
-esis	abnormal state/condition	ur**esis**
es/o (Am.)	within/inwards	**eso**deviation
esophag/o (Am.)	esophagus/gullet	**esophago**stomy
esthesi/o (Am.)	sensation	an**esthesio**logy
estr/o (Am.)	estrogen/female/estrus	**estro**genic
ethm/o	ethmoid bone	**ethm**oidonasal
eti/o (Am.)	causation	**etio**logy
eu-	good/normal/easily	**eu**tocia
eury-	wide/broad	**eury**cephalic
ex-	out/out of/away from	**ex**ophthalmos
exo-	out/away from/outside	**exo**gastic
-externa	external	otitis **externa**
extr/a/o	outside of/beyond	**extra**hepatic
faci/o	face	**facio**maxillary
falc/i	falx/sickle shaped structure	**falci**form
fasci/o	fascia/fibrous tissue e.g. covering muscles	**fascio**tomy
febr/o	fever	**febr**ile
fec/o (Am.)	feces/waste	**fec**al
femor/o	femur/thigh	**femor**al
-ferent	carrying/to carry/to bear	ef**ferent**
fer/o	to carry/to bear	urini**fer**ous
ferr/o	iron	**ferro**protein
fet/i/o (Am.)	fetus	**feto**metry
fibrill/o	muscular twitching	**fibrill**ation
fibrin/o	fibrinogen	**fibrino**lytic
fimbri/o	fringe	**fimbri**ate
fibr/o	fibre	**fibr**osis
fibul/o	fibula	**fibulo**calcaneal
fil/o	thread	**filo**pressure
fissur-	split/cleft	**fissur**al
fistul/o	tube/pipe	**fistul**a
flagell/o	flagellum/whip	**flagell**osis
flav/o	yellow	**flavo**protein
-flect	bend	re**flect**
-flex-	bend	**flex**ion
fluor/o	fluorescent/luminous/flow	**fluoro**scopy
foet/o	foetus (Am. fet/o)	**foet**al
follicul/o	small sac/follicle	**follicul**itis
fore-	before/in front of	**fore**brain

-form	having form/structure of	epilepti**form**
foss/o	depression	**foss**a
fove/o	pit	**fove**a
fraen/o	fraenum or fraenulum/restraining structure e.g. fraenulum of the lip	**fraen**al
fren/o (Am.)	frenum or frenulum/restraining structure e.g. frenulum of the lip	**fren**oplasty
front/o	front/forehead	**front**otemporal
-fuge	agent that suppresses/gets rid of	lacti**fuge**
fund/o	bottom/base (of an organ)	**fund**us
fung/i	fungus	**fung**icide
furc/o	branching	bi**furc**ation
galact/o	milk	**galacto**poiesis
gamet/o	gametes/sperm or eggs	**gameto**genesis
gangli/o	ganglion/swelling/plexus	**gangli**form
ganglion/o	ganglion/swelling/plexus	**ganglion**ectomy
gastr/o	stomach	**gastro**pathy
-gen	agent that produces/precursor	pepsino**gen**
-genesis	capable of causing/pertaining to formation	spermato**genesis**
-genic	pertaining to formation/originating in	oestro**genic**
genicul/o	knee	**genicul**ar
geni/o	chin	**geni**oglossal
genit/o	genitals/reproductive organs/produced by birth	**genit**al
gen/o	cause/produce/originate	**geno**phobia
-genous	arising from/produced by/producing	andro**genous**
ger/i/o	old age/the aged	**ger**iatric
geront/o	old age/the aged	**geront**ology
gingiv/o	gum	**gingiv**itis
gli/a/o	glue-like (pertains to neuroglial supporting cells of CNS)	**gli**oma
-globin	protein	myo**globin**
-globulin	protein	immuno**globulin**
glomerul/o	glomerulus of kidney	**glomerul**itis
gloss/o	tongue	**gloss**ectomy
gluc/o	sugar/sweet	**gluco**neogenesis
glyc/o	sugar/sweet	**glyco**protein
glycogen/o	glycogen, a polysaccharide	**glycogen**osis
glycos-	sugar (obsolete variant of glucose)	**glycos**uria
gnath/o	jaw	**gnatho**plasty
-gnomy	science or means of judging	patho**gnomy**
-gnos-	to know/known or knowledge/judgment	**gnos**ia
-gnosia	condition of knowing /receiving/recognizing	hyper**gnosia**
-gnosis	to know/known or knowledge/judgment	pro**gnosis**
gonad/o	gonads (ovaries or testes)	**gonad**otrophin
gonecyst/o	seminal vesicle	**gonecysto**lith
goni/o	angle/corner	**gonio**scopy
gon/o	seed/semen/knee	**gono**coccus
gony/o	knee	**gony**oncus
-grade	to go	retro**grade**
-gram	X-ray/tracing/recording/one thousandth of a kilogram (g)	mammo**gram**
granul/o	granule/granular	**granul**oma
-graph	usually recording instrument /a recording/X-ray/ mathematical curve representing data	electrocardio**graph**
-graphy	technique of recording/making X-ray	electrocardio**graphy**
-gravida	pregnancy/pregnant woman	primi**gravida**
gravid/o	pregnancy	**gravido**cardiac
gyn-	woman	**gyn**andrism
gynaec/o	woman (Am. gynec/o)	**gynaeco**logy

gynec-	woman	**gynec**oid
gynec/o (Am.)	woman	**gynec**ological
gyn/o	woman	**gyn**opathy
-gyric	pertaining to circular motion	oculo**gyric**
haern/a/o	blood (Am. hem/a)	**haema**dynamometer
haemat/o	blood (Am. hemat/o)	**haemat**ology
haemoglobin/o	haemoglobin (Am. hemoglobin)	**haemoglobin**uria
halit/o	breath	**halit**osis
hallux	great toe	**hallux** rigidus
hapl/o	single/simple	**hapl**opia
hapt/o	touch	**hapto**meter
hecto-	one hundred	**hecto**gram
helc/o	ulcer	**helc**osis
heli/o	sun	**heli**osis
helic/o	helix/spiral form	**helic**oid
helmint/h/o	worms	ant**helminth**ic
hem/a/o (Am.)	blood	**hemo**cytoblast
hemat/o (Am.)	blood	**hemat**ology
hemi-	half/on one side	**hemi**plegia
hepatic/o	hepatic bile duct	**hepatico**stomy
hepat/o	liver	**hepato**cyte
hept/a	seven	**hepta**chromic
herni/o	hernia	**herni**orrhaphy
heter/o	other/another/different	**hetero**sexual
hex-	six/hold/being	**hex**ose
hidr/o	sweat/perspiration	**hidr**osis
histi/o	type of macrophage (histiocyte)	**histio**cytosis
hist/o	tissue	**histo**logy
hol/o	entire/whole	**holo**crine
homeo-	alike/resembling/unchanging/constant	**homeo**stasis
homo-	the same	**homo**zygous
humer/o	humerus	**humero**radial
hyal/o	glass-like	**hyal**oid
hydatid/i/o	hydatid cyst	**hydatid**osis
hydr/a/o	water	**hydro**nephrosis
hygr/o	moisture	**hygro**blepharic
hymen/o	hymen	**hymeno**tomy
hy/o	hyoid bone	**hyo**mandibular
hyp(h)-	under	**hyp**hidrosis
hyper-	above normal/excessive/over	**hyper**chromia
hypn/o	sleep	**hypno**tic
hypo-	below normal/under	**hypo**thyroidism
hyster/o	uterus/womb	**hyster**ectomy
-ia	condition of/abnormal condition/disease	poly**uria**
-ial	pertaining to	bronch**ial**
-ian	specialist	physic**ian**
-iasis	abnormal condition/process or condition resulting from/disease	lith**iasis**
-iatrics	medical specialty	paed**iatrics** (Am. ped**iatrics**)
iatr/o	medical treatment/doctor	**iatr**ogenic
-iatry	treatment by a doctor/specialty (of doctor)	psych**iatry**
-ible	capable of/able	flex**ible**
-ic[1]	pertaining to	gast**ric**
-ic[2]	used in pharmacology to mean a drug or drug action	diure**tic**
-ical	pertaining to/dealing with	cytolog**ical**
ichthy/o	dry/scaly/fish like	**ichthy**osis
-ician	person associated with/specialist	techn**ician**

-ics	art or science of	gene**tics**
-ictal	pertaining to seizure/attack	pre**ictal**
icter/o	jaundice	**icter**ogenic
-ide	binary chemical compound	glyco**side**
idi/o	self/one's own/peculiar to an organism	**idio**pathic
-igo	attack/abnormal condition	ver**tigo**
il-	in/none	**il**legitimate
-ile	capable of/able	contrac**tile**
ile/o	ileum	**ileo**colitis
ili/o	ilium/flank	**ilio**femoral
im-	in/none/not	**im**potence
immun/o	immune/immunity	**immuno**logy
in-	in/none/not	**in**cision
-in	used as suffix for various chemicals	glycer**in**
incud/o	anvil/incus (ear ossicle)	**incudo**malleal
-ine	pertaining to/also used as suffix for chemicals derived or thought to be derived from ammonia	am**ine**
infer/o	inferior/below/beneath	**infero**lateral
infra-	below/inferior to	**infra**mammary
inguin/o	groin	**inguin**al
insulin/o	insulin/Islet of Langerhan's	**insulino**genesis
inter-	between	**inter**costal
-interna	internal	otitis **interna**
intestin/o	intestine	**intestin**al
intra-	within/inside	**intra**nasal
intro-	into/within/inwards	**intro**flexion
intus-	in/into	**intus**susception
iod/o	iodine	**iod**ism
-ion	action/condition resulting from action	abla**tion**
-ior	pertaining to	poster**ior**
ips/e/i/o	the same/self	**ips**ilateral
ir-	in/none/not	**ir**reducible
irid/i/o	iris	**irido**plegia
ir/o	iris	**ir**itis
ischi/o	ischium	**ischio**coccygeal
isch/o	condition of holding back/reducing/suppress	**isch**aemia (Am. **isch**emia)
-ism	process/state or condition	prosta**tism**
-ismus	process/state or condition	strab**ismus**
is/o-	same/equal	**iso**graft
-ist	specialist	optometr**ist**
-ite	end product	metabol**ite**
-itis	inflammation	tonsill**itis**
-ity	state/condition	sever**ity**
-ium	metallic elements	calc**ium**
-ive[1]	pertaining to/tendency	adhes**ive**
-ive[2]	used in pharmacology to mean a drug or drug action	antituss**ive**
-ize	use/subject to/to make	neutral**ize**
-ject	throw	pro**ject**ile
jejun/o	jejunum	**jejuno**stomy
juxta-	adjoining/near	**juxta**position
kal/i	potassium	**kali**uresis
kary/o	nucleus	**karyo**gram
kerat/o	horny/epidermis/cornea	**kerato**plasty
keratin/o	keratin (a protein present in skin, hair and nails)	**keratin**ous
ket/o/n	ketones/carbonyl group	**keton**uria
kin/e/o	motion/movement	**kin**esis
kinesi/o	motion/movement	**kinesi**ology

-kinesis	a motion/movement	irido**kinesis**
kinet/o	motion/movement	**kineto**cardiography
kilo-	one thousand	**kilo**calorie
-kymia	condition of involuntary twitching of muscle/ a wave of contraction in a muscle	myo**kymia**
kyph/o	crooked/hump	**kyph**osis
labi/o	lip	**labio**plasty
labyrinth/o	labyrinth of ear	**labyrinth**itis
lachrym/o	tear/tear ducts/lacrimal apparatus	**lachrym**al
lacrim/o	tear/tear ducts/lacrimal apparatus	**lacrimo**nasal
lact/i/o	milk	**lacti**ferous
laevo-	left (Am. levo-)	**laevo**cardia
-lalia	condition of talking	dys**lalia**
lamell/a	thin leaf or plate	**lamell**ar
lamin/o	lamina/thin plate/part of vertebral arch	**lamin**ectomy
lapar/o	abdomen/flank	**laparo**tomy
-lapaxy	empty/wash out/evacuate	litho**lapaxy**
laryng/o	larynx	**laryng**ectomy
later/o	side	**latero**torsion
lei/o	smooth	**leio**dermia
leiomy/o	smooth muscle	**leiomy**oma
lent/i	lens	**lenti**conus
-lepsy	seizure/fit	epi**lepsy**
lept/o	thin/fine/slender	**lepto**meningitis
leuc/o	white	**leuco**cyte (Am. **leuko**cyte)
leuk/o	white	**leuk**oblast
levo- (Am.)	left	**levo**cardia
-lexia	condition of speech/words	dys**lexia**
lien/o	spleen	**lieno**cele
-ligation	tying off of a vessel with a suture	vaso**ligation**
lingu/a/o	tongue/tongue-shape	**linguo**gingival
lip/o	fat/fatty tissue	**lip**oma
-listhesis	splitting	spondylo**listhesis**
-lith	stone	uretero**lith**
-lithiasis	abnormal condition of stones	uretero**lithiasis**
lith/o	stone	**litho**trite
lob/o	lobe	**lob**ar
lochi/o	vaginal discharge (lochia)	**lochio**rrhagia
loc/o	place	**loc**us
logad-	white of the eye	**logad**ectomy
-logist	specialist who studies	cardio**logist**
log/o	words/speech/study/thought	**logo**phasia
-logy	study of	laryngo**logy**
loph/o	ridge/tuft	**loph**odont
lord/o	bend forward	**lord**osis
lumb/o	loin/lower back	**lumbo**costal
lump-	lump/swelling	**lump**ectomy
lute/o	yellow/corpus luteum of ovary	**luteo**trophic
lymph/a/o	lymph	**lymph**oma
lymphaden/o	lymph node (aden/o – gland)	**lymphaden**itis
lymphangi/o	lymph vessel	**lymphangio**graphy
lyo-	water soluble/solvent/dissolve	**lyo**phil
-lys/o	break down/disintegration/dissolve	**lys**in
-lysis	break down/disintegration/dissolve	auto**lysis**
-lytic	pertaining to break down/disintegration	haemo**lytic** (Am. hemo**lytic**)
macro-	large	**macro**phage
macul/o	spot/blotch	**maculo**papular

mal-	bad/diseased or impaired	**mal**nutrition
-malacia	condition of softening	myo**malacia**
malac/o	softening	**malac**ic
malign-	bad/harmful	**malign**ant
malle/o	hammer/malleus (ear ossicle)	**malle**otomy
mamill/i/o	nipple	**mamilli**plasty
mamm/a/o	breast/mammary gland	**mammo**graphy
mammill/i/o	nipple	**mammill**itis
mandibul/o	mandible	**mandibulo**plasty
man/o	pressure	**mano**metry
manus-	hand	**manus** extensa
mast/o	breast/mammary gland	**mast**algia
mastoid/o	nipple shaped/mastoid process of the temporal bone	**mastoid**ectomy
maxill/o	maxilla	**maxillo**facial
meat/o	meatus/opening/external orifice e.g. of the urethra	**meat**otomy
medi/o	middle/midline	**medi**al
-media	middle	otitis **media**
medull/o	inner part/medulla	adrenal **medulla**
mega-	abnormally large	**mega**colon
megal/o	abnormally large	**megal**oglossia
-megaly	enlargement	acro**megaly**
melan/o	melanin/dark pigment	**melan**oma
melit/o	sugar/honey	**melit**uria
mel/o	limb/cheek	**mel**agra
melon/o	cheek	**melono**plasty
mening/i/o	membranes (of CNS)	**mening**itis
menisc/o	meniscus/crescent-shaped	**menisco**cyte
men/o	menses/menstruation/monthly flow	**men**orrhagia
ment/o	chin/mind	**mento**plasty
mes/o	middle/intermediate	**meso**derm
meta-	change in form/position/after	**meta**plasia
metacarp/o	metacarpus	**meta**carpal
metatars/o	metatarsal	**metatars**algia
-meter	measuring instrument/a measure	audio**meter**
metr/a/i/o	uterus/womb	endo**metri**osis
-metrist	person who measures	audio**metrist**
-metry	process of measuring	audio**metry**
micro-	small/one millionth	**micro**glia
mid-	middle	**mid**brain
-mileusis	to carve	kerato**mileusis**
milli-	one thousandth	**milli**litre
mi/o	make smaller/less	**mi**opia
mito-	thread-like/mitosis	**mito**tic
mono-	one/single	**mono**somy
-morph	shape/form	ecto**morph**
morph/o	shape/form	**morpho**genesis
mort/o	death	**mort**al
-motor-	moving/action/set in motion	oculo**motor**
muc/o	mucus	**muc**ous
multi-	many	**multi**gravida
muscul/o	muscle	**musculo**cutaneous
my-	(from myein) to close/squint	**my**opia
mycet/o	fungus	**mycet**oid
myc/o	fungus	broncho**myc**osis
myel/o	bone marrow/spinal cord	**myel**oma
myelomat/o	bone marrow/spinal cord	**myelomat**osis
my/o	muscle	**myo**globin
myocardi/o	myocardium (heart muscle)	**myocardio**pathy
myom/at/o	muscle tumour	**myomat**osis

myos/o	muscle	**myos**itis
myring/o	eardrum/tympanic membrane	**myringo**tome
myx/o	mucus	**myx**adenitis
nano-	one billionth (10^{-9})	**nano**metre
narc/o	stupor/numbness	**narco**tic
nas/o	nose	**naso**pharyngitis
-natal	pertaining to birth	ante**natal**
nat/o	birth	neo**nato**logy
natr/i	sodium	**natri**uresis
necr/o	death/dead tissue	**necr**osis
neo-	new	**neo**plasia
nephr/o	kidney	**nephr**itis
neur/o	nerve (rarely tendon)	**neuro**logy
neutr/o	neutral	**neutro**phil
noc/i	harm	**noci**ceptor
noct/i	night/darkness	**noct**uria
nod/o	knot/swelling	**nod**ule
nom/o	distribute/law/custom	**nomo**topic
non-	without/no	**non** compos mentis
normo-	normal	**normo**cytosis
nos/o	disease	**noso**logy
not/o	back	**noto**chord
nucle/o	nucleus	**nucleo**protein
nulli-	none	**nulli**para
nyctal/o	night/darkness	**nyctal**opia
nyct/o	night/darkness	**nyct**algia
-nyxis	perforation/pricking/puncture	kerato**nyxis**
obstetric-	pertaining to midwifery	**obstetric**ian
occipit/o	occiput, posterior region of the skull	**occipito**cervical
occlus/o	shut/close up	**occlus**ion
octa/i/o-	eight	**octi**gravida
ocul/o	eye	bin**ocul**ar
odont/o	tooth/teeth	orth**odont**ics
-oedema	swelling due to fluid (Am. edema)	myx**oedema**
oes/o	within (Am. es/o)	**oeso**gastritis
oesophag/o	oesophagus/gullet (Am. esophago)	**oesophago**stomy
oestr/o	oestrogen (a female sex-hormone)/oestrus (Am. estr/o)	**oestro**genic
-oid	resembling	lip**oid**
-ola	small	arteri**ola**
-ole	small	arteri**ole**
olecran/o	elbow/olecranon (bony projection of ulna)	**olecran**arthropathy
ole/o	oil	**oleo**granuloma
olfact/o	sense of smell/smell	**olfact**ory
olig/o	deficiency/few/little	**olig**uria
-olisthesis	slipping	spondylo**listhesis**
-oma	tumour/swelling	sarc**oma**
oment/o	omentum (peritoneal fold of stomach)	**omento**plasty
om/o	shoulder	**omo**clavicular
omphal/o	umbilicus/navel	**omphalo**genesis
onc/o	tumour/mass	**onco**logy
-one	hormone	progester**one**
onych/o	nail	**onycho**dystrophy
oo-	egg	**oo**cyte
oophor/o	ovary	**oophor**ectomy
-op-	seeing/looking at	presby**op**ia
ophthalm/o	eye	**ophthalmo**scope
-ophthalmos	eye	ex**ophthalmos**

-opia	condition of vision/defective vision	ambly**opia**
opistho-	backward	**opisth**ognathism
-opsia	condition of vision/defective vision	hemiachromat**opsia**
-opsy	to view/process of viewing	bi**opsy**
optic/o	vision/eye/optic nerve	**optic**al
opt/o	vision/eye	**opt**ometry
orbit/o	orbit (bony cavity) of eye	**orbito**nasal
-or	person or agent	don**or**
orchid/o	testis	**orchido**pathy
orch/i/o	testis	**orchio**plasty
-orexia	condition of appetite	an**orexia**
organ/o	organ	**organo**genesis
or/o	mouth	**or**al
orth/o-	straight/normal/correct	**orth**optics
-ory	pertaining to	sens**ory**
os-	bone/a mouth/orifice	**os** uteri
osche/o	scrotum	**oscheo**plasty
-ose	carbohydrate/sugars/starches/full of/pertaining to	gluc**ose**
-osis	abnormal condition/disease of/abnormal increase	leucocyt**osis** (Am. leukocyt**osis**)
osm/o	odour/smell/osmosis	**osmo**dysphoria
osse/o	bone	**osse**ous
oss/i	bone	**oss**icle
ossicul/o	ear ossicles/bones	**ossicul**ectomy
ost/e/o	bone	**osteo**arthritis
ot/o	ear	**ot**ology
oul/o	scar/gum	**oul**ectomy
-ous	pertaining to	urinifer**ous**
ovari/o	ovary	**ovario**tomy
ov/i/o	egg/ovum	**ovi**duct
-oxia	condition of oxygen	hyp**oxia**
ox/i/o	oxygen	**oxi**metry
oxy-	oxygen /sharp /quick	**oxy**tocic
pachy-	thick	**pachy**dermia
paed/o	child (Am. ped/o)	**paed**iatric
palae/o	old/primitive (Am. pale/o)	**palaeo**cortex
palat/o	palate	**palato**plasty
pale/o (Am.)	old/primitive	**paleo**cortex
palm/o	palm	**palm**ar
palpebr/a	eyelid	**palpebr**itis
pan-	all	**pan**carditis
pancreatic/o	pancreatic duct	**pancreatico**enterostomy
pancreat/o	pancreas	**pancreato**lysis
pannicul/o	fatty layer e.g. of abdomen	**pannicul**itis
pant/o	all/entire	**pant**atrophy
papill/i/o	nipple like/optic disc	**papillo**retinitis
para-	beside/near	**para**nephric
-para(re)	to bear/bring forth offspring (woman who has borne viable young)	primi**para**
parathyr/o	parathyroid gland	**parathyro**trophic
parathyroid/o	parathyroid gland	**parathyroid**ectomy
-paresis	slight paralysis	juvenile **paresis**
parotid/o	parotid gland	**parot**itis
-parous	pertaining to production of live young	nulli**parous**
-partum	birth/labour	post **partum**
patell/o	patella/knee cap	**patello**femoral
-pathia	condition of disease	psycho**pathia**
pathic	pertaining to disease	idio**pathic**

path/o	disease	**patho**logist
-pathy	disease/emotion	gastro**pathy**
-pause	stopping	meno**pause**
pect-	chest/breast/thorax	**pect**us
pector/o	chest/breast/thorax	**pector**al
pedicul/o	lice	**pedicul**osis
ped/i/o (Am.)	foot/(child)	**ped**iatrics
pelli-	skin/hide	**pelli**cle
pelv/i/o	pelvis	**pelvi**meter
-penia	lack of/condition of deficiency	erythro**penia**
pen/i	penis	**pen**itis
pepsin/o	digestion/pepsin	**pepsino**gen
pept-	digestion/pepsin	**pept**ic
per-	through/completely/excessive	**per**cutaneous
peri-	around	**peri**corneal
pericardi/o	pericardium	**pericardi**tis
perine/o	perineum	**perineo**rrhaphy
periton/e/o	peritoneum	**periton**itis
petr/o	stone/rock	osteo**petr**osis
-pexis	surgical fixation/fix in place/storing	glyco**pexis**
-pexy	surgical fixation/fix in place/storing	arthro**pexy**
phac/o	lens	**phaco**scopy
phae/o	dusky/dark (Am. phe/o)	**phaeo**chromocyte
-phagia	condition of eating/swallowing	poly**phagia**
phag/o	eating/consuming	**phago**cyte
-phagy	eating or swallowing	copro**phagy**
phak/o	lens	**phak**itis
phalang/o	phalange/finger/toe	**phalang**eal
phall/o	penis	**phall**ic
phaner/o	visible/manifesting	**phanero**genic
pharm/ac/o	drug/medicine	**pharmaco**logy
pharyng/o	pharynx	**pharyng**itis
-phasia	condition of speaking/speech	dys**phasia**
phas/i/o	speech	a**phasio**logy
phe/o	dusky/dark	**pheo**chromocyte (Am.)
-phil	love/affinity for/cell type with affinity for	neutro**phil**
-philia	condition of love / affinity for	haemo**philia** (Am. hemo**philia**)
-phily	condition of love / affinity for	necro**phily**
phleb/o	vein	**phleb**ectomy
-phobia	condition of fear	hydro**phobia**
-phonia	condition of having voice	a**phonia**
phon/o	sound/voice	**phono**cardiograph
-phore	a carrier	chromato**phore**
-phoresis	movement in a specified way/bearing/ carrying/driving ions	electro**phoresis**
-phoria	condition of mental state/feeling/bearing/ deviation of the eyes	eu**phoria**
phor/o	mental state/bearing/carrier (e.g. of disease)	**phoro**logy
phosph/o	phosphate/phosphorus/phosphoric acid	**phospho**lipid
phot/o	light	**photo**sensitive
phrenic/o	diaphragm/mind/phrenic nerve	**phrenic**ectomy
phren/i/o	diaphragm/mind/phrenic nerve	**phreno**gastric
-phthisis	wasting away	neuro**phthisis**
-phyma	tumour/boil/swelling	rhino**phyma**
phys/i/o	nature/physical things/physiology	**physio**therapy
-physis	growth	hypo**physis**
-phyt/e/o	plant/fungus	dermato**phyte**
pico-	small/a quantity multiplied by 10^{-12}	**pico**gram

pil/i/o	hair	**pilo**sebaceous
pineal/o	pineal gland	**pineal**ocyte
pituitar-	pituitary gland	hypo**pituitar**ism
placent/o	placenta	**placento**graphy
-plakia	condition of broad/flat (patch)	leuko**plakia**
-plania	condition of wandering e.g. a cell moving position	leucocyto**plania** (Am. leukocyto**plania**)
plan/o	flat	**plano**cellular
plant/i	sole of foot	**plant**ar
-plasia	condition of growth/formation (increase in number of cells)	hyper**plasia**
-plasm	formative substance	cyto**plasm**
plasma-	plasma cell/fluid of blood	**plasma**therapy
plasm/o	anything moulded, shaped or formed/ formative substance/growth	**plasmo**cyte
-plastic	pertaining to formation	neo**plastic**
-plasty	surgical repair/reconstruction	kerato**plasty**
platy-	flat	**platy**onychia
-plegia	condition of paralysis/stroke	para**plegia**
pleo-	more	**pleo**cytosis
plethysm/o	volume	**plethysmo**graph
pleur/o	pleural membranes/rib/side	**pleuro**dynia
plex/o	network of nerves, blood or lymph vessels	**plex**us
-plexy	strike/paralyze	apo**plexy**
-ploid(y)	chromosome sets in a cell	di**ploid**
pluri-	several/more	**pluri**glandular
-pnea (Am.)	breathing	a**pnea**
pneum/a/o	gas/air, also lung/breath	**pneumo**thorax
pneumat/o	gas/air/breath	**pneumato**metry
pneumon/o	lung/air	**pneumon**ectomy
-pnoea	breathing (Am. pnea)	dys**pnoea**
pod/o	foot	**pod**iatry
pogon/o	beard	**pogon**iasis
-poiesis	formation	erythro**poiesis**
poikil/o	varied/irregular	**poikilo**cyte
polio-	grey matter (of CNS)	**polio**myelitis
pollex	thumb	**pollex** flexus
poly-	many/too much	**poly**uria
polyp/o	polyp/small growth	**polyp**ectomy
pont/o	pons (part of metencephalon of brain)	**ponto**cerebellar
por/o	passage/pore	osteo**por**osis
port/o	portal vein	**port**ography
post-	after/behind	**post**-ganglionic
poster/o	back of body/behind/posterior to	**postero**superior
posth/o	prepuce/foreskin	balano**posth**itis
-prandial	meal	post**prandial**
-praxia	condition of purposeful movement/conduct	a**praxia**
pre-	before/in front of	**pre**tracheal
preputi/o	prepuce/foreskin	**preputio**tomy
presby/o	old man/old age	**presby**opia
primi-	first	**primi**gravida
pro-	before/favouring/in front of	**pro**drome
proct/o	rectum/anus	**proct**algia
progest/o	progesterone	**progesto**gen
prostat/o	prostate gland	**prostat**ism
prosth/o	adding (replacement part)	**prosth**odontics
proto-	first	**proto**diastole
protoz/o	protozoa	**protozo**iasis
proxim/o	near	**proxim**al

prurit/o	itching	**pruri**tic
pseudo-	false	**pseudo**piegia
psych/o	mind	**psych**osis
-ptosis	falling/displacement/prolapse	blepharo**ptosis**
-ptotic	pertaining to falling/displacement/prolapse/ affected with a ptosis	nephro**ptotic**
ptyal/o	saliva	**ptyalo**graphy
-ptysis	spitting/coughing up	pyo**ptysis**
pub/o	pubis	**pub**ovesical
puerper/o	puerperium/time of childbirth	**puerper**al
pulm/o	lung	**pulmo**-aortic
pulmon/o	lung	**pulmon**ary
pupill/o	pupil	**pupillo**metry
purul/o	pus-filled	**purul**oid
pustul/o	infected pimple/pustule	**pustul**osis
pyel/o	pelvis/trough of kidney	**pyelo**lithotomy
pyle/o	portal (vein)	**pyle**phlebitis
pylor/o	pylorus	**pylor**ic
py/o	pus	**pyo**genic
pyret/o	heat/fire/burning/fever	**pyret**ic
pyr/o	heat/fire/burning/fever	**pyro**gen
quadr/i/u-	four	**quadri**plegia
quinque-	five	**quinque**cuspid
quint-	five	**quint**an
rachi/o	spine	**rachio**pathy
radic/o	nerve root	**radico**tomy
radicul/o	nerve root	**radicul**itis
radi/o	radiation/X-ray/radius	**radio**therapy
re-	back/contrary/again	**re**position
rect/o	rectum	**recto**sigmoid
ren/i/o	kidney	**reno**graphy
reticul/o	net like/reticulum	**reticulo**cytosis
retin/o	retina	**retino**blastoma
retro-	backwards/behind	**retro**verted
rhabd/o	rod/rod-shaped	**rhabd**oid
rhabdomy/o	striated muscle	**rhabdomy**oma
rhe/o	electric current/flow of fluid	**rheo**logy
rheumat/o	rheumatism	**rheumat**ism
rhin/o	nose	**rhino**plasty
rhiz/o	root/nerve root	**rhizo**tomy
rhod/o	red	**rhod**opsin
rhytid/o	wrinkle	**rhytido**plasty
roentgen/o	X-ray/Roentgen rays	**roentgeno**graphy
rostr/i	superior/a rostrum/beak	**rostr**al
-rrhage	bursting forth/excessive flow	haemo**rrhage** (Am. hemo**rrhage**)
-rrhagia	condition of bursting forth/excessive flow	oto**rrhagia**
-rrhaphy	suture/suturing/stitching	teno**rrhaphy**
-rrhea (Am.)	excessive discharge/flow	rhino**rrhea**
-rrhexis	breaking/rupturing	ovario**rrhexis**
-rrhoea	excessive discharge/flow (Am. -rrhea)	rhino**rrhoea**
(r)rhythm/o	rhythm	ar**rhythm**ia
rubr-	red	**rub**or
rug/o	wrinkle/fold/ridge	**rug**a
facchar/o	sugar/sweet	**saccharo**lytic
sacr/o	sacrum	**sacro**coccygeal

salping/o	Eustachian (auditory) tube/Fallopian tube	**salpingo**stomy
sanguin/o	blood/bloody	**sanguino**lent
sapr/o	decay/decayed matter	**sapr**odontia
sarc/o	fleshy/connective tissue	**sarc**oid
-sarcoma	malignant (fleshy) tumour	Karposi's **sarcoma**
sarcomat/o	sarcoma (malignant fleshy tumour e.g. of connective tissues)	**sarcomat**osis
scapul/o	scapula	**scapulo**clavicular
scat/o	faeces/faecal matter (Am. feces)	**scato**logy
-schisis	cleaving/splitting/parting	palato**schisis**
schist/o	cleaving/splitting/parting	**schisto**cephalus
schistosom/o	parasitic worm of genus Schistosoma	**schistosom**iasis
schiz/o	split/cleft/divided	**schizo**trichia
scint/i	spark/flash of light	**scinti**scan
scirrh/o	hard	**scirrh**us
scler/o	hard/sclera (white of eye)	**sclero**tome
-sclerosis	hardening	arterio**sclerosis**
scoli/o	crooked/twisted	**scoli**osis
-scope	instrument to view/examine	endo**scope**
-scopist	specialist who uses viewing instrument	endo**scopist**
-scopy	visual examination/examination	endo**scopy**
scot/o	darkness	**scot**opia
scotom/o	scotoma/blind spot	**scotoma**graph
scrot/o	scrotum	**scroto**cele
seb/o	sebum/sebaceous gland	**sebo**lith
-sect(ion)	cut	caesarean **section**
secundi-	second	**secundi**gravida
semi-	half/partly	**semi**comatose
semin/i	semen	**semin**oma
sen/i	old	**sen**ile
sens/o	sense	**senso**motor
sensor/i	sense/sensation	**sensor**ium
-sepsis	infection	a**sepsis**
septi-	seven	**septi**para
septic/o	sepsis/infection/putrefaction	**septic**aemia (Am. **septic**emia)
sept/o	septum e.g. nasal septum	**septo**tomy
sequestr-	sequestrum, a portion of dead bone	**sequestr**ectomy
ser/o	serum	**sero**positive
sex/i	six	**sexi**digital
sialaden/o	salivary glands	**sialaden**itis
sial/o	saliva/salivary glands	**sialo**graphy
sider/o	iron	**sidero**penia
sigmoid/o	sigmoid colon	**sigmoido**scopy
silic/o	glass/silica	**silic**osis
sinistr/o	left/left side	**sinistro**cardia
sin/o	sinus	**sino**atrial
sinus-	sinus	**sinus** venosus
sinus/o	sinus	**sinus**itis
-sis	abnormal condition/state of	symbio**sis**
sit/o	food	**sito**phobia
somatic/o	body	**somatico**splanchnic
somat/o	body	**somato**trophic
somn/i/o	sleep	**somn**ial
son/o	sound	ultra**sono**graphy
-spadia(s)	condition of drawing out	hypo**spadia**
-spasm	involuntary contraction of muscle	blepharo**spasm**
spasm/o	spasm	**spasmo**dyspnoea
spermat/o	sperm	**spermato**genesis
sperm/i/o	sperm	**spermi**cidal

sphen/o	sphenoid bone/wedge shaped	**spheno**mandibular
spher/o	sphere-shaped/round	**sphero**phakia
sphincter/o	sphincter/ring-like muscle	**sphinctero**plasty
sphygm/o	pulse	**sphygmo**manometer
-sphyx-	pulsing	a**sphyx**ia
spirill/o	spiral-shaped bacteria of genus Spirillum	**Spirillum** minus
spir/o	to breathe	**spiro**metry
spirochaet/o	spirochaete (a spiral-shaped bacterium)	**spirochaet**e
spirochet/o (Am.)	spirochete (a spiral-shaped bacterium)	**spirochet**e
splanchn/i/o	viscera/splanchnic nerve	**splanchn**ic
splen/o	spleen	**splen**ectomy
spondyl/o	vertebra/vertebrae/spinal column	**spondyl**itis
spongi/o	sponge	**spongi**form
spor/o	spore	**sporo**mycosis
squam/o	scale/scale-like	**squam**ous
-stalsis	contraction	peri**stalsis**
stapedi/o	stirrup/stapes (ear ossicle)	**stapedio**tenotomy
staphyl/o	resembling bunch of grapes/clusters/uvula	**staphylo**cocci
-stasis	stopping/controlling/cessation of movement	haemo**stasis** (Am. hemo**stasis**)
-stat	agent/device that prevents change/stops	cryo**stat**
-static	pertaining to stopping/controlling/standing	haemo**static** (Am. hemo**static**)
-staxis	dripping/a dropping e.g. of blood	epi**staxis**
stear/i/o	fat	**steari**form
steat/o	fat	**steat**oma
sten/o	narrow/constricted	**steno**coriasis
-stenosis	abnormal narrowing	urethro**stenosis**
sterc/o	faeces (Am. feces)	**sterco**lith
ster/e/o	solid/three dimensional	**stereo**scopic
stern/o	sternum	**sterno**costal
steth/o	chest/breast	**stetho**scope
-sthenia	condition of strength/full power	mya**sthenia**
sthen/o	strength/full power	a**sthen**ic
stomat/o	mouth	**stomat**itis
stom/o	mouth/mouth-like opening	**stom**al
-stomy	to form a new opening or outlet/communication/ an opening	colo**stomy**
strab/o	squinting	**strab**ismus
strat/i	layer	**strat**iform
strept/o	twisted chain	**strepto**cocci
striat/o	mark/stripe	**striat**ed
styl/o	stake/styloid process (of temporal bone)	**stylo**mastoid
sub-	under	**sub**cutaneous
sud/or/i	sweat/perspiration	**sudor**esis
super/o	superior/above/excess	**supero**lateral
supra-	above/over/excess	**supra**hepatic
sy-	with/together	**sy**stole
sym-	with/together	**sym**melia
sympathic/o	sympathetic nervous system/nerves	**sympathico**tropic
symphysi/o	symphysis (fibro-cartilaginous joint) e.g. symphysis pubis	**symphysio**tomy
syn-	together/in association	**syn**chronous
syndesm/o	ligament/connective tissue	**syndesm**ectomy
syndrom/o	running together	**syndrom**ic
-synechia	condition of adhering together	blepharo**synechia**
synovi/o	synovial fluid/membranes	**synovi**al
syphil/o	syphilis	**syphil**oma
syring/o	tube/cavity	**syringo**myelia
system/o	system	**system**ic

tachy-	fast	**tachy**cardia
tact-	touch	**tact**ile
tal/o	ankle/ankle bone	**tal**ar
tars/o	tarsus/ankle/eyelid edge	**tars**algia
-taxia	condition of ordered movement	a**taxia**
tax/o	ordered movement/arrangement/classification	**tax**ology
tectori/o	covering/roof-like	**tectori**al
tel-	tela or web	**tel**angiectasis
tele-	far away/operating at a distance	**tele**cardiography
telo-	end	**telo**phase
tendin/o	tendon	**tendin**oplasty
tend/o	tendon	**tend**otome
ten/o	tendon	**ten**orrhaphy
tenont/o	tendon	**tenonto**phyma
ter-	three	**ter**valent
terat/o	monster/deformed fetus	**terato**genic
testicul/o	testicle/testis	**testicul**ar
test/o	testicle/testis	**testo**sterone
tetra-	four	**tetra**ploid
thalam/o	thalamus (part of cerebral cortex)	**thalamo**tomy
than/at/o	death	**thanato**phobia
thec/o	sheath	**thec**al
thel/e/o	nipple	**thele**plasty
-therapy	treatment	physio**therapy**
-thermia	condition of heat	hypo**thermia**
therm/o	heat	**therm**ography
-thermy	heat	cystodia**thermy**
thio-	sulphur	**thio**cyanate
thoracico-	thorax	**thoracico**-abdominal
thorac/o	thorax	**thoraco**tomy
-thorax	thorax/chest	pneumo**thorax**
thromb/o	thrombus/clot	**thromb**osis
thrombocyt/o	platelet	**thrombocyto**penia
thymic/o	thymus gland	**thymico**lymphatic
thym/o	thymus gland	**thym**ic
thyr/o	thyroid gland	**thyro**trophic
thyroid/o	thyroid gland	hypo**thyroid**ism
tibi/o	tibia	**tibio**fibular
-tic[1]	pertaining to	necro**tic**
-tic[2]	used in pharmacology to mean a drug or drug action	antiepilep**tic**
tine/o	gnawing worm/ringworm	*Tinea pedis*
-tion	state or condition/process	resec**tion**
-tocia	condition of birth/labour	eu**tocia**
toc/o	labour/birth	**toco**logy
-tome	cutting instrument	myringo**tome**
tom/o	slice/section	**tomo**graphy
-tomy	incision into	laparo**tomy**
-tonia	condition of tension/tone	a**tonia**
ton/o	stretching/tension/tone	**tono**meter
tonsill/o	tonsil	**tonsill**ectomy
top/o	place/particular area	**topo**logy
tort/i	twisted	**tort**icollis
-toxic	pertaining to poisoning	nephro**toxic**
toxic/o	poison	**toxico**logy
tox/i/o	poison	**tox**ic
trabecul/o	trabecula/anchoring strand of connective tissue/ trabecular meshwork of the eye	**trabecul**ectomy
trachel/o	neck/uterine cervix	**trachelo**plasty

trache/o	trachea	**tracheo**stomy
trans-	across	**trans**urethral
-trauma	injury/wound	baro**trauma**
-tresia	condition of an opening/perforation	a**tresia**
tri-	three	**tri**cuspid
trichin/o	*Trichinella spiralis* (parasitic nematode worm)	**trichin**iasis
trich/o	hair	**trich**osis
trigon/o	trigone/triangular space e.g. at the base of the bladder	**trigon**itis
-tripsy	act of crushing	litho**tripsy**
-triptor	instrument designed to crush or fragment e.g. using shock waves	litho**triptor**
-trite	instrument designed to crush or fragment	litho**trite**
-trophic	pertaining to nourishment/stimulation	adreno**trophic**
troph/o	nourishment/food/stimulation	**tropho**blast
-trophy	nourishment/development/increase in cell size	a**trophy**
-tropia	condition of turning/deviation	hyper**tropia**
-tropic	affinity for/stimulating/changing in response to a stimulus/turning towards	thyro**tropic**
-tubal	pertaining to a tube	ovario**tubal**
turbin/o	top-shaped/turbinate bone (nasal concha)	**turbin**ectomy
tuss/i	cough	anti**tuss**ive
tympan/o	tympanic membrane/middle ear	**tympano**plasty
typhl/o	caecum (Am. cecum)	**typhlo**cele
-ula	small/little	ling**ula**
ulcer/o	ulcer/sore/local defect in a surface	**ulcero**genic
-ule	small	ven**ule**
uln/o	ulna	**ulno**radial
ul/o/e	scar/gingiva (gums)	**ul**oid
ultra-	beyond	**ultra**sonography
-ulum	small	coag**ulum**
-ulus	small	sacc**ulus**
-um	thing/structure/noun ending/a name	ov**um**
un-	not/opposite of/release from	**un**differentiated
ungu/o	nail	**ungu**al
uni-	one	**uni**lateral
uran/o	palate	**urano**rrhaphy
urat/o	urates/salt of uric acid (found in calculi)	**urat**uria
urea-	urea	**urea**poiesis
ur/e/o	urine/urinary tract	**uro**logy
-uresis	excrete in urine/urinate	lith**uresis**
ureter/o	ureter	**uretero**stenosis
urethr/o	urethra	**urethro**scopy
-uria	condition of urine/urination	poly**uria**
urin/a/o	urine	**urino**meter
urticar/i	nettle rash/hives	**urticar**ia
-us	thing/structure/noun ending/a name	bronch**us**
uter/o	uterus	**utero**tubal
uve/o	uvea (pigmented parts of eye)	**uve**itis
uvul/o	uvula	**uvulo**ptosis
vagin/o	vagina	**vagin**itis
vag/o	vagus nerve	**vago**tomy
valv/o	valve	**valvo**tomy
valvul/o	valve	**valvulo**tome
varic/o	dilated veins/varicose vein	**varico**phlebitis
vascul/o	vessel	**vascul**ar
vas/o	vessel/vas deferens	**vas**ectomy

venacav/o	vena cava/great vein	**venacavo**graphy
ven/e/i/o	vein	**vene**section
vener/o	sexual intercourse	**vener**eal
ventricul/o	ventricle of heart or brain	**ventriculo**graphy
ventr/i/o-	belly side of body	**ventro**dorsal
verm/i	worm	**vermi**cide
-version	turning	retro**version**
vertebr/o	vertebra	**vertebr**al
vesic/o	bladder/blister	**vesico**prostatic
vesicul/o	seminal vesicle	**vesicul**itis
vestibul/o	vestibule/space leading to the entrance of a canal e.g. in the ear	**vestibulo**tomy
vibri/o	comma-shaped bacterium of genus Vibrio	**vibrio**cidal
vibr/o	vibration	**vibro**cardiogram
vir/o/u	virus/virion	**viro**lactia
viscer/o	viscera/internal organs (esp. abdomen)	**viscero**peritoneal
vit/o	life	**vit**al
vitre/o	glass/vitreous body of eye	**vitreo**retinal
viv/i	life	**vivi**section
vol/o	palm	**vol**ar
vulv/o	vulva	**vulv**itis
xanth/o	yellow	**xanth**oma
xen/o	strange/foreign	**xeno**graft
xer/o	dry	**xer**ophthalmia
xiph/i/o	xiphoid process	**xiphi**costal
-y	process/condition/noun ending/a name	apoplex**y**
-yl-	substance	but**yl**ene
zo/o	animal	**zo**oid
zyg/o	joined	**zygo**dactyly
zygomatic/o	zygomatic arch	**zygomatico**temporal
-zyme	fermentation/enzyme	lyso**zyme**
zym/o	fermentation/enzyme	**zym**osis